FROM INFLAMMATION TO CANCER

Advances in Diagnosis and Therapy for Gastrointestinal and Hepatological Diseases

FROM INFLAMMATION TO CANCER

Advances in Diagnosis and Therapy for Gastrointestinal and Hepatological Diseases

Editors

Chi Hin Cho

The Chinese University of Hong Kong, China

Jun Yu

The Chinese University of Hong Kong, China

World Scientific

NEW JERSEY • LONDON • SINGAPORE • BEIJING • SHANGHAI • HONG KONG • TAIPEI • CHENNAI

Published by

World Scientific Publishing Co. Pte. Ltd.
5 Toh Tuck Link, Singapore 596224
USA office: 27 Warren Street, Suite 401-402, Hackensack, NJ 07601
UK office: 57 Shelton Street, Covent Garden, London WC2H 9HE

British Library Cataloguing-in-Publication Data
A catalogue record for this book is available from the British Library.

FROM INFLAMMATION TO CANCER
Advances in Diagnosis and Therapy for Gastrointestinal and Hepatological Diseases

ISBN 978-981-4343-59-6

Typeset by Stallion Press
Email: enquiries@stallionpress.com

Printed in Singapore by Mainland Press Pte Ltd.

Foreword

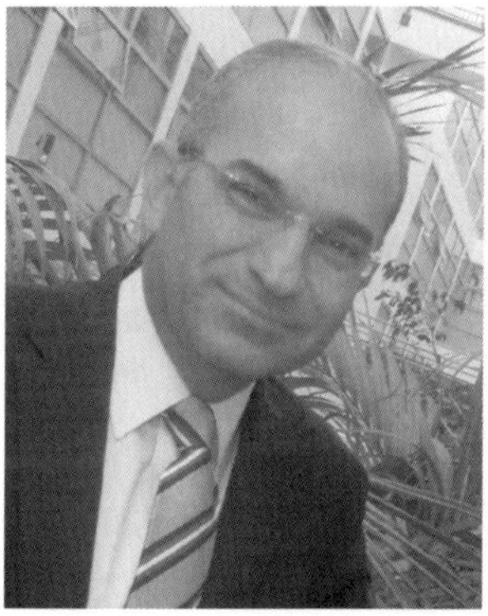

Inflammation is often regarded by biologists as an adaptation of the organism to the slings and arrows of outrageous fortune. To clinicians, however, inflammation is a means to an end: healing. Unfortunately, this healing may never occur especially if the initial injury, be it microbial, chemical or physical, persists. This protracted inflammation, which is termed chronic, can cause considerable damage to the host and may even kill it. The role of chronic inflammation in cancer was perhaps first described by Marjolin in 1828 but it is the German physician and father of modern pathology Rudolf Ludwig Virchow whose name is more commonly associated with this observation. It is now well established that almost all organs in the body that suffer from chronic inflammation are at increased risk of cancer. The gastrointestinal tract in particular bears the lion's share of this inflammation-induced cancer burden. Modern science has allowed the molecular mechanisms involved in inflammation-induced cancer to be elucidated and the next few years will witness a huge translational benefit from this knowledge. From a public health perspective, acceptance of the role of inflammation in cancer, through rigorous well-conducted science, will act as a stimulus for implementing strategies to reduce it. Thus, strategies to combat chronic infections, adopt healthy anti-inflammatory diets, encourage regular physical activity and perhaps the development of safe and cheap chemopreventive agents will all act to reduce the huge burden of cancer on society.

For most scientists and clinicians it is essential to keep abreast of the latest advances in this story. The book by Cho and Yu is an excellent compendium of the latest knowledge in this subject, as it pertains to the gastrointestinal tract and liver. It is written by experts in the field and spans the basic and clinical disciplines effortlessly and comprehensively. It is focused on mechanistic insight and translational relevance, precisely the combination that is essential in advancing this field. This book represents state-of-the-art knowledge on many aspects of inflammation-induced cancer and should be essential reading for researchers, both basic and clinical, gastroenterologists, oncologists, internists, and indeed any cancer scientists. It is essential to inspire the next generation of researchers to continue the fight against cancer and this book offers many inspiring success stories. I have no doubt that it will have a major impact in the field and this will ultimately benefit cancer patients and society at large.

Emad M El-Omar
BSc (Hons), MB ChB, MD (Hons), FRCP (Edin), FRSE
Professor of Gastroenterology / Honorary Consultant Physician
Editor in Chief, GUT
Division of Applied Medicine
Institute of Medical Sciences
School of Medicine & Dentistry
Aberdeen University
Foresterhill, Aberdeen AB25 2ZD
UK
E-mail: e.el-omar@abdn.ac.uk

About the Editors

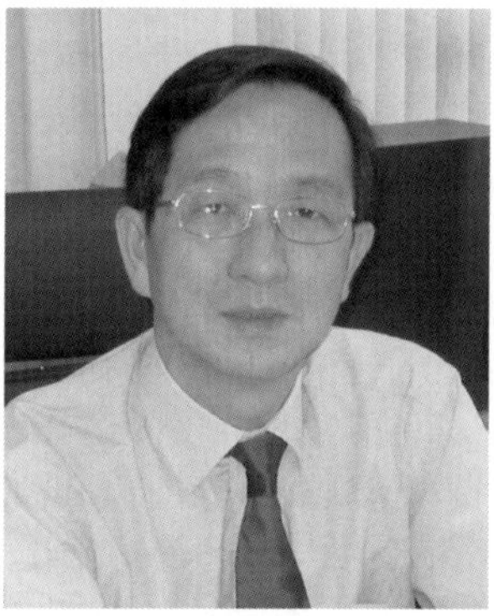

Prof. C. H. CHO

Prof. C. H. CHO

Prof. C. H. Cho started his academic career from 1978 in Canada. He moved on to Taiwan in 1981 and returned to Hong Kong in 1984. Currently, Prof. Cho is the Professor of Pharmacology and Associate Director of the School of Biomedical Sciences, Faculty of Medicine, The Chinese University of Hong Kong. He was the Chairman of the Department of Pharmacology from 2007 to 2009 in the same University and Chair Professor of Pharmacology in the University of Hong Kong from 2000 to 2006. He has been President of the Gastrointestinal Pharmacology Section of the International Union of Basic and Clinical Pharmacology since 2006. Prof. Cho is a member of editorial boards, associate editor and editor of more than 25 national and international journals in the areas of biomedical sciences, pharmacology and gastroenterology.

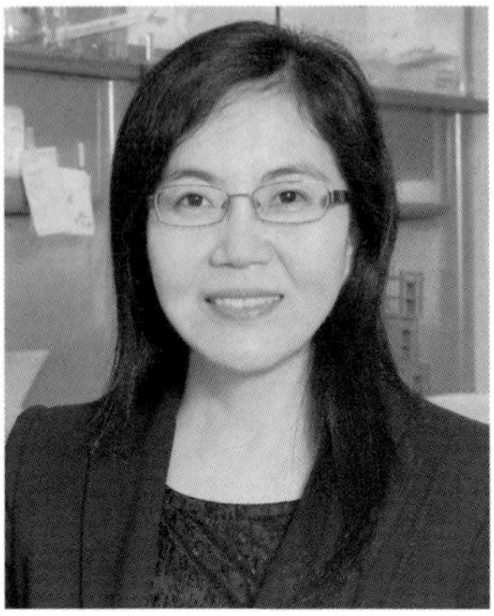

Prof. Jun YU

Prof. Jun YU

Prof. Jun Yu completed her MD and PhD at Tongji Medical University and then she embarked on her career as a gastrointestinal specialist in the Department of Gastroenterology and Hepatology, the Second affiliated Hospital, Beijing University. She undertook postdoctoral research in the Department of Gastroenterology and Hepatology at the University of Dresden and University of Magdeburg, Germany and subsequently in the Department of Medicine and Therapeutics, CUHK. She worked as a Senior Research Officer at Storr Liver Unit, Westmead Hospital, University of Sydney. She returned to Hong Kong in 2005 and currently she is a Professor at Institute of Digestive Disease and Department of Medicine and Therapeutics, The Chinese University of Hong Kong. Her research interests are mainly on (1) identification of the epigenetic and genetic alterations in relation to the mechanisms of pathogenesis, early diagnosis and prognostic prediction of gastrointestinal cancers, and (2) murine non-alcohol steatohepatitis (NASH) in relation to the mechanisms of development of experimental NASH, and treatment response.

List of Main Contributors

Prof. Chi Hin Cho, BPharm, PhD
School of Biomedical Sciences
Faculty of Medicine
The Chinese University of Hong Kong
Hong Kong, China

Dr. Carmen CM Cho, MB BS, FRCR
Department of Imaging and Interventional Radiology
Prince of Wales Hospital
The Chinese University of Hong Kong
Hong Kong, China

Assoc. Prof. Chi-Jen Chu, MD
Division of Gastroenterology
Department of Medicine
Taipei Veterans General Hospital
Taipei, Taiwan

Prof. Michael J. Duffy, PhD
Nuclear Medicine Laboratory
St Vincent's University Hospital
Dublin, Ireland

Assoc. Prof. Guy D. Eslick, PhD, FACE, FFPH
The Whiteley-Martin Research Centre
Discipline of Surgery, The University of Sydney
Sydney Medical School, Nepean Hospital
Sydney, Australia

Prof. Geoffrey C. Farrell, MD, FRACP
Department of Gastroenterology and Hepatology
The Canberra Hospital
Australian National University
Canberra, Australia

Prof. Hongchuan Jin, MD, PhD
Biomedical Research Center
Sir Runrun Shaw Hospital
Zhejiang University
Hangzhou, China

Prof. Yutaka Kondo, MD, PhD
Division of Molecular Oncology
Aichi Cancer Center Research Institute
Nagoya, Japan

Prof. Rupert WL Leong, MD
Gastroenterology and Liver Services
Sydney South West Area Health Service
Concord Hospital
Sydney, Australia

Prof. Liwei Lu, PhD
Department of Pathology
Faculty of Medicine
The University of Hong Kong
Hong Kong, China

Prof. John M. Luk, DrMedSc
Department of Pharmacology and Department of Surgery
National University Health System
Cancer Science Institute of Singapore
National University of Singapore
Institute of Molecular and Cell Biology, A*STAR
Singapore

Prof. Naofumi Mukaida, MD, PhD
Division of Molecular Bioregulation
Cancer Research Institute
Kanazawa University
Kanazawa, Japan

Dr. Ioannis A. Voutsadakis, MD, PhD
Centre Pluridisciplinaire d'Oncologie
Centre Hospitalier Universitaire Vaudois
Lausanne, Switzerland

Prof. Hongying Wang, MD, PhD
State Key Laboratory of Molecular Oncology
Cancer Institute and Cancer Hospital
Chinese Academy of Medical Sciences
Peking Union Medical College
Beijing, China

Dr. Xin Wei Wang, PhD
Liver Carcinogenesis Section
Laboratory of Human Carcinogenesis
Centre for Cancer Research
National Cancer Institute
Bethesda, USA

Prof. WS Fred Wong, BPharm, PhD
Department of Pharmacology, Yong Loo Lin Science of Medicine
Immunology Program, Life Science Institute
National University of Singapore
Singapore

Prof. Jun Yu, MD, PhD
Institute of Digestive Disease
Department of Medicine and Therapeutics
Faculty of Medicine
The Chinese University of Hong Kong
Hong Kong, China

Contents

Section I
Inflammation and Cancer

Chapter 1

General Introduction

Chung Wah Wu and Jun Yu*

Institute of Digestive Disease and
Department of Medicine and Therapeutics,
The Chinese University of Hong Kong,
Hong Kong, China

Gastrointestinal (GI) cancers are among the top cancer types in terms of incidence and mortality worldwide. The underlying infection and inflammation play a major role in the development of GI cancers. In this chapter, the etiology and epidemiology association between major GI cancers and associated inflammation diseases will be discussed, including the association between inflammatory bowel diseases and colorectal cancer (CRC); Barrett's esophagus and esophageal cancer; hepatitis virus infection or steatohepatitis and hepatocellular carcinoma (HCC); *Helicobacter pylori* (*H. pylori*) infection and gastric cancer (GC).

Introduction

Cancer is one of the world's leading causes of death. Every year, 14% of the world's population die of cancer. The relationship between inflammation and cancer has long been recognized. This is based on the findings that tumors often arise at sites of chronic inflammation. Infiltration of inflammatory cells and upregulation of chemokines and cytokines are frequently present in tumors, implicating a strong association between the inflammation mechanism and tumorigenesis. Epidemiological studies have shown that chronic inflammation

* Corresponding author. E-mail: junyu@cuhk.edu.hk

increases the risk of numerous cancers, including the most common ones such as lung cancer, gastric cancer and liver cancer. The processes of inflammation and tumorigenesis share many common molecular pathways such as the nuclear factor-κB (NF-κB) pathway, RAS–RAF signaling pathway, prostaglandin-synthesis pathway, etc. This has made possible the use of some anti-inflammatory drugs as potential anti-cancer agents. For example, cyclooxygenase 2 (COX2) inhibitor, a class of nonsteroidal anti-inflammatory drug, is able to reduce the risk and mortality rate of certain cancers.

How inflammation and cancer are linked

The connection between inflammation and cancer can be best described by two pathways: the extrinsic pathway and the intrinsic pathway. An extrinsic pathway is driven by inflammatory conditions which present before a malignant change and can subsequently increase cancer risk at the inflammatory site. Examples of the extrinsic pathway include the inflammatory conditions brought by gastric reflux and hepatitis virus infection, which increase the risk for GC and HCC, respectively. The intrinsic pathway is activated by genetic events that cause neoplasia, for example, the activation of oncogenes, the aberrant gain or loss of chromosome and the inactivation of tumor suppressor genes. Cells transformed in this way produce inflammatory mediators, creating an inflammatory microenvironment even though there is no underlying inflammation condition. In intrinsic pathway, the genetic alteration is the direct cause of both tumorigenesis and inflammation, and the inflammation condition could further enhance tumorigenesis.

Inflammation conditions that are linked to specific GI cancers

Bowel cancer

CRC is the fourth most common cancer in men and the third in women and the fourth most common cause for cancer-related deaths worldwide. The lifetime risk of CRC is approximately 6% and of colorectal adenoma approximately 50%. The progression from adenoma to colorectal carcinoma usually takes 5–10 years, characterized by accumulation of genetic abnormality in colon epithelial cells. The risk of colorectal cancer increases with age. In developed countries, more than 90% of cases are diagnosed in individuals older than 50 years old. Risk is also increased with certain inherited genetic mutations such as *familial adenomatous polyposis* (FAP) and hereditary nonpolyposis colorectal cancer (HNPCC), a personal or family history of CRC or polyps, and chronic inflammatory bowel disease.

Inflammatory bowel disease (IBD) represents a group of inflammatory conditions of the small intestine and colon. The cause of IBD is not exactly known. There is evidence that the disease is caused by a combination of factors, including intrinsic genetic predisposition, environmental factors and auto-inflammation. Crohn's disease (CD) and ulcerative colitis (UC), the main forms of IBD, are different in the location and nature of inflammation. CD can affect any part of the gastrointestinal tract from mouth to anus, although a majority of the cases start in the terminal ileum, whereas UC is restricted to the colon and the rectum. Microscopically, UC is restricted to the mucosa, while CD can affect the whole bowel wall. Although CRC complicating UC and CD only accounts for 1–2% of all CRC cases in the general population, CRC is a serious consequence of IBD, as it accounts for one in six of all deaths in IBD patients.

UC or CD patients have increased risk for CRC. Based on a study carried out in UK, the cumulative risk for developing CRC was 8% at 22 years from onset of symptoms for Crohn's colitis and 7% at 20 years from onset of symptoms for ulcerative colitis, representing an 18- and 19-fold increase in cancer risk, respectively, when compared with the background population of matched demographic data.[1]

Carcinomas complicating CD or UC have been found to have similar pathological features. In a study based on 80 CRC patients complicating CD or UC, cancers in UC and CD occurred at a median of 15 and 18 years after onset of IBD. The tumors were multiple in 11% of CD patients and 12% of UC patients and occurred with the presence of dysplasia in 73% and 79% of CD and UC patients, respectively.[2] Histological features of the tumors developed in connection with the two diseases were similar. For example, tumors were predominantly present in chronically inflamed areas of the bowel, suggesting that chronic inflammation, as a common process of the two diseases, is an important underlying mechanism leading to carcinogenesis in IBD. And unlike sporadic CRC where dysplastic lesions arise in one or two focal areas of the colon, the dysplasia in colitic mucosa is usually multifocal.

Small bowel cancer is extremely rare compared with cancers of the large bowel. Although few small bowel cancers have been reported in CD, patients with CD show an increased risk of developing this type of cancer. Studies based on European cohorts have revealed that CD patients are 16 to 66 times more likely to develop small bowel cancer than the background population.[1,3–5]

The adenoma to carcinoma process of sporadic CRC development and the neoplastic transformation in IBD share many common intrinsic molecular alterations such as the loss of function of adenomatosis polyposis coli (APC) protein, p53 mutations and aberrant methylation of mismatch repair genes; however, there are several differences in the sequence of molecular events between them. For example, APC loss of function, an early event common in sporadic CRC, is less frequent and usually occurs late in the colitis associated dysplasia–carcinoma sequence. On the contrary, p53 mutations, usually a late event in the adenoma–carcinoma sequence, occur early in non-dysplastic mucosa of colitis patients.

Barrett's esophagus and esophageal cancer

Esophageal cancer is the ninth most common cancer in the world, of which adenocarcinoma and squamous cell cancer are the major subtypes. Esophageal adenocarcinoma accounts for 50–80% of all esophageal cancers, which arises from glandular cells that are present at the junction of the esophagus and stomach. The incidence of esophageal adenocarcinoma is increasing by 10% annually in western countries while that of esophageal squamous carcinoma remains unchanged. Esophagus adenocarcinoma confers a very poor prognosis, even in patients undergoing curative resection, with a mean 5-year survival rate of less than 20%.[6]

Gastroesophageal reflux disease (GERD) and Barrett's esophagus are common precursors to esophageal adenocarcinoma. GERD is a chronic symptom induced by the abnormal reflux in the esophagus, resulting in mucosal damage and esophagitis. Barrett's esophagus is an intermediate step in the progression from reflux esophagitis to esophageal adenocarcinoma, characterized by metaplasia in which the squamous epithelium of the distal esophagus is replaced by columnar epithelium and mucus-secreting goblet cells. Approximately 10% to 20% patients with the chronic reflux develop Barrett's esophagus. The incidence of adenocarcinoma in Barrett's esophagus with dysplasia is about 30–125 times higher than that of the general population.[7] Patients with longer segments of Barrett's esophagus are more prone to the esophageal adenocarcinoma than those with short segments.

Evidence suggests that bile acids in the refluxate play a key role in inducing Barrett's esophagus. Increased bile acid exposure can increase esophageal mucosal damage and the severity of Barrett's esophagus. The predominant bile acids detected in patients with esophagitis and Barrett's esophagus were cholic, taurocholic, and glycocholic acids and a significantly greater proportion of secondary bile acids produced by bacteria such as taurodeoxycholic and deoxycholic acid.[8] Bile acid exposure can cause chronic inflammation. Normally, the inflammation of esophageal squamous epithelium heals by the regeneration of new squamous cells. In Barrett's esophagus, healing occurs through replacement of damaged cells by columnar epithelium and mucus-secreting goblet cells. These new cells are more resistant to the toxic agents causing the chronic inflammation than the normal esophageal squamous tissue. Persistent inflammation gives rise to increased release of pro-inflammatory mediators including cytokines, chemokines, prostaglandins, and reactive oxygen/nitrogen species. These factors create a microenvironment that facilitates neoplastic transformation and potentiates the progression of cancer.

Viral infections and hepatocellular carcinomas

Liver cancer is the fifth most common cancer in men and the eighth in women, and the third leading cause of cancer death in men and the sixth among women. The prognosis of HCC is very poor with a five-year survival rate below 9%. Areas with higher incidence of chronic hepatitis B virus (HBV) and hepatitis C virus (HCV) infections such as Asia and west and central Africa have a higher incidence of HCC. More than 80% of HCC cases occur in developing countries. China alone accounts for nearly 55% of the total cases.

Cirrhosis is the major risk factor for progression to HCC. It is initiated from liver fibrosis, which is a wound healing process in response to various kinds of hepatic insults. Fibrosis is characterized by connective tissue production and deposition; it progresses at variable rates depending on the cause of insults, environmental and host factors. Cirrhosis, an advanced stage of liver fibrosis, is accompanied by distortion of the hepatic vasculature, leading to compromised exchange between hepatic sinusoids and hepatocytes. Alcoholic liver disease and hepatitis C are the most common causes of cirrhosis in the Western world, while hepatitis B prevails in most parts of Asia and west and central Africa. HCV infection and nonalcoholic steatohepatitis (NASH) are also important etiology of cirrhosis.

HBV and HCV infections are responsible for the majority of hepatocellular carcinomas, accounting for over 80% of all HCC worldwide. There are an estimated 400 million people chronically infected with HBV worldwide, among which up to 40% will develop complications of cirrhosis and HCC. Approximately 70–80% of HBV-related HCC occurs in cirrhotic livers, whereas the remainder of the HCC occurs in the absence of cirrhosis. Case-control studies have shown that chronic HBV carriers possess 100-fold increased risk of HCC compared with the general population.

HBV infection induces HCC through both intrinsic and extrinsic pathways. For intrinsic pathways, HBV can integrate its DNA into the host genome, causing numerous mutations and chromosome instability. The accumulation of genetic mutation can directly induce tumorigenesis and create a microenvironment that favors tumor growth. Extrinsically, the adaptive immune response, particularly virus-specific killer T cells, contributes to most of the liver injuries associated with HBV infection by killing infected hepatocytes and producing antiviral cytokines. Antigen-nonspecific inflammatory cells can worsen killer T cell-induced immunopathology. Activated platelets at the site of infection also facilitate inflammatory processes by interacting with leukocytes and by secreting chemokines, cytokines and inflammatory mediators.

Chronic HCV infection is another major risk factor for the development of HCC. There are approximately 170 million people infected with HCV worldwide, and around 20% of the HCV-infected patients case will progress to cirrhosis. Once HCV-related cirrhosis is established, HCC develops at an annual rate of 1% to 4% and rates of up to 7% have been reported in Japan. HCC risk was increased 17-fold in HCV-infected patients compared with HCV-negative controls.[9] Unlike HBV, HCV, a positive stranded RNA virus that lacks reverse transcriptase activity, is not able to integrate into the host genome. HCV mainly induces HCC through extrinsic pathways by inducing hepatic cell injury and chronic inflammation.

Non-alcoholic fatty liver disease (NAFLD) is a spectrum of liver diseases caused by the excess fat accumulation in liver, which ranges from simple steatosis to steatohepatitis and finally cirrhosis. NASH is an advanced stage of NAFLD, characterized by a mixed inflammatory lobular infiltrate, liver cell injury, and variable fibrosis. The transformation from simple steatosis to NASH depends on the presence of oxidative stress. During β-oxidation of excess fatty acid, reactive oxygen species (ROS) are generated. ROS can lead to elevated lipid peroxides that form adducts with cellular nucleophiles, such as proteins and nucleic acids, resulting in cell damage and the subsequent initiation of an inflammatory response. Chronic inflammatory response can lead to fibrosis and cirrhosis. Clinically, NASH is highly associated with obesity, insulin resistance and type II diabetes. Up to 20% of patients with NASH may progress to cirrhosis, and 40% of cirrhosis patients will die from liver related disease including HCC.

In a retrospective cohort study, 420 patients diagnosed with NAFLD in Minnesota were followed up for a mean duration of 7.6 years.[10] Twenty-one of them (5%) were diagnosed with cirrhosis, and 2 among them developed HCC. Seven out of the 420 patients died of liver-related disease, one among them died of HCC, as compared with the general population of Minnesota in which liver disease only accounts for less than 1% of all death.[10] Once cirrhosis and HCC are established in NASH patients, it becomes difficult to recognize histopathological features of NASH. However, the causative association between NASH and HCC could also be identified through clinical and demographic factors. For example, among HCC patients who had no identifiable cause for chronic liver disease such as alcoholic and viral hepatitis, there is a higher prevalence of obesity and diabetes.[11]

Similar to NAFLD, alcoholic liver disease (ALD) encompasses a spectrum of liver injury, ranging from simple steatosis to steatohepatitis and cirrhosis. Continued alcohol use at 40 g per day increased the risk of progression to cirrhosis to 30%, and fibrosis or cirrhosis to 37%.[12] A central pathway of generating oxidative stress in alcohol exposed hepatocytes is through the alcohol inducible cytochrome P450 2E1 (CYP2E1), an endoplasmic monooxygenase that oxidizes ethanol. During its catalytic cycle, CYP2E1 readily releases ROS as a result of incomplete transfer of electrons to molecular oxygen and subsequently induces the recruitment of inflammatory response. It has been reported that HCC risk is increased in a linear fashion with daily intake of more than 60 g.[9] However, with the concomitant presence of HCV infection, there was an additional 2-fold increase in HCC risk compared with that observed with alcohol use alone.

H. pylori infection and gastric cancer

GC is the second leading cause of cancer death in men and the fourth among women worldwide. It develops from a stepwise progression from chronic gastritis, atrophic gastritis, intestinal metaplasia, dysplasia and subsequently to cancer. A series of changes in gastric carcinogenesis is often initiated by *H. pylori* infection. *H. pylori* is a bacterium that colonizes the stomach. It is not exactly known how *H. pylori* is transmitted, but the most likely route of spread is from person to person through fecal-oral or oral-oral routes. Possible environmental sources include water contaminated with human waste. In the absence of antibiotic-induced eradication, infection with this gram negative bacterium induces a chronic immune response that persists for the life of the host. Colonization of *H. pylori* in gastric mucosa is associated with inflammatory cell infiltration into the gastric mucosa, resulting in gastritis. Different *H. pylori* strains induce varying degrees of gastritis, reflecting their individual abilities to interact with the host. One strain-specific *H. pylori* constituent that increases cancer risk is the cytotoxin-associated gene (*cag*) pathogenicity island, a genetic locus that encodes a type IV secretion system that could lead to a loss of cellular polarity.

Around 59% of gastric cancer cases in developing countries and 63% of cases in developed countries can be attributed to *H. pylori* infection. Studies from Asia have shown that individuals who test positive for

Table 1. Inflammatory diseases are able to increase the risk of gastrointestinal cancers.

Type of GI cancer	Rank of mortality rate in male	Rank of mortality rate in female	Inflammatory disease	Cause of inflammation	Percentage of cancer cases with the inflammation	Increased risk of cancer caused by inflammation (by folds)
Colon Cancer	4	5	Crohn's disease	Anto-inflammatory	1%–2%	18
			Ulcerative colitis	Anto-inflammatory	1%–2%	19
Small bowel Cancer	Unknown	Unknown	Crohn's disease	Anto-inflammatory	Unknown	16–66
Esophageal Cancer	5	7	Barrett's esophagus	Bile acid	Unknown	30–125
Liver Cancer	3	6	HBV infection	HBV	80%	5–15
			HCV infection	HCV	80%	17
			Alcoholic steatohepatitis	Alcohol	Unknown	Unknown
			Non-alcoholic steatohepatitis	Metabolic syndromes	Unknown	Unknown
Gastric Cancer	2	4	*H. pylori* infection	*H. pylori*	~60%	>2

H. pylori have at least a two-fold increased risk of developing gastric cancer compared with those who test negative.[13–14] The association between *H. pylori* and gastric cancer is especially strong for young patients less than 30 years of age.[15] A large prospective study from Japan showed that no individuals who were negative for *H. pylori* developed gastric cancer during the long-term follow-up;[13] Consistently, a study from Taiwan found that all gastric cancers only developed in patients infected with *H. pylori*.[16] These findings suggest that infection with this bacterium plays an important part in gastric-cancer development. However, eradication of *H. pylori* was not found to be an effective remedy. Clinical evidence showed eradication of *H. pylori* had not prevented the development of gastric cancer.[17–19] In fact, most patients may have been infected with *H. pylori* in childhood and various degrees of mucosal damage had already been established before any intervention. Eradication of the bacterium was also found to result in GERD, esophagitis and weight gain in adults.[20–22]

Conclusion

Infections and inflammatory responses are linked to 15–20% of all cancer deaths.[23] Notably, inflammation conditions in gastrointestinal cancers are important precursors to malignancy. There are many triggers of chronic inflammation that increase cancer risk. Microbial infections play particular prominent roles in GI cancer. Thus, further understanding of the underlying inflammatory mechanisms that lead to the cancer will provide the opportunity of developing anticancer drugs and allow early intervention of cancer formation.

References

1. Gillen CD, Walmsley RS, Prior P *et al.* (1994) Ulcerative colitis and Crohn's disease: A comparison of the colorectal cancer risk in extensive colitis. *Gut* **35**:1590–2.
2. Choi PM, Zelig MP. (1994) Similarity of colorectal cancer in Crohn's disease and ulcerative colitis: Implications for carcinogenesis and prevention. *Gut* **35**:950–4.

3. Fireman Z, Grossman A, Lilos P *et al.* (1989) Intestinal cancer in patients with Crohn's disease. A population study in central Israel. *Scand J Gastroenterol* **24**:346–50.
4. Munkholm P, Langholz E, Davidsen M, Binder V. (1993) Intestinal cancer risk and mortality in patients with Crohn's disease. *Gastroenterology* **105**:1716–23.
5. Persson PG, Karlen P, Bernell O *et al.* (1994) Crohn's disease and cancer: A population-based cohort study. *Gastroenterology* **107**:1675–9.
6. Urba S. (2004) Esophageal cancer: Preoperative or definitive chemoradiation. *Ann Oncol* **15**(Suppl 4):iv93–6.
7. Wild CP, Hardie LJ. (2003) Reflux, Barrett's oesophagus and adenocarcinoma: Burning questions. *Nat Rev Cancer* **3**:676–84.
8. Nehra D, Howell P, Williams CP *et al.* (1999) Toxic bile acids in gastro-oesophageal reflux disease: Influence of gastric acidity. *Gut* **44**:598–602.
9. Donato F, Tagger A, Gelatti U *et al.* (2002) Alcohol and hepatocellular carcinoma: The effect of lifetime intake and hepatitis virus infections in men and women. *Am J Epidemiol* **155**:323–31.
10. Adams LA, Lymp JF, St Sauver J *et al.* (2005) The natural history of nonalcoholic fatty liver disease: A population-based cohort study. *Gastroenterology* **129**:113–21.
11. Regimbeau JM, Colombat M, Mognol P *et al.* (2004) Obesity and diabetes as a risk factor for hepatocellular carcinoma. *Liver Transpl* **10**:S69–73.
12. Teli MR, Day CP, Burt AD *et al.* (1995) Determinants of progression to cirrhosis or fibrosis in pure alcoholic fatty liver. *Lancet* **346**:987–90.
13. Uemura N, Okamoto S, Yamamoto S *et al.* (2001) *Helicobacter pylori* infection and the development of gastric cancer. *N Engl J Med* **345**:784–9.
14. Yamagata H, Kiyohara Y, Aoyagi K *et al.* (2000) Impact of *Helicobacter pylori* infection on gastric cancer incidence in a general Japanese population: The Hisayama study. *Arch Intern Med* **160**:1962–8.
15. Huang JQ, Sridhar S, Chen Y *et al.* (1998) Meta-analysis of the relationship between *Helicobacter pylori* seropositivity and gastric cancer. *Gastroenterology* **114**:1169–79.
16. Hsu PI, Lai KH, Hsu PN *et al.* (2007) *Helicobacter pylori* infection and the risk of gastric malignancy. *Am J Gastroenterol* **102**:725–30.

17. Leung WK, Lin SR, Ching JY *et al.* (2004) Factors predicting progression of gastric intestinal metaplasia: Results of a randomised trial on *Helicobacter pylori* eradication. *Gut* **53**:1244–9.
18. Sung JJ, Lin SR, Ching JY *et al.* (2000) Atrophy and intestinal metaplasia one year after cure of *H. pylori* infection: A prospective, randomized study. *Gastroenterology* **119**:7–14.
19. Wong BC, Lam SK, Wong WM *et al.* (2004) *Helicobacter pylori* eradication to prevent gastric cancer in a high-risk region of China: A randomized controlled trial. *JAMA* **291**:187–94.
20. Azuma T, Suto H, Ito Y *et al.* (2001) Gastric leptin and *Helicobacter pylori* infection. *Gut* **49**:324–9.
21. Furuta T, Shirai N, Xiao F *et al.* (2002) Effect of *Helicobacter pylori* infection and its eradication on nutrition. *Aliment Pharmacol Ther* **16**:799–806.
22. Hamada H, Haruma K, Mihara M *et al.* (2000) High incidence of reflux oesophagitis after eradication therapy for *Helicobacter pylori*: Impacts of hiatal hernia and corpus gastritis. *Aliment Pharmacol Ther* **14**:729–35.
23. Balkwill F, Mantovani A. (2001) Inflammation and cancer: Back to Virchow? *Lancet* **357**:539–45.

Chapter 2

General Mechanisms of Inflammation

Liwei Lu* and Min Yang

Department of Pathology, The University of Hong Kong, Hong Kong, China

Inflammation is a host defense against invading pathogens, damaged tissue and cellular irritates such as toxins in local tissue. The well-known clinical signs of inflammation include redness, swelling, warmth and pain at the site of infection or trauma. The increase in vascular diameter leads to increased local blood flow, hence manifested as redness and warmth; followed by the adhesion of leukocytes to the local blood vessel walls. Consequently the increase of vascular permeability in local blood vessels gives rise to swelling or edema and pain. In general, the initiated inflammatory responses result in the recruitment of various types of immune cells to eliminate foreign pathogens, clear damaged cells and trigger tissue-repairing processes. Both macrophages and neutrophils in the innate immune system constitute a first line of host defense against invading pathogens. When these cells become activated after phagocytosing pathogens, they can further activate other immune cells including dendritic cells and T cells. Moreover, many types of immune cells can recognize pathogenic invaders via a diversity of receptors for pathogen-associated molecular patterns (PAMPs) expressed on the surface of various microbes, which plays an important role for the induced adaptive immunity during an inflammatory response at local sites. In addition to infection-triggered inflammatory response, there is increasing evidence indicating that inflammation is also present and contributes to cancer cell proliferation, angiogenesis and metastasis.

*Corresponding author. E-mail: liweilu@hkucc.hku.hk

Thus, further understanding of the mechanistic modulation of inflammatory response may lead to the development of novel strategies for cancer treatment. Here, we review the general process and immune mechanisms of inflammation.

Categories of inflammation

According to the duration of its response, inflammation can be classified into acute inflammation and chronic inflammation. Acute inflammation is of relatively short duration, lasting from minutes to a few days, and its main characteristics are the exudation plasma proteins and leukocyte migration to the inflamed location. At the site of infection or injury, inflammation is initiated by the response of macrophages and neutrophils to pathogens. Pathogens that overcome the phagocytic process are also faced with other host defense measures, including soluble factors such as acute phase proteins, complement proteins and cytokines. The outcomes of acute inflammation are either resolved or it progresses to chronic inflammation. As an inflammatory response with a prolonged duration, chronic inflammation is often caused by persistent infections such as tuberculosis (TB), prolonged exposure to toxic agents, and auto-immune diseases such as arthritis rheumatism, which is characterized by extensive infiltration with mononuclear cells, including macrophages, lymphocytes, mast cells, eosinophils and plasma cells in local tissues, reflecting persistent reaction to invading pathogens or injuries. Consequently, this leads to a delayed type (type IV) hypersensitivity reaction, including T cell activation, cytokine and chemokine secretion, and accumulation of macrophages at the site of infection or injury. The sustained release of pro-inflammatory cytokines and factors starts to damage the surrounding healthy tissue. The outcomes of chronic inflammation include tissue destruction or fibrosis. Chronic inflammation can often lead to granuloma formation, which is characterized by the accumulation of numerous activated macrophages, epithelioid cells and multinucleated giant cells in tissue. Chronic inflammation usually accompanies persistent microbial infections, burns, auto-immune diseases, severe allergies, transplants and cancers. It becomes evident that chronic inflammation contributes significantly to the tissue damage as well as wasting in many types of cancers.

Under certain circumstances, the term "sterile inflammatory response" is used to refer to the innate immune response to tissue damages mediated by non-microbial insults such as trauma or ischemia. In this chapter, we focus on reviewing the general process of acute inflammation.

Inflammatory process

Upon the breaching of physical barriers, such as the skin and mucosal epithelia of the respiratory, gastrointestinal and reproductive tracts, invading pathogens or tissue injuries trigger the response of host defense. The inflammatory reactions usually include the initiation of inflammation which is caused by infection, trauma, allergy or even autoimmunity *via* the release of inflammatory mediators from various types of immune cells into the tissues. These inflammatory mediators increase the vascular permeability, adhesion of endothelial cells and influx of leucocytes into the site of inflammation to combat infection or tissue injury. Subsequently, the gradual termination of the inflammatory response and tissue repair are achieved by anti-inflammatory mediators and products of clotting system to repair the wound or damaged tissue. During the process, both macrophages and neutrophils non-specifically engulf and degrade foreign particles, and secrete soluble mediators that recruit the immune cells of the adaptive system to the site of tissue injury.

Initiation of inflammation

During the early phase of the inflammation, activated macrophages secrete cytokines such as interleukin-1 (IL-1), tumor necrosis factor-α (TNF-α) and IL-6. In addition to their ability to induce fever, these cytokines can trigger hepatocytes to produce acute phase proteins, especially C-reactive protein (CRP), a well-recognized non-specific marker for inflammation. CRP binds to phosphocholine expressed on the surface of dead or dying cells as well as bacteria, which activates the complement system. The binding of complement component C3b to foreign substances and damaged cells enhances phagocytosis by macrophages that express a receptor for C3b. Thus, CRP plays an important role in an early defense system against infection.

Among many inflammatory mediators, IL-1 has been recognized as a master mediator initiator of inflammation by its key function in neutrophil recruitment, lymphocyte activation and induction of inflammatory cytokines. As listed in Table 1, various inflammatory mediators exert different functions in triggering inflammation. For example, the lipid mediators such as prostaglandins, leukotrienes and platelet-activating factor (PAF) are rapidly produced by monocytes and macrophages through enzymatic pathways. Collectively, they promote activated macrophages to release chemoattractant cytokines for attracting leukocytes from the blood

Table 1. Major mediators for the inflammatory response.

Type	Mediators	Function
Cytokines	IL-1 IL-6 TNF-α	Induce fever; increase acute-phase proteins; activate inflammation and coagulation
Acute-phase proteins	C-reactive protein	Activate complement system
Lipid Mediators	Prostaglandins Leukotrienes Platelet activating factor (PAF)	Promote releasing of chemoattractant cytokines; increase vascular permeability, smooth muscle contraction
Chemokines	C-C subgroup (IL-8, IP-10, SDF-l) C-X-C subgroup (RANTES, MCP)	Control lymphocyte adhesion, chemotaxis and activation; regulate leukocyte traffic
Complement system	C5a C3a	Increase vascular permeability; induce the expression of adhesion molecules; attract neutrophils and monocytes; promote mast cells to release granules
Kinin System	Bradykinin	Increase vascular permeability; promote the influx of plasma proteins, cause pain
Coagulation system	Fibrin peptides Heparin	Form a clot to prevent microorganisms from entering the bloodstream

flow. Moreover, lipid inflammatory mediators can induce platelet activation, smooth muscle contraction, vascular dilation, neutrophil degranulation and eosinophil chemotaxis. Although heparin is an anticoagulant, it also interacts with chemokines to mediate the migration of inflammatory cells.

It has become clear that the complement system also triggers the inflammatory response. The complement system, an important component of innate immune response, consists of over 30 proteins in the blood plasma and can be sequentially activated by proteolytic cleavage or other modifications. In general, complements can be activated through three pathways: (1) The classical pathway is initiated by binding of antibodies to soluble antigens forming the immune complex or to antigenic epitopes on the surface of pathogens; (2) The alternative pathway is triggered by certain ligands on the surface of pathogen to directly bind complement component C3b; (3) The complement system can be activated by the third distinctive lectin pathway, independent of both antibodies and C1 complex, via mannose-binding lectin (MBL). Human MBL, belonging to the collectin family with multiple carbohydrate recognition domains, is able to bind to surface sugar groups expressed on a variety of pathogens, which play a crucial role in the innate recognition of pathogens. Moreover, MBL can also recognize the carbohydrate structures expressed on aberrant or damaged host cells, indicating an increasingly recognized critical function for MBL to maintain homeostasis in health and disease. Once the complement cascade is activated, the major functions of complements include: lysis of pathogens by activating the membrane attack complex; enhancement of phagaocytosis (opsonization); clearance of immune complex from the blood circulation; enhancement of antigen presentation to lymphocytes; enhancement of B cell activation as well as attraction of neutrophils to the site of infection (chemotaxis) for local inflammation induction. Notably, the classical pathway represents an important example of the linkage between innate and adaptive immune responses during the host defense. Similarly, the kinin system is an enzymatic cascade, starting when the Hageman factor, a plasma clotting factor, is activated after tissue damage. The activation of Hageman factor leads to the cleavage of kininogen for producing bradykinin. As a potent inflammatory mediator, bradykinin can increase vascular permeability and vasodilation and induce smooth muscle contraction. The coagulation system represents another enzymatic cascade triggered by the damage of blood vessels, which generates a large amount of thrombin to activate the clotting process for preventing bleeding as well as the spread of invading pathogens. All these components of the innate immune system act in concert to provide an effective protection from invading pathogens or tissue injuries.

Influx of leukocytes

During the inflammatory response, leukocytes following a gradient of chemoattractants can migrate through endothelium to the site of infection or injury. During the process, endothelial cells are activated and express selectins and other cell adhesion molecules to capture leukocytes and assist them for extravasation into the site of inflammation.

Over 60 trillion endothelial cells cover as much as 4,000 square meters in our human body. In the inflammatory response, endothelial cells act as sentinel cells. The extensive coverage of endothelial cells offers effective detection of bacteria once they enter into the bloodstream. Moreover, recent studies indicate that endothelial cells from different organs express surface CD14, Toll-like receptor 2(TLR2), TLR4, TLR9 and MD2 and the MyD88 (TLR signaling adaptor myeloid differentiation primary-response protein 88) and respond to various TLR ligands. Therefore, endothelial cells, acting as sentinel cells, are critically involved in host defense against infection.

During an inflammatory response, leukocytes are attracted to migrate to the inflamed sites. Selectins expressed on endothelial cells mediate the initial tethering and rolling of leukocytes and a combination of chemokines and intergrins further mediates the firm adhesion, which then allows leukocytes to emigrate out of the vasculature (Figure 1). Selectins are a family of calcium-dependent, type I transmembrane glycoproteins consisting of E-selectin (CD62E), P-selectin (CD62P) and L-selectin. P-selectin is constitutively expressed and stored in secretory granules. Surface expression of P-selectin on venular endothelium is substantially increased upon stimulation by inflammatory mediators. E-selectin is not presynthesized in endothelial cells, which is expressed on the surface of endothelial cells as quickly as 2 h after TNF-α stimulation both *in vivo* and *in vitro* while its expression declines within 24 h. The overlapping functions between E-selectin and P-selectin enhance the leukocyte recruitment during inflammation. Unlike the expression of P-selectin and E-selectin on endothelial cells, L-selectin is expressed on many leukocyte subsets, which allows for the optimal interactions between leukocytes and endothelial cells.

In addition to selectins, other adhesion molecules such as vascular cell adhesion molecule 1 (VCAM1) that are expressed by activated endothelium also promote leukocyte migration. Moreover, activated complement proteins, especially the anaphylatoxin C5a, also contribute to the trafficking of leukocytes.

Effector mechanisms

In general, neutrophils in the blood are the first batch of cells attracted to the site of infection. The infiltration of neutrophils into the tissue usually peaks within the first few hours of an acute inflammatory response, which is then followed by monocytes. Infiltrated monocytes further differentiate into macrophages in the tissue. The major functions of neutrophils and macrophages are to engulf and kill pathogens through both oxidative and non-oxidative mechanisms. The interaction between neutrophils and endothelial cells is crucial for completion of the extravasation process. Neutrophils can be rapidly recruited to inflamed sites during an innate immune response to infection. To achieve the successful extravasation, neutrophils must first tether to the vascular endothelium and then roll along the endothelium before they are firmly arrested at affected sites. Upon the completion of extravasation, neutrophils leave the vasculature and migrate to the distinct sites of infection (Figure 1). In this process, the family of selectin molecules, especially P-selectin and E-selectin expressed by endothelial cells, facilitate the initial tethering and rolling of neutrophils in the postcapillary venules of the peripheral vasculature. At the same time, chemotactic factors also greatly increase the expression of L-selection on neutrophils. Furthermore, the adhesion molecules LFA-1 and Mac-1 expressed on neutrophils interact with ICAM-1 and ICAM-2 on the endothelial cells, an essential step for the migration of neutrophils

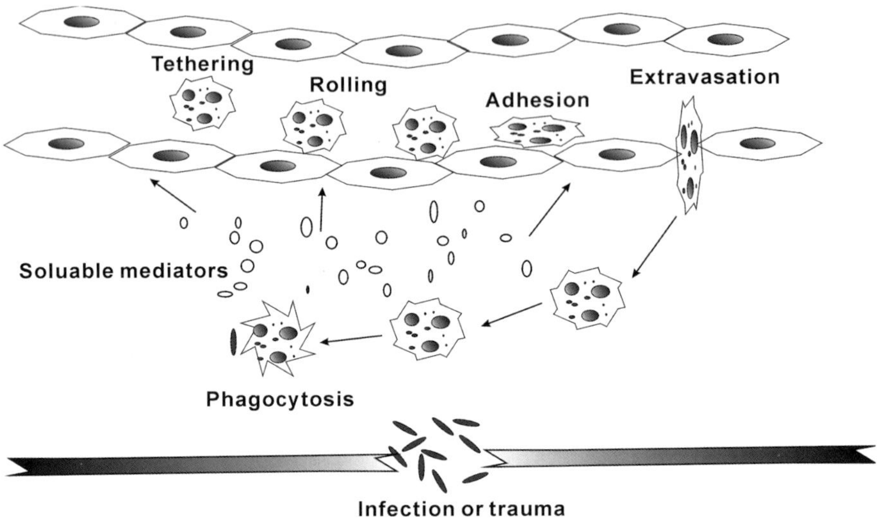

Figure 1. Leukocyte migration during an inflammatory response. Inflammatory mediators activate endothelial cells by increasing the vessel permeability and expressing adhesion molecules to capture leukocytes to make them tether, roll, and adhere to the endothelium and finally migrate through junctions between the endothelial cells into the local tissues that are damaged by invading pathogens or trauma. Activated neutrophils and macrophages engulf and destroy pathogens such as bacteria by phagocytosis.

from the blood flow to the site of tissue injury. Neutrophils possess a range of toxic molecules that contribute to the killing of bacteria. Neutrophils capture and engulf bacteria and internalize them into phagolysosomes. The phagolysosomes are constituted by proteins including NADPH oxidase that generates reactive oxygen species, proteases including elastase and cathepsin G and antimicrobial proteins such as defensins and bacterial/permeability-increasing protein. Moreover, recent findings suggest that neutrophil extracellular traps (NETs) consisting of chromatin coated with proteases might improve the efficiency of bacteria capturing in the blood. Unlike neutrophils, lymphocytes undergo a distinct extravasating process through the interactions of their homing receptors with tissue-specific adhesion molecules on high-endothelial venules in lymphoid organs and other secondary lymphoid tissues. Notably, effector lymphocytes can also undergo the transendothelial migration in the inflamed tissue.

Extensive studies have demonstrated that sensing and detection of the pathogens by the innate immune system are largely dependent upon the functional interaction between pattern-recognition receptors (PRRs) and the pathogen-associated molecule. The largest family of PRRs is the membrane-associated TLRs, which have an external leucine-rich repeat recognition domain and an intracellular Toll-IL-1 receptor signaling domain. As essential sensors of invading pathogens, TLRs are transmembrane receptors that transduce signaling by homo- or hetero-dimerization after binding to their ligands. The cell-surface TLPs, including TLR-1, -2, -4, -5, -6, recognize ligands expressed on bacterial cell walls such as lipopolysaccharide (LPS), lipoteichoic acid (LTA) and peptidoglycan. In contrast, the endosomal TLRs, such as TLR-3, -7, -8, -9, recognize intracellular components such as nucleic acids for detection of various viruses. Other PRRs including nucleotide-binding domain leucine-rich repeat containing receptors (NLRs), RIG-like RNA helicases (RLHs) and C-type lectin receptors (CLRs) have also been recently characterized for their specific recognition of PAMPs on microbes. NLR family members have been found to form multiprotein complexes, namely inflammasomes, with the cysteine protease caspase-1 and the adaptor protein ASC (apoptosis-associated speck-like protein containing a CARD). The central effector molecule in inflammasome is caspase-1, which can activate the enzymatic cleavage of cytosolic IL-1β, IL-18 and IL-33. Upon the activation of the caspase-1 in response to inflammatory stimuli, the production and secretion of inflammatory cytokines IL-1β, IL-18 and IL-33 by macrophages play critical roles in host defense against infectious pathogens and cellular perturbations. There is compelling evidence that inflammation is closely associated with many human diseases. Therefore, further elucidation of the mechanisms underlying the activation of inflammasome will provide new insights in understanding the initiation and control of an inflammatory response. The design of effective and specific drugs to target inflammasome and its function holds the great potential for new therapeutic approaches for inflammatory diseases as well as chronic autoimmune conditions.

Although the innate immune response is the front line defense in dealing with infections, the generation of an adaptive immune response serves an essential step for fighting against invading pathogens. The first stage to induce the adaptive immunity is the acquisition of antigens by professional antigen-presenting cells (APCs). APCs process antigens in peripheral tissues and migrate to the draining lymph nodes and present antigens to T cells. Following the recognition of antigens, activated T cells undergo division and acquire potent effector functions. Upon activation by APC, $CD4^+$ T cells can differentiate into T follicular helper T cells and cytokine-producing effector T cells including Th1 and Th2 cells. Recent studies have demonstrated a significant role for $Foxp3^+$ regulatory T cells (Treg) in maintaining peripheral tolerance and suppressing auto-immune inflammatory reactions. Treg cells can effectively inhibit inflammatory response and induce immune tolerance via the production of inhibitory cytokines or in a cell contact-dependent manner. Many autoimmune disorders are manifested as chronic inflammatory diseases in which the balance between the regulatory and inflammatory arms of the immune system is deregulated. Recent studies suggest that the local inflammatory microenvironment, including activated APC, secreted cytokines, as well as metabolic or damaged cell components, can affect the generation and function of Treg cells. It has become evident that Treg cell plasticity and function largely depend upon local IL-2 production and the molecular milieu at the site of inflammation. Thus, it is possible that inhibitory cytokines such as IL-10 and TGF-β produced by Treg cells or other immune cells promote infectious tolerance. T helper 17 (Th17) cells are a relatively new $CD4^+$ T cells subset producing the proinflammatory cytokine IL-17, which promote tissue inflammation in host defense responses against infection and in autoimmune diseases. The presence of T cells, in particular Th17 cells, has been documented in various human carcinomas as well as animal models of cancer. Although IL-17 can be also produced by infiltrated neutrophils and other tissue cells, there is emerging evidence that Th17 cells can promote dendritic cell recruitment and enhance $CD8^+$ cytotoxic T cell activation in the tumor site, which indicates the potential application of using Th17 cells as cellular therapy for cancers or chronic infections. Thus, an acute inflammatory response associated with anti-tumor immunity might help fight against various tumors. Further studies will provide new insight into the complex relationship between inflammation and cancer.

In the secondary lymphoid organs, antigen-specific T cells migrate to the B cell follicles and help to activate B cells. Subsequently, B cells proliferate and differentiate into antibody-secreting plasma cells and memory B cells. B cells can recognize both soluble and membrane-associated antigens. B-cell activation is initiated by stimulating B-cell receptor (BCR) through a specific antigen. Extensive studies have assessed the role of various BCR-associated signaling and membrane molecules in B-cell responses. Within seconds of the antigen interaction with the BCR, there is phosphorylation of tyrosine residues located within ITAM of the transducer elements Igα and Igβ. Thus antigen recognition triggers the sequential binding to ITAMs and the activation of protein tyrosine kinases (PTK), such as lyn (a member of the src kinases family) and syk that is recruited by previously phosphorylated ITAM. The outcome of BCR engagement is influenced by several factors, including concentration of the antigen, the affinity of BCR for antigen, a cohort of co-receptors, intracellular enzymes and adaptor molecules. It has been shown in B cells that they have abnormal antigen receptors-mediated early signal transduction events in inflammatory auto-immune diseases. Recent studies suggest that membrane-associated antigen is more potent in B-cell activation *in vivo*. The fate of activated B cells can be classified into two differentiation pathways. On the one hand, B cells can differentiate into extrafollicular plasmablasts that are essential for rapid antibody production and early protective immune responses; on the other hand, activated B cells enter the germinal centers (GC). Within GC, mature B cells undergo clonal expansion, somatic hypermutaion of V_H genes, class switch recombination at the IgH locus and further selection for high affinity maturation of BCR and subsequently differentiate into memory B cells and plasma cells. This reaction ultimately produces plasma cells that secrete high affinity antibody with predominantly switched isotypes. If newly generated plasma cells receive survival signals from stromal cells in the microenvironment such as bone marrow or spleen, they may survive for many months as long-lived plasma cells, which provide a long-lasting protection from secondary challenge with the same antigen. In a humoral immune response, follicular dendritic cells (FDC)-B cell interactions in GCs play a crucial role in full activation of B cells. FDC-B cell interactions usually require two distinct but synergistic signals. The first signal, delivered through the BCR, is provided by the antigen itself and is responsible for the specificity of the antibody secreted. The second signal is derived from the B cell coreceptor complex consisting of CD19, CD21 and CD81. B-cell co-receptor complex is essential for the rapid trapping of complement-coated antigens by B cells, and is critical for early protective antibody responses to lethal pathogens that rapidly multiply and quickly overwhelm the immune system. Secreted antibodies by plasma cells are soluble molecules circulating in the blood where they act as effector molecules of the humoral immunity. The major functions of antibodies secreted by plasma cells include neutralization that eliminates the pathogens or their pathogenecity, opsonization that enhances antigen phagocytosis by macrophages and neutrophils, complement activation that leads to the cytolysis of pathogens, and antibody-dependent cell-mediated cytotoxicity that destroys antibody-bound target cells. In a tightly regulated fashion, both effector T and B cells are the central players involved in the resolution of inflammation necessary for containing the infections, especially the systemic infection.

Termination of inflammation and tissue repair

During the late stage of inflammation, anti-inflammatory mediators and tissue repair system become activated to control the infection and tissue injury, which includes various kinds of inhibitors for pro-inflammatory cytokines such as soluble receptors (sTNFαR, sIL-R, etc.), anti-inflammatory cytokines (IL-4, IL-10 and TGF-β) as well as antibodies arising from the adaptive immune response. Upon the control of inflammation by anti-inflammatory mediators, the wound healing system becomes activated. Enzymes of the clotting system such as plasmin enter damaged tissues and assist the formation of blood clot to commence wound healing. In addition to its key role in limiting inflammatory response, TGF-β has been shown to promote proliferation of fibroblasts and deposition of extracellular matrix proteins for tissue repairing. Moreover, various immune cells including myofibroblasts and macrophages can produce collagen to repair damaged tissues. The effective immune responses are essential for the regulation of both duration and intensity of the acute inflammation, which are further implicated in the control of tissue damage and repair for healing.

Regulatory mechanisms of inflammation

This complex inflammatory response represents the host defense for its adaption to cell loss or tissue damage, which requires the delicate coordination of many functional programs operated at multiple levels, including responsiveness of immune cells to inflammatory stimuli, production of cytokines and other mediators and modulation of transcriptional controls on gene expression and signal transductions. Recent studies have revealed that the inflammatory gene expression profile consists of a number of coordinately regulated set of genes encoding key functional molecules in an inflammatory response. For example, TLR ligands have been identified as the inducers of acute inflammation in macrophages. After only a few hours of stimulation by LPS, macrophages, upon the transcriptional response, express a complex set of genes controlling phagocytosis, cytokine and chemokine production, cell migration and activation, tissue remodeling. Among the best characterized transcriptional response, three categories of transcription factors including NF-κB, IFN-regulatory factors (IRFs) and cAMP-responsive-element-binding protein 1 (CREB1) are known to possess key functions in inflammation.

Recent studies have implicated microRNAs in the regulation of innate and adaptive immune responses as well as inflammatory networks in various cell and tissue types. MicroRNAs are short non-coding RNAs that posttranscriptionally modulate the expression of multiple target genes and are thus implicated in a large array of cellular and developmental processes. Since it is apparent that most protein-coding genes are subjected to the regulation by microRNAs, this highlights the potent effect of these small molecules on gene expression pattern and its regulatory network. Thus, it is possible that the inflammatory response can be modulated or controlled by synthesizing mRNAs encoding proteins that promote or inhibit inflammation. Together, post-transcriptional mechanisms that modify mRNA stability or translation can provide more rapid and flexible control of the inflammatory process, which may prove to be particularly important in coordinating the initiation and resolution of inflammation or containing the severe systemic infection.

Conclusion

The relationship between the inflammation caused by bacteria or trauma and host defense by our immune system represents a well-regulated balance. To successfully infect the host, invading pathogens evade the multifaced innate immune system to overcome the immune surveillance. At the initiation stage of inflammation, innate immunity acts as a front line of host defense, among which a major function of recruited immune cells is phagocytosis of the invading pathogen. When the innate defense mechanisms fail to prevent an infection, the adaptive immune response is mobilized for lymphocyte activation, cytokine secretion and increased production of inflammatory mediators. Thus, the regulated inflammatory response offers an effective protection following infection or tissue damage by restricting the cellular damage to the local affected sites. Future studies on the regulatory mechanisms in the inflammation response would enable the potential manipulation of various immune components of inflammation.

References

1. Stutz A, Golenbock DT, Latz E. (2009) Inflammasomes: Too big to miss. *J Clin Invest* **119**:3502–11.
2. Hickey MJ, Kubes P. (2009) Intravascular immunity: The host-pathogen encounter in blood vessels. *Nat Rev Immunol* **9**:364–75.
3. Petri B, Phillipson M, Kubes P. (2008) The physiology of leukocyte recruitment: An *in vivo* perspective. *J Immunol* **180**:6439–46.
4. Millington OR, Zinselmeyer BH, Brewer JM *et al.* (2007) Lymphocyte tracking and interactions in secondary lymphoid organs. *Inflamm Res* **56**:391–401.
5. Batista FD, Harwood NE. (2009) The who, how and where of antigen presentation to B cells. *Nat Rev Immunol* **9**:15–27.

Chapter 3

Genetic and Epigenetic Alterations in Inflammation-Related Cancers — General Mechanisms of Cancers

Yasuyuki Okamoto and Yutaka Kondo*

Division of Molecular Oncology,
Aichi Cancer Center Research Institute,
Nagoya 464-8681, Japan

While the connection between inflammation and tumorigenesis was suggested a long time ago, key factors linking these two processes remain to be completely understood. A defining characteristic of the malignant tumor cell is its inappropriate growth and strong invasive and metastatic capability. Studies have shown that during chronic inflammation, several factors were released from the inflammatory cells, and genetic and epigenetic abnormalities were accumulated in the progenitor cells, which may be sufficient to confer malignant growth properties. This chapter mainly focuses on and discusses the fundamental mechanisms linking chronic inflammation and tumorigenesis.

Introduction

In the 19th century, Rudolf Virchow had suggested the close association between cancer and inflammation as the reason for the infiltration of lymphoreticular cells into cancer tissue.[1] In the last decade, molecular researches have revealed some molecular mechanisms that underlie links between inflammation and carcinogenesis. Two lines have been shown in this relationship (Figure 1).[2]

* Corresponding author. E-mail: ykondo@aichi-cc.jp

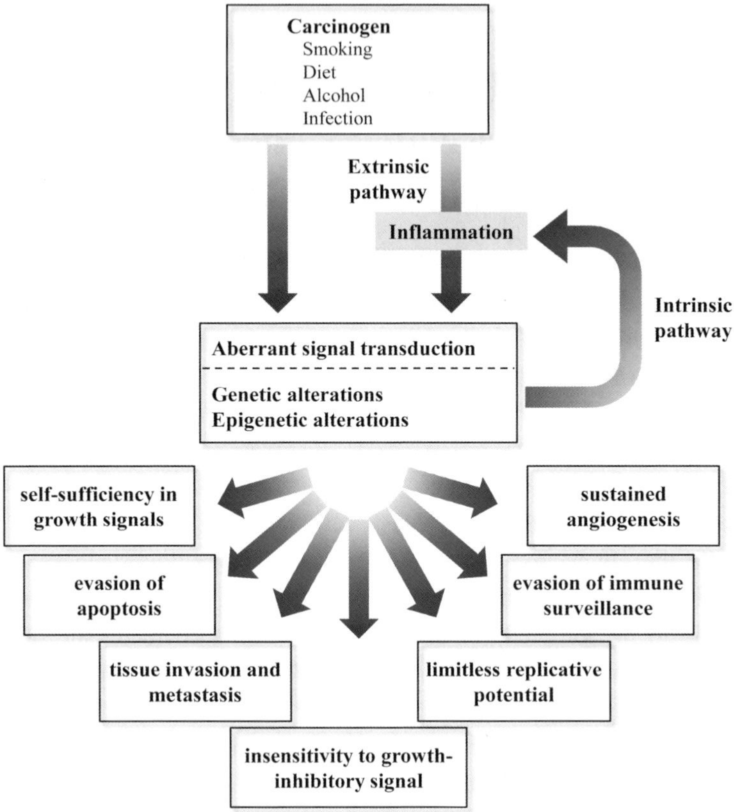

Figure 1. Overview of carcinogenic pathways connecting inflammation and cancers. Two pathways, the intrinsic pathway and the extrinsic pathway, exist in inflammation-related carcinogenesis.[2] These pathways might link to the defining characteristics of malignant tumors, such as self-sufficiency in growth signals, insensitivity to growth-inhibitory signal, evasion of programmed cell death (apoptosis), limitless replicative potential, sustained angiogenesis, tissue invasion and metastasis, and evasion of immune surveillance.[11,12]

First, chronic inflammation increases the risk of cancer. The causes of inflammation in gastrointestinal tract and accessory digestive glands are varied, such as infection, autoimmune disorders, or toxic chemicals. *Helicobacter pylori*, which inhabits various areas of the stomach, particularly the antrum, causes a chronic inflammation that links to the gastric cancer or mucosa-associated lymphoid tissue (MALT) lymphoma.[3] Hepatitis B virus or hepatitis C virus infection leads to chronic hepatitis and causes hepatocellular carcinoma.[4] Inflammatory bowel diseases are also known to increase the risk of colon cancer.[5] These causes are closely associated with the activation of the "extrinsic pathway." In contrast to an increase in the risk of cancer by chronic inflammation, non-steroidal anti-inflammatory drugs decrease the risk of colon carcinogenesis.[6–8]

Second, inflammation, which is caused by oncogenic stress, induces cancer development. Genetic and epigenetic alterations affect the expression of inflammatory genes and lead to recruitment of inflammatory cells (intrinsic pathway). For example, the mutations of RAS family proteins promote RAS-RAF signaling pathway, which activates inflammatory chemokines and cytokines and results in more aggressive tumor formation.[9,10] Thus, genetic or epigenetic alterations cause both inflammation and tumor formation.[2] Consequently, inflammatory cells characterize the tumor microenvironment and play an important role in tumor development and progression.

A fundamental question in cancer biology is which molecular signatures are required for acquisition of malignant behavior (Figure 1). To acquire the characteristics of malignant behavior, seven hallmarks have been indicated: self-sufficiency in growth signals, insensitivity to growth-inhibitory signal, evasion of programmed cell death (apoptosis), limitless replicative potential, sustained angiogenesis, tissue invasion and metastasis, and evasion of immune surveillance.[11,12] In addition, the importance of the five types of stress during tumor formation has been proposed: metabolic stress, proteotoxic stress, mitotic stress, oxidative stress and DNA damage stress.[13] Together, a combination of these sets of hallmarks confers the cells malignant phenotype. Since inflammation may induce genetics and epigenetics alterations, aberrant activation of chemokines and cytokines, aberrant production of reactive oxygen species (ROS), and other stresses, a complex network of these factors may lead to tumor formation (Figure 2). In this chapter, we discuss the general mechanisms of malignant tumor formation in gastrointestinal tract and accessory digestive glands.

Signaling pathways

A common finding in chronic inflammatory diseases is the activation of growth factor expression and signaling (Figure 3).[2,14] Such growth factors

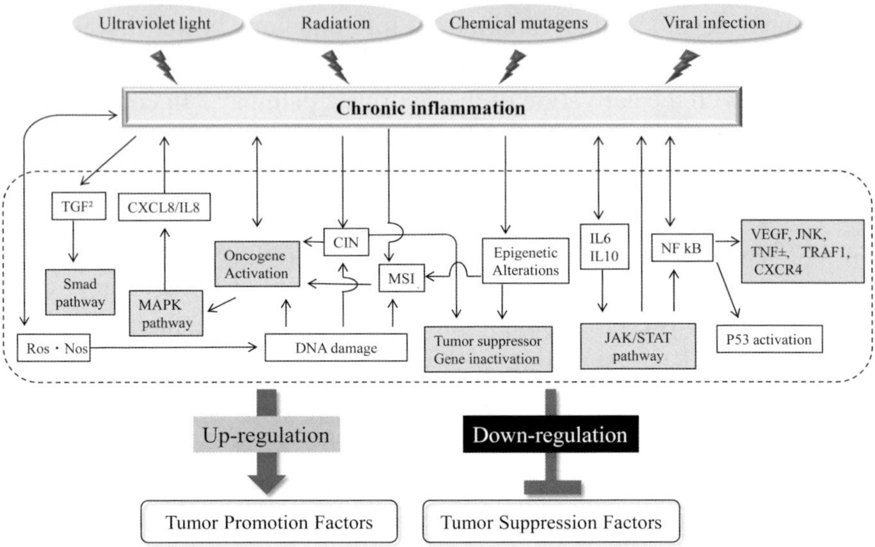

Figure 2. Schematic diagram of inflammation-associated factors. Chronic inflammation, caused by infection, or toxic chemicals, affects the various inflammatory mediators such as ROS/NOS, cytokine, chemokine, and NF-κB. These mediators alter gene activities through direct or indirect mechanisms such as mutation, CIN, MSI, and epigenetic alterations, and contribute to activation of oncogenes and inactivation of tumor suppressor genes. Furthermore, the genetic alterations induce chronic inflammations through inflammatory mediators and signaling pathway such as MAPK pathway and JAK/STAT pathway. The inflammatory mediator and genetic alterations interact with each other, propagating tumor microenvironment.

by chronic stimulation may contribute to neoplastic transformation through a series of molecular and functional changes. In addition, the presence of inflammatory cells in the tumor and their chemical mediators in the cancerous tissues affects cancer behavior through cell cycle, angiogenesis, or cell adhesion.

NF-κB

NF-κB is an important coordinator of innate immunity and inflammation. NF-κB provides a mechanistic link between inflammation and cancer, and plays a key role in both the extrinsic the pathway and intrinsic

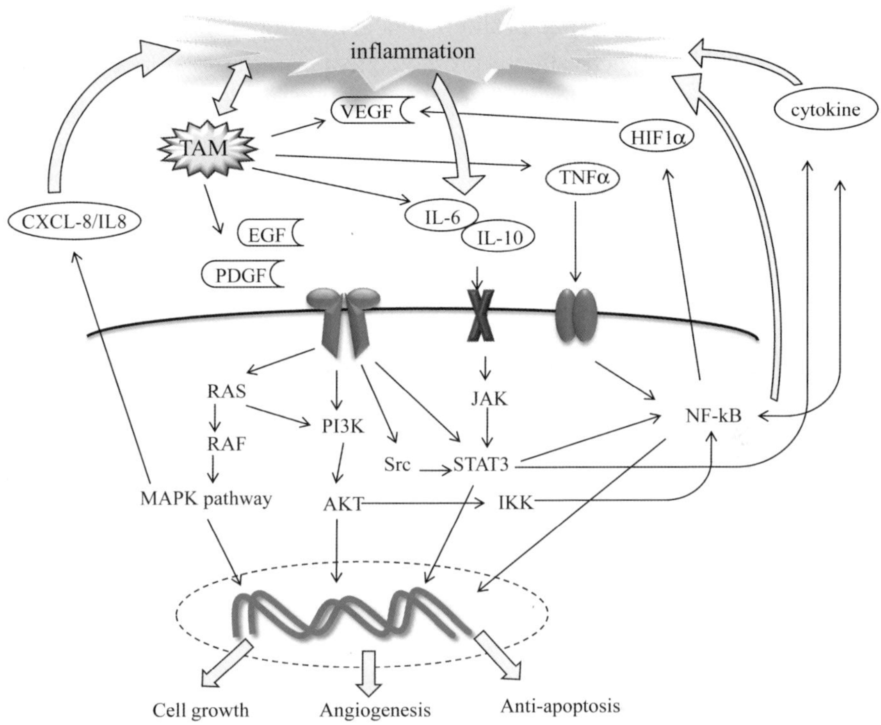

Figure 3. Interaction between signaling pathway and inflammation. Tyrosine kinase receptor is activated by growth factors (VEGF, PDGF, and EGF) from inflammatory cells, such as TAMs. The activation of tyrosine kinase receptor leads to the recruitment of RAS, which through RAF activation, results in a cascade of serine/threonine kinase phosphorylation (MAPK kinase and extracellular signal-regulated kinase). Phospho-extracellular signal-regulated kinase is then translocated into the nucleus where it activates transcription factors related to proliferation and survival as well as transcription factors of CXCL-8. Expression of CXCL8 initiates the intrinsic pathways. PI3K/Akt pathway is promoted by tyrosine kinase receptor activity or RAS activity. Activated Akt transiently associates with IKK and induces the activation of NF-κB. NF-κB is also activated by STAT3 and various chemokine such as TNF-a. NF-κB activate intrinsic pathways, inducing the expression of inflammatory cytokines, such as HIF1a.

pathway.[15] NF-κB drives the expression of inflammatory cytokines, such as interleukin-8 (CXCL-8/IL-8), CXCL1, and hypoxia-inducible factor 1 alpha (HIF1α) ,which are important for the synthesis of inflammatory mediator.[16,17] Further, in cancer and epithelial cells exposed to carcinogens,

NF-κB leads cell survival and proliferation, activating cyclin D1 and c-Myc. In cancer cell, NF-κB activation is promoted by pro-inflammatory cytokines, such as tumor necrosis factor alpha (TNFα) and interleukin-1 (IL-1). NF-κB can also be activated as a result of genetic alteration, such as RAS mutation through phosphatidylinositol 3 kinase (PI3K)/AKT pathway. Activation of NF-κB in the gastrointestinal tract leads to induction of proinflammatory cytokines, which maintain inflammation. Intestinal NF-κB activation has been found in patients with Crohn's diseases and ulcerative colitis. In colitis-associated cancer model, it was shown that depletion of IKKB from intestinal epithelial cells led to a decrease in tumor incidence without affecting the inflammation level.[18,19] Thus the IKKB/NF-κB pathway induced by inflammation plays a key role in promoting tumorigenesis. Furthermore, NF-κB is highly interconnected with Janus kinase (JAK) — signal transducer and activator of transcription (STAT) pathway. There are striking parallels between NF-κB and STAT3. Both proteins are not continuously activated in cancer and are essential for transducing cytoplasmic signals from extracellular stimuli.

STAT3

STAT3 signaling is a major intrinsic pathway for cancer inflammation because of its frequent activation in malignant cells and plays a key role in regulating many genes crucial for cancer inflammation.[20] STAT signaling pathways were originally discovered in the context of normal cytokine signaling. STAT3 is inducible by interleukin-6 (IL-6) signaling as well as other cytokines.[21,22] These cytokines drive the JAK and STAT3 activation, leading tumor cell survival through the up-regulation of anti-apoptotic genes. In addition to being downstream of cytokines, STAT3 is activated by growth factor receptors, including epidermal growth factor receptor (EGFR), vascular epidermal growth factor receptor (VEGFR) and HER2, and non-receptor tyrosine kinases, such as proto-oncogene tyrosine-protein kinase SRC. Notably, the activation of STAT3 signaling pathway is transmitted to stromal inflammatory cells in the tumor microenvironment. This is because STAT3 is a transcription factor regulating numerous genes encoding cytokines, chemokines and growth factors in tumor cells, the associated receptors of which in turn activate STAT3 in stromal cells.

Thus, a STAT3-feedforward loop is established between tumor cells and non-transformed cells in the microenvironment, which also includes immune cells.[17,23]

RAS

The RAS subfamily of proteins are the most frequently mutated dominant oncogenes in human cancer. They induce intrinsic pathways to promote inflammatory cytokine and chemokines through the RAS-RAF signaling pathway.[9,24] Generally, activated RAS regulates multiple cellular functions through several effectors. The best characterized effectors are the mitogen-activated protein kinase (MAPK) signaling molecules. Phosphoric extracellular signal-regulated kinase (ERK) is translocated into the nucleus through MAPK pathway, inducing cell proliferation and survival. RAS signal also activates PI3K, downstream of which the AKT pathway is linked to NF-κB, coordinator between cancer and inflammation. The inflammatory mediator interleukin-8 (CXCL-8/IL-8), which is a potent chemotactic factor for neutrophils and is closely associated with the initiation of an inflammatory response, is a transcriptional target of RAS signaling.[10] Therefore, the induction of CXCL-8/IL-8 by oncogenic RAS could provide a mechanism by which neoplastic cells recruit immune cells to the tumor site. Clinical studies have demonstrated that the tumorigenic potential of human colon and pancreatic has been shown to directly correlate with the amount of CXCL-8/IL-8 expression.[25,26]

TNF-α

Tumor necrosis factor (TNF) is a cytokine involved in systemic inflammation and is a member of a group of cytokines that stimulate the acute phase reaction. TNF-α appears to have a bilateral character in the tumorigenesis. Initially, TNF-α was known to be a regulator of immune cells and inhibit tumorigenesis. However, now TNF-α is also known to play a role in promoting tumor cell growth at the early stages.[27] TNF is produced mainly from macrophages, while they are also produced from a variety of other cell types, including lymphoid cells, endothelial cells, and malignant cells. When chronically produced in the tumor microenvironment, TNF-α is a major mediator of cancer-related inflammation.[28–30] TNF-receptor (TNFR) activation leads to recruitment of intracellular adaptor proteins that activate multiple signal transduction pathways. Downstream of TNF-signal is related to the NF-κB signaling and the MAPK signaling, promoting tumor cell growth and activating the intrinsic pathway.[31]

TAM

Tumor-associated macrophage (TAM) is the principal leukocyte subset driving an amplification of the inflammatory response in the tumor microenvironment.[2] A meta-analysis demonstrated that over 80% of studies show a correlation between macrophage density and poor patient prognosis.[32] Thereafter several reports have supported this conclusion. For example, the density of macrophages in hepatocellular carcinoma patients after curative resection was strongly associated with disease recurrence and poor survival.[33] TAM assists tumor cells to progress in many ways, which result in the acquisition of malignant phenotype. For example, TAMs accumulate in hypoxic regions of tumors and stimulate angiogenesis by expressing factors such as vascular endothelial growth factor (VEGF). TAMs produce various growth factors and chemokines: epidermal growth factor (EGF), platelet-derived growth factor receptor (PDGFR), IL-6 and TNF-α. These productions contribute to the tumor in acquiring hallmarks of cancer. TAMs also promote tumor invasion by producing proteases, such as urokinase-type plasminogen activator (uPA) and matrix metalloproteinase 9 (MMP-9) that break down the basement membrane and remodel the stromal matrix, which lead to tumor cell invasion.[34,35]

Genetic instability

Tumor cell phenotype is the consequence of a relatively high level of genetic instability that is caused by the defects in checkpoint signaling. Two distinct pathways of genetic instability have been described: the chromosomal instability (CIN) and microsatellite instability (MSI).[36,37] These genetic instabilities with sequential mutational damage in a set of important tumor-related genes confer growth and survival advantages to the tumor cells.

Tumor cells with CIN show an imbalance in chromosome number (aneuploidy), regional chromosomal amplifications, and loss of heterozygosity (LOH). Although it has been known that proteins of the mitotic checkpoints are dysregulated in most cancers with CIN, precise molecular mechanisms underlying CIN remain to be elucidated.[38,39] DNA damage accumulates as a result of exposure to exogenous stress (ultraviolet light, radiation and chemical mutagens) and endogenous reactive metabolites including reactive oxygen and nitrogen species (ROS and NOS).[40] Another source of DNA damage is from errors that occur during normal DNA metabolism or aberrant DNA processing reactions, including DNA replication, recombination, and repair. Since DNA damage may induce mutations in cells, which could lead to carcinogenesis, cells possess multiple mechanisms to repair DNA damage and prevent such mutations. Normal cells require precise regulation of cell cycle and check point.

Dysregulation of G1 check point has been well studied in human cancers (Figure 4). CDKN2B (p15), CDKN2A (p16) and CDKN1A (p21) are known as cyclin-dependent kinase (CDK) inhibitor.[41] The Cyclin D binds to CDK4, and makes the active cyclin D-CDK4 complex. Cyclin D-CDK4 complex in turn phosphorylates the retinoblastoma protein (Rb). The phosphorylated Rb separates from the E2F-Rb complex, consequently activating E2F. Activated E2F induce the expression of cyclin E, which makes a complex with CDK2 and foster the cell cycle progression (Figure 4). Thus, activation of p16 and p53 (inducing p21 activation) could suppress E2F and drive the cells into quiescence (enter into G0 phase). Through the inactivation of p16 or p53 and RASSF1A, cancer cells acquire insensitivity to growth-inhibitory signal. Thus, inactivating mutation in these genes links to defects in checkpoint signaling leading to abnormal chromosome numbers. Interestingly, one of the mechanisms for inactivation of these genes is associated with epigenetic alterations (Figure 4). Integrated network between genetic and epigenetic alterations appears to confer the driving force for tumor formation.

Products of the *mitotic arrest-deficient* (*MAD*) gene and the *budding uninhibited by benzimidazoles* (*BUB*) are the important cell cycle checkpoint factors that control sister chromatid separation (Figure 4).[42,43] In some cancers displaying CIN, the loss of mitotic checkpoint was associated with

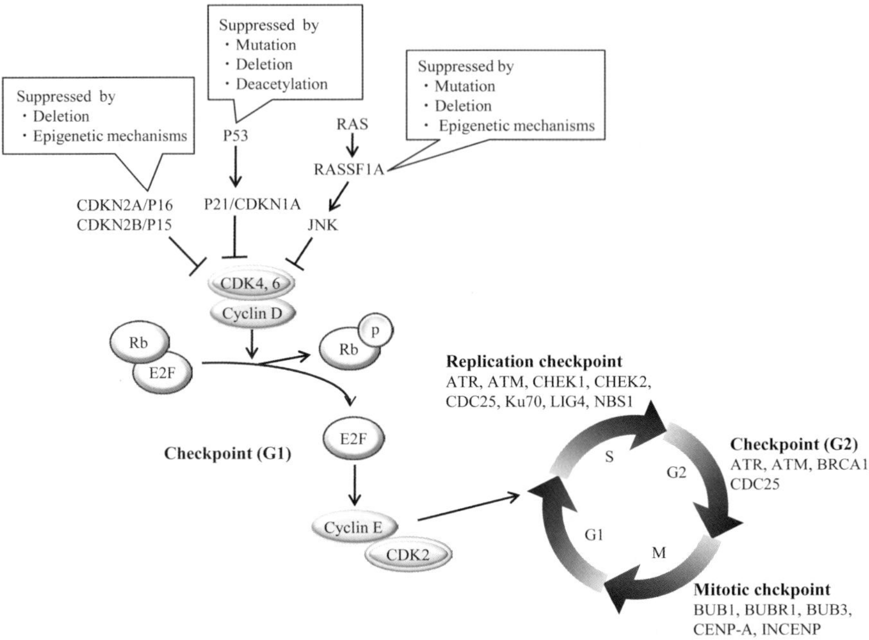

Figure 4. Schematic diagram of cell cycle checkpoints associated with tumorigenesis. Cell cycle checkpoints are shown with a corresponding list of genes in relation to cell cycle phases. When DNA damage accumulates as a result of exposure to exogenous stress, checkpoints machineries regulate the cell cycle to repair DNA damage and prevent genetic abnormalities. Disruption of the checkpoints proteins by gene mutations and/or epigenetic abnormalities may lead aneuploidy, regional chromosomal amplifications, and LOH.

the mutational inactivation of the *BUB1* and *BUBR1* genes.[44,45] Proteins with regulation of kinetochore function, such as centoromere-associated protein A (CENP-A) and INCENP, have been found to be overexpressed in human colon cancers.[46,47] Mutations or amplification of other DNA checkpoint genes have been identified in cancers. Mutations in the *ataxia telangiectasia mutated* (*ATM*) and *ataxia telangiectasia and Rad3-related* (*ATR*) have been implicated to be involved in tumor formation.[48] Mutations in genes that encode for other DNA repair proteins are associated with an increased risk of human cancers, including *BRCA1*, *BRCA2*, *CHEK1*, and *CHEK2*, which are all involved in the regulation of double-strand DNA breaks.[43,49–51]

Microsatellites are genomic regions in which short DNA sequences or a single nucleotide is repeated. Although mutations occur in some microsatellites because of the misalignment of their repetitive subunits during DNA replication, such mutations are usually repaired by the DNA mismatch repair (MMR) in normal cells.[52] Mutations or epigenetic silencing of MMR members (*MLH1*, *MSH2*, and *MSH6*) is associated with increased MSI and with hereditary and sporadic human cancers. The pathogenesis from MSI is found in many tumor types, but has been studied mostly in familial colorectal cancers, hereditary nonpolyposis colon cancer (HNPCC) that is caused by a germ-line mutation in any of the mismatch-repair genes. Some mechanisms for inactivation of MMR protein are linked to inflammation in human malignancies. Expression of *MLH1* is silenced by aberrant promoter DNA methylation. Studies in colon cancers have indicated a close relationship between MSI and CpG island methylator phenotype (CIMP, described below).[53] It has been suggested that chronic inflammation may link to DNA methylation of *MLH1*.[54] Other MMR proteins, MSH2 and MSH6, are suppressed by HIF-1α, which is induced in cancer cell by inflammatory cytokines.[55] Moreover, ROS directly suppress the activity of MMR on inducing frameshift mutation.[56] MSI has also been documented in the nonneoplastic inflammatory lesions, pancreatitis and ulcerative colitis and metaplasia in stomach, suggesting an early event in some cancers.[54,57–60]

As is described above, genetic instability is sometimes associated with epigenetic alterations, since some important proteins that are involved in checkpoint or MMR pathways are the target of epigenetic silencing mechanism (Figure 4). Thus, an integrated network between genetic and epigenetic alterations appears to confer the driving force for tumor formation.

Epigenetic alterations

The relationship between promoter DNA methylation and inflammation has been documented in many types of cancers.[4,61–63] Epigenetic abnormities play a key role in carcinogenesis. The epigenetic alterations are associated with gene silencing, sometimes together with point mutations and deletions, serving as a mechanism leading to the inactivation of tumor suppressor genes and cancer-related genes in human cancers. Dysregulation of these target genes, which compromise multiple carcinogenic pathways, is connected with essential tumor properties such as tumor cell proliferation, anti-apoptosis, neo-angiogenesis, invasive behavior and chemotherapy resistance.[64,65] Two epigenetic alterations, DNA methylation and histone modification, have been well studied in human cancers.

DNA methylation

Promoter DNA methylation is widely recognized as an epigenetic modification. DNA methylation occurs in the cytosine-guanine sequence (CpG) in the DNA strand in mammals. While approximately 70% of CpG dinucleotides are methylated and scattered throughout the genome, short unmethylated CpG-rich regions (up to 2 kb) are found and called "CpG islands (CGI)".[66,67] CGI is more likely to be associated with the 5′ regions of genes (>50%), where DNA methylation takes place to maintain the repressive chromatin state and stably silence promoter activity.[68]

A close association between aberrant DNA methylation and inflammation is suggested.[14,69] Indeed, aberrant DNA methylation is frequently observed even in noncancerous tissues of patients with inflammation-associated cancers, such as liver cancers, ulcerative colitis–associated colon cancers, and gastric cancers.[4,61,70,71] In gastric cancer, *Helicobacter pylori* (*H. pylori*) infection in the stomach is known to induce aberrant DNA methylation, which appears to increase the risk of gastric cancer.[61] By contrast, the immunosuppressive drug blocked the induction of aberrant methylation caused by *H. pylori* infection in Mongolian gerbils.[72] In the glutathione peroxidase 1 (Gpx1) and Gpx2 double knockout mouse model, which represents the inflammatory bowel disease predisposing to intestinal cancer, increased production of reactive oxygen species (ROS) induced aberrant DNA methylation.[73]

Recent studies have shown the existence of an accumulation of high rates of aberrant promoter DNA methylation in a subset of cancers, including colon cancer, gastric cancer, pancreatic cancer, and glioblastoma, known as CIMP.[74–77] CIMP-positive tumors represent a clinically and etiologically distinct group that is characterized by epigenetic instability. Colorectal cancer (CRC) is the most comprehensively studied cancer in terms of CIMP. CIMP-positive CRCs exhibit characteristic genetic and clinical features, including high rates of *BRAF* and *KRAS* mutations, low rates of p53 mutations, a specific histology (mucinous, pooly differentiated), proximal location, and characteristic clinical outcomes.[53] Further, the existence of different classes of CIMP tumors (e.g., CIMP1/CIMP-high and CIMP2/CIMP-low) has been suggested recently, raising the possibility that sporadic CRCs arise from distinct parallel pathways, in which the type of genetic and epigenetic instability ultimately explain the characteristic carcinogenesis pathways altered.[78,79] Given these distinct clinicopathological features, CIMP-related carcinogenesis may proceed through a specific pathway in which the epigenetic alterations that occur in pre-malignant cells determine subsequent genetic alterations, thereby fostering the progression of these clones.[80] Although aberrant DNA methylation in promoter CGIs has been comprehensively studied in human cancers, the mechanisms regulating the establishment of *de-novo* DNA methylation as well as causing CIMP tumors remain poorly understood. Further studies may clarify the mechanism of how DNA methylation aberrantly occurs in certain CGIs during tumorigenesis.

Histone modifications

The N-terminal domains of all core histones (H2A, H2B, H3, and H4) are subject to chemical modifications, such as acetylation, methylation, ubiquitylation, and phosphorylation at certain residues.[81] These post-translational modifications can either activate or repress transcription, depending on the type of chemical modification and its location in the histone protein. This modification pattern of histone has been linked to chromatin structure and gene function during development as well as tumorigenesis.[80,82] Early studies have shown that the link between DNA methylation and histone modifications is mediated by a group of proteins with methyl DNA binding activity, including MECP2, MBD1, and KAIZO, which localize to DNA-methylated promoters and recruit a protein complex that contains histone deacetylases (HDACs) and histone methyltransferases, suggesting that DNA methylation induces chromatin structural changes through alteration of histone modifications.[83–85]

Recently it has been shown that histone modifications cooperate with DNA methylation to affect gene inactivation in some tumor suppressor genes.[86–89] DNA methylation and histone modifications might interact with each other and establish stable gene silencing.[87,90,91]

Perspectives

Although the link between inflammation and cancer is generally understood, several open questions still remain. It is still unclear whether inflammation is a sufficient factor for the development of cancer. Since it may be true that the longer the inflammation persists, the higher is the risk of associated carcinogenesis, multiple factors must be involved during the establishment of inflammation-related cancers, although some factors may be indirectly associated with inflammation. We may also recognize that given the underlying nature of the inflammation, a set of the gene products identified in analyses of expression in inflammation-related cancers are likely to be associated with the proliferative state and that pharmacologic chemicals targeting such molecules may therefore represent a general targeting of proliferating cells. Nevertheless, further knowledge about cancer-related inflammation can be linked to the useful and potent approaches to prevent and treat cancer.

References

1. Balkwill F, Mantovani A. (2001) Inflammation and cancer: Back to Virchow? *Lancet* **357**:539–45.
2. Mantovani A, Allavena P, Sica A *et al.* (2008) Cancer-related inflammation. *Nature* **454**:436–44.
3. Polk DB, Peek RM, Jr. (2010) *Helicobacter pylori*: Gastric cancer and beyond. *Nat Rev Cancer* **10**:403–14.
4. Kondo Y, Kanai Y, Sakamoto M *et al.* (2000) Genetic instability and aberrant DNA methylation in chronic hepatitis and cirrhosis — A comprehensive study of loss of heterozygosity and microsatellite instability at 39 loci and DNA hypermethylation on 8 CpG islands in microdissected specimens from patients with hepatocellular carcinoma. *Hepatology* **32**:970–9.

5. Waldner MJ, Neurath MF. (2009) Colitis-associated cancer: The role of T cells in tumor development. *Semin Immunopathol* **31**:249–56.
6. Chan AT, Ogino S, Fuchs CS. (2007) Aspirin and the risk of colorectal cancer in relation to the expression of COX-2. *N Engl J Med* **356**:2131–42.
7. Flossmann E, Rothwell PM. (2007) Effect of aspirin on long-term risk of colorectal cancer: Consistent evidence from randomised and observational studies. *Lancet* **369**:1603–13.
8. Koehne CH, Dubois RN. (2004) COX-2 inhibition and colorectal cancer. *Semin Oncol* **31**:12–21.
9. Guerra C, Schuhmacher AJ, Canamero M *et al.* (2007) Chronic pancreatitis is essential for induction of pancreatic ductal adenocarcinoma by K-Ras oncogenes in adult mice. *Cancer Cell* **11**:291–302.
10. Sparmann A, Bar-Sagi D. (2004) Ras-induced interleukin-8 expression plays a critical role in tumor growth and angiogenesis. *Cancer Cell* **6**:447–58.
11. Hanahan D, Weinberg RA. (2000) The hallmarks of cancer. *Cell* **100**:57–70.
12. Kroemer G, Pouyssegur J. (2008) Tumor cell metabolism: Cancer's Achilles' heel. *Cancer Cell* **13**:472–82.
13. Luo J, Solimini NL, Elledge SJ. (2009) Principles of cancer therapy: Oncogene and non-oncogene addiction. *Cell* **136**:823–37.
14. Grivennikov SI, Greten FR, Karin M. (2010) Immunity, inflammation, and cancer. *Cell* **140**:883–99.
15. Rayet B, Gelinas C. (1999) Aberrant rel/nfkb genes and activity in human cancer. *Oncogene* **18**:6938–47.
16. Rius J, Guma M, Schachtrup C *et al.* (2008) NF-kappaB links innate immunity to the hypoxic response through transcriptional regulation of HIF-1alpha. *Nature* **453**:807–11.
17. Kujawski M, Kortylewski M, Lee H *et al.* (2008) Stat3 mediates myeloid cell-dependent tumor angiogenesis in mice. *J Clin Invest* **118**:3367–77.
18. Greten FR, Eckmann L, Greten TF *et al.* (2004) IKKbeta links inflammation and tumorigenesis in a mouse model of colitis-associated cancer. *Cell* **118**:285–96.
19. Ouyang W, Li J, Ma Q *et al.* (2006) Essential roles of PI-3K/Akt/IKKbeta/NFkappaB pathway in cyclin D1 induction by arsenite in JB6 Cl41 cells. *Carcinogenesis* **27**:864–73.

20. Bollrath J, Greten FR. (2009) IKK/NF-kappaB and STAT3 pathways: Central signalling hubs in inflammation-mediated tumour promotion and metastasis. *EMBO Rep* **10**:1314–9.
21. Darnell JE, Jr., Kerr IM, Stark GR. (1994) Jak-STAT pathways and transcriptional activation in response to IFNs and other extracellular signaling proteins. *Science* **264**:1415–21.
22. Heinrich PC, Behrmann I, Muller-Newen G *et al.* (1998) Interleukin-6-type cytokine signalling through the gp130/Jak/STAT pathway. *Biochem J* **334** (Pt 2):297–314.
23. Yu H, Kortylewski M, Pardoll D. (2007) Crosstalk between cancer and immune cells: Role of STAT3 in the tumour microenvironment. *Nat Rev Immunol* **7**:41–51.
24. Sumimoto H, Imabayashi F, Iwata T *et al.* (2006) The BRAF-MAPK signaling pathway is essential for cancer-immune evasion in human melanoma cells. *J Exp Med* **203**:1651–6.
25. Li A, Varney ML, Singh RK. (2001) Expression of interleukin 8 and its receptors in human colon carcinoma cells with different metastatic potentials. *Clin Cancer Res* **7**:3298–304.
26. Shi Q, Abbruzzese JL, Huang S *et al.* (1999) Constitutive and inducible interleukin 8 expression by hypoxia and acidosis renders human pancreatic cancer cells more tumorigenic and metastatic. *Clin Cancer Res* **5**:3711–21.
27. Moore RJ, Owens DM, Stamp G *et al.* (1999) Mice deficient in tumor necrosis factor-alpha are resistant to skin carcinogenesis. *Nat Med* **5**:828–31.
28. Pikarsky E, Porat RM, Stein I *et al.* (2004) NF-kappaB functions as a tumour promoter in inflammation-associated cancer. *Nature* **431**:461–6.
29. Balkwill F. (2006) TNF-alpha in promotion and progression of cancer. *Cancer Metastasis Rev* **25**:409–16.
30. Sethi G, Sung B, Aggarwal BB. (2008) TNF: A master switch for inflammation to cancer. *Front Biosci* **13**:5094–107.
31. Aggarwal BB. (2003) Signalling pathways of the TNF superfamily: A double-edged sword. *Nat Rev Immunol* **3**:745–56.
32. Bingle L, Brown NJ, Lewis CE. (2002) The role of tumour-associated macrophages in tumour progression: Implications for new anticancer therapies. *J Pathol* **196**:254–65.
33. Zhu XD, Zhang JB, Zhuang PY *et al.* (2008) High expression of macrophage colony-stimulating factor in peritumoral liver tissue is associated with poor

survival after curative resection of hepatocellular carcinoma. *J Clin Oncol* **26**:2707–16.
34. Hildenbrand R, Dilger I, Horlin A *et al.* (1995) Urokinase and macrophages in tumour angiogenesis. *Br J Cancer* **72**:818–23.
35. Giraudo E, Inoue MHanahan D. (2004) An amino-bisphosphonate targets MMP-9-expressing macrophages and angiogenesis to impair cervical carcinogenesis. *J Clin Invest* **114**:623–33.
36. Kinzler KW, Vogelstein B. (1996) Lessons from hereditary colorectal cancer. *Cell* **87**:159–70.
37. Lengauer C, Kinzler KW, Vogelstein B. (1997) Genetic instability in colorectal cancers. *Nature* **386**:623–7.
38. Pino MS, Chung DC. (2010) The chromosomal instability pathway in colon cancer. *Gastroenterology* **138**:2059–72.
39. Negrini S, Gorgoulis VG, Halazonetis TD. (2010) Genomic instability — an evolving hallmark of cancer. *Nat Rev Mol Cell Biol* **11**:220–8.
40. Nathan C. (2002) Points of control in inflammation. *Nature* **420**:846–52.
41. Polager S, Ginsberg D. (2009) p53 and E2f: Partners in life and death. *Nat Rev Cancer* **9**:738–48.
42. Rajagopalan H, Nowak MA, Vogelstein B *et al.* (2003) The significance of unstable chromosomes in colorectal cancer. *Nat Rev Cancer* **3**:695–701.
43. Sieber OM, Heinimann K, Tomlinson IP. (2003) Genomic instability — the engine of tumorigenesis? *Nat Rev Cancer* **3**:701–8.
44. Bardelli A, Cahill DP, Lederer G *et al.* (2001) Carcinogen-specific induction of genetic instability. *Proc Natl Acad Sci U S A* **98**:5770–5.
45. Cahill DP, Lengauer C, Yu J *et al.* (1998) Mutations of mitotic checkpoint genes in human cancers. *Nature* **392**:300–3.
46. Chittenden TW, Howe EA, Culhane AC *et al.* (2008) Functional classification analysis of somatically mutated genes in human breast and colorectal cancers. *Genomics* **91**:508–11.
47. Adams RR, Eckley DM, Vagnarelli P *et al.* (2001) Human INCENP colocalizes with the Aurora-B/AIRK2 kinase on chromosomes and is overexpressed in tumour cells. *Chromosoma* **110**:65–74.
48. Khanna KK, Jackson SP. (2001) DNA double-strand breaks: Signaling, repair and the cancer connection. *Nat Genet* **27**:247–54.
49. Deng CX. (2006) BRCA1: Cell cycle checkpoint, genetic instability, DNA damage response and cancer evolution. *Nucleic Acids Res* **34**:1416–26.

50. Bolderson E, Richard DJ, Zhou BB *et al.* (2009) Recent advances in cancer therapy targeting proteins involved in DNA double-strand break repair. *Clin Cancer Res* **15**:6314–20.
51. Zhang H, Tombline G, Weber BL. (1998) BRCA1, BRCA2, and DNA damage response: collision or collusion? *Cell* **92**:433–6.
52. Lynch HT, de la Chapelle A. (2003) Hereditary colorectal cancer. *N Engl J Med* **348**:919–32.
53. Issa JP. (2004) CpG island methylator phenotype in cancer. *Nat Rev Cancer* **4**:988–93.
54. Fleisher AS, Esteller M, Harpaz N *et al.* (2000) Microsatellite instability in inflammatory bowel disease-associated neoplastic lesions is associated with hypermethylation and diminished expression of the DNA mismatch repair gene, hMLH1. *Cancer Res* **60**:4864–8.
55. Koshiji M, To KK, Hammer S *et al.* (2005) HIF-1alpha induces genetic instability by transcriptionally downregulating MutSalpha expression. *Mol Cell* **17**:793–803.
56. Chang CL, Marra G, Chauhan DP *et al.* (2002) Oxidative stress inactivates the human DNA mismatch repair system. *Am J Physiol Cell Physiol* **283**:C148–54.
57. Leung WK, Kim JJ, Kim JG *et al.* (2000) Microsatellite instability in gastric intestinal metaplasia in patients with and without gastric cancer. *Am J Pathol* **156**:537–43.
58. Cravo ML, Albuquerque CM, Salazar de Sousa L *et al.* (1998) Microsatellite instability in non-neoplastic mucosa of patients with ulcerative colitis: Effect of folate supplementation. *Am J Gastroenterol* **93**:2060–4.
59. Brentnall TA, Chen R, Lee JG *et al.* (1995) Microsatellite instability and K-ras mutations associated with pancreatic adenocarcinoma and pancreatitis. *Cancer Res* **55**:4264–7.
60. Brentnall TA, Crispin DA, Bronner MP *et al.* (1996) Microsatellite instability in nonneoplastic mucosa from patients with chronic ulcerative colitis. *Cancer Res* **56**:1237–40.
61. Maekita T, Nakazawa K, Mihara M *et al.* (2006) High levels of aberrant DNA methylation in Helicobacter pylori-infected gastric mucosae and its possible association with gastric cancer risk. *Clin Cancer Res* **12**:989–95.
62. Nakajima T, Maekita T, Oda I *et al.* (2006) Higher methylation levels in gastric mucosae significantly correlate with higher risk of gastric cancers. *Cancer Epidemiol Biomarkers Prev* **15**:2317–21.

63. Eads CA, Lord RV, Kurumboor SK *et al.* (2000) Fields of aberrant CpG island hypermethylation in Barrett's esophagus and associated adenocarcinoma. *Cancer Res* **60**:5021–6.
64. Baylin SB, Herman JG, Graff JR *et al.* (1998) Alterations in DNA methylation: a fundamental aspect of neoplasia. *Adv Cancer Res* **72**:141–96.
65. Jones PA, Baylin SB. (2002) The fundamental role of epigenetic events in cancer. *Nat Rev Genet* **3**:415–28.
66. Bestor TH, Gundersen G, Kolsto AB *et al.* (1992) CpG islands in mammalian gene promoters are inherently resistant to de novo methylation. *Genet Anal Tech Appl* **9**:48–53.
67. Cross SH, Bird AP. (1995) CpG islands and genes. *Curr Opin Genet Dev* **5**:309–14.
68. Illingworth R, Kerr A, Desousa D *et al.* (2008) A novel CpG island set identifies tissue-specific methylation at developmental gene loci. *PLoS Biol* **6**:e22.
69. Edwards RA, Witherspoon M, Wang K *et al.* (2009) Epigenetic repression of DNA mismatch repair by inflammation and hypoxia in inflammatory bowel disease-associated colorectal cancer. *Cancer Res* **69**:6423–9.
70. Issa JP, Ahuja N, Toyota M *et al.* (2001) Accelerated age-related CpG island methylation in ulcerative colitis. *Cancer Res* **61**:3573–7.
71. Toyota M, Itoh F, Kikuchi T *et al.* (2002) DNA methylation changes in gastrointestinal disease. *J Gastroenterol* **37**(Suppl 14):97–101.
72. Niwa T, Tsukamoto T, Toyoda T *et al.* (2010) Inflammatory processes triggered by Helicobacter pylori infection cause aberrant DNA methylation in gastric epithelial cells. *Cancer Res* **70**:1430–40.
73. Hahn MA, Hahn T, Lee DH *et al.* (2008) Methylation of polycomb target genes in intestinal cancer is mediated by inflammation. *Cancer Res* **68**:10280–9.
74. Toyota M, Ahuja N, Ohe-Toyota M *et al.* (1999) CpG island methylator phenotype in colorectal cancer. *Proc Natl Acad Sci USA* **96**:8681–6.
75. Toyota M, Ahuja N, Suzuki H *et al.* (1999) Aberrant methylation in gastric cancer associated with the CpG island methylator phenotype. *Cancer Res* **59**:5438–42.
76. Ueki T, Toyota M, Sohn T *et al.* (2000) Hypermethylation of multiple genes in pancreatic adenocarcinoma. *Cancer Res* **60**:1835–9.
77. Noushmehr H, Weisenberger DJ, Diefes K *et al.* (2010) Identification of a CpG island methylator phenotype that defines a distinct subgroup of glioma. *Cancer Cell* **17**:510–22.

78. Shen L, Toyota M, Kondo Y *et al.* (2007) Integrated genetic and epigenetic analysis identifies three different subclasses of colon cancer. *Proc Natl Acad Sci U S A* **104**:18654–9.
79. Ogino S, Kawasaki T, Kirkner GJ *et al.* (2006) CpG island methylator phenotype-low (CIMP-low) in colorectal cancer: Possible associations with male sex and KRAS mutations. *J Mol Diagn* **8**:582–8.
80. Baylin SB, Ohm JE. (2006) Epigenetic gene silencing in cancer — a mechanism for early oncogenic pathway addiction? *Nat Rev Cancer* **6**:107–16.
81. Strahl BD, Allis CD. (2000) The language of covalent histone modifications. *Nature* **403**:41–5.
82. Jenuwein T, Allis CD. (2001) Translating the histone code. *Science* **293**:1074–80.
83. Nan X, Ng HH, Johnson CA *et al.* (1998) Transcriptional repression by the methyl-CpG-binding protein MeCP2 involves a histone deacetylase complex. *Nature* **393**:386–9.
84. Hendrich B, Bird A. (1998) Identification and characterization of a family of mammalian methyl-CpG binding proteins. *Mol Cell Biol* **18**:6538–47.
85. Bird A. (2002) DNA methylation patterns and epigenetic memory. *Genes Dev* **16**:6–21.
86. Kondo Y, Shen L, Yan PS *et al.* (2004) Chromatin immunoprecipitation microarrays for identification of genes silenced by histone H3 lysine 9 methylation. *Proc Natl Acad Sci USA* **101**:7398–403.
87. Feldman N, Gerson A, Fang J *et al.* (2006) G9a-mediated irreversible epigenetic inactivation of Oct-3/4 during early embryogenesis. *Nat Cell Biol* **8**:188–94.
88. Ohm JE, McGarvey KM, Yu X *et al.* (2007) A stem cell-like chromatin pattern may predispose tumor suppressor genes to DNA hypermethylation and heritable silencing. *Nat Genet* **39**:237–42.
89. Schlesinger Y, Straussman R, Keshet I *et al.* (2007) Polycomb-mediated methylation on Lys27 of histone H3 pre-marks genes for de novo methylation in cancer. *Nat Genet* **39**:232–6.
90. Kondo Y. (2009) Epigenetic cross-talk between DNA methylation and histone modifications in human cancers. *Yonsei Med J* **50**:455–63.
91. Widschwendter M, Fiegl H, Egle D *et al.* (2007) Epigenetic stem cell signature in cancer. *Nat Genet* **39**:157–8.

Chapter 4

From Inflammation to Cancer: The Molecular Basis

Hongchuan Jin*

Biomedical Research Center, Sir Runrun Shaw Hospital, Medical School of Zhejiang University, Hangzhou, China

The link between inflammation and cancer has been recognized for a long time. Instead of a simple summation of molecular events in single cells, carcinogenesis results from the complex interaction of cancer-stem cells and tumor-permissive microenvironment. The tumor-permissive microenvironment is featured by the suppression of cell-mediated immune response, pro-angiogenesis and inhibition of apoptosis. A number of soluble bioactive factors including various cytokines and growth factors, produced by tumor cells or non-tumor cells, contribute to the formation of such an inflammatory microenvironment by the persistent activation of multiple intracellular signaling pathways such as NF-κB and STAT3 pathways.

Carcinogenesis is a multi-stage process resulting from the accumulation of many genetic and epigenetic changes. However, it is more than a simple summation of molecular events in single cells. The role of inflammatory microenvironment in carcinogenesis was well recognized, eventually revolutionizing our strategies to cancer treatment and prevention.

* Email: jinhc@srrsh.com

Inflammation and cancer: a brief overview of history

As early as two millennia ago, Claudius Galen noticed the link between inflammation and cancer. He expanded Hippocrates' basic theory of cancer as an excess of black bile (melancholia), a concept that survived intact through the Middle Ages and was only superseded at the end of the eighteenth century. Based on the phenotypic similarities, he concluded that cancer was a swelling resulting from an inflammation when it has been cooled excessively.[1]

Later in 1863, the German pathologist Rudolf Virchow postulated that chronic inflammation was a precondition for tumorigenesis based on his observations that leucocytes presented in neoplastic tissues and inflammation-inducing agents, either infective or noninfective, can usually promote cell proliferation.[2–4] He realized that cancer development is a stepwise process and that cancer is usually converted by polypous alterations resulting from 'normal' inflammatory hyperplasia.

Today, the causal relationship between inflammation and cancer is widely accepted. First, many cancers indeed arise from chronic inflammation. For example, hepatocellular carcinoma often develop in cirrhotic liver after a long history of chronic hepatitis. Second, removal of pathogen or eradication of inflammation could suppress carcinogenesis. Eradication of *Helicobacter pylori*, the gram-negative bacterium identified as the major etiological factor in gastric adenocarcinoma, can significantly decrease the incidence of gastric carcinogenesis.[5] Similarly, vaccination to prevent viral infection and ensuing chronic inflammation substantially reduced the incidence of tumors like hepatocellular and cervical carcinoma.[6,7] Third, inflammation-suppressive agents such as non-steroidal anti-inflammatory drugs (NSAIDs) can prevent cancer development.[8] These observations suggested that common mechanisms are active in both inflammation and cancer tissues. In contrast to inflammation, which is usually self-limiting, uncontrolled cell proliferation and invasion are persistent in tumor microenvironment, eventually causing the growth of tumor. Indeed, tumors were recognized as over-healing wounds or wounds that fail to heal.[9]

Current model of tumorigenesis: interplay between tumor stem cells and tumor-permissive microenvironment

Some cancers (group I cancers) originated from tissues with chronic inflammation while the rest (group II cancers) developed without any clear epidemiological basis for inflammation (Table 1). Cancers originating from the gastrointestinal tract are the most representative type of group I cancers. For example, chronic hepatitis induced by hepatitis B and C virus account for more than 80% of hepatocellular carcinoma worldwide. Chronic ulcerative colitis can greatly increase the risk of colorectal carcinogenesis. Other group I cancers include endocrine cancers such as breast and prostate cancers, often showing a subtle association with inflammation. This is because the endocrine system could interact directly with the immune response.[10] Nevertheless, epidemiological evidence exists that both breast and prostate cancer occur more frequently in the presence of chronic mastitis and prostatitis, respectively.[11,12]

The group II cancers include brain tumors such as retinoblastoma and testicular cancers. Most of these tumors originated from immunologically privileged tissues where immune responses are largely suppressed. In addition, the genetic alterations are frequently dominated in this group of cancers. Actually the first tumor suppressor gene Rb (Retinoblastoma) was identified in child retinoblastoma.[13] Moreover, the loss-of-heterozygosity (LOH) of neurofibromatosis type I and II genes contributes to the development of neurofibromatosis type I and II, respectively. Metastatic tumors could also be included in group II cancers since they can grow into

Table 1. Two groups of cancers based on the contribution of inflammation.

Cancers with a history of inflammation	Cancers without a clear history of inflammation
Hepatocellular carcinoma	Lymphoma
Colorectal carcinoma	Brain tumors
Gastric carcinoma	Testicular carcinoma
Cervical cancer	
Lung cancer	Leukemia
Breast cancer	Metastatic cancers
Prostate cancer	

tumors in microenvironments without any history of inflammation. Although the inflammation program in tumor microenvironment was eventually activated in an exaggerated and prolonged manner in most of carcinoma tissues, the mechanism underlying the initiation of group I and II cancers might have subtle differences (Figure 1).

Stem cells not only are responsible for the tissue homeostasis, but also play important roles in carcinogenesis since stem cells but not terminal differentiated cells were believed to be the target cells to accumulate enough genetic and epigenetic changes for malignant transformation.[14] In addition, stem cells are important to remodel the microenvironment, allowing transformed stem cells to survive and grow into tumors.

The microenvironments in chronic inflammatory tissues are rich with growth factors and cytokines important to promote cell proliferation, wound repair, and tissue regeneration. Furthermore, there are some DNA damage-inducing agents such as reactive oxygen and nitrogen species (RONS) that can cause genomic alterations, promoting the accumulation of mutations in cancer stem cells and the consequent perpetuation of tumor growth.[15]

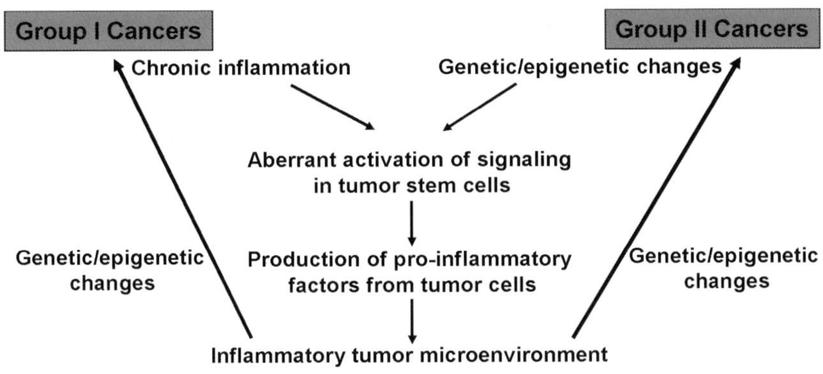

Figure 1. Cancers can be separated into two groups based on the role of inflammation on the initiation of carcinogenesis. In group I cancers such as gastric cancer and hepatocellular carcinoma, chronic inflammation eventually creates a tumor-permissive microenvironment to select tumorigenic stem cells from non-transformed cells. In contrast, in group II cancers, cancer stem cells initiated the transformation program as well as inflammatory response and eventually educated the microenvironment to be tumor-permissive.

Inflammatory microenvironments are filled with immune cells that normally should play a role in tissue homeostasis and tumor surveillance. However, chronic inflammation may eventually create an environment that would favor the survival and expansion of transformed cells. Meanwhile, tumor-initiating cells during their progression can not only circumvent inhibitory signals from immune cells but also suppress the anti-tumor immune response, eventually transforming the inflammation microenvironment into tumor-permissive microenvironment, the niche for cancer stem cells.

During the progression of group II cancers, the aberrant activation of oncogenes sufficient for the transformation of cancer stem cells can also coordinate inflammatory transcriptional programs.[16–21] These oncogene-coordinated inflammatory responses can promote angiogenesis and recruit cells of myelomonocytic origin to remodel the microenvironment with tumor-initiating cells, eventually facilitating the formation of an inflammatory microenvironment essential for tumor progression. For example, active Ras can result in the upregulation of inflammatory cytokine interleukin-8 (IL-8) which in turn promotes inflammatory response, angiogenesis, and eventually tumor growth.[18] Another oncogene MYC, which encodes a transcription factor and is deregulated in many human tumors, can activate a transcriptional program to elicit the production of several cytokines important for the remodeling of inflammatory microenvironment such as IL-1β.[22]

Tumor microenvironment

Tumor-permissive microenvironment is featured by the suppression of cell-mediated immunity, pro-angiogenesis, and inhibition of apoptosis. Through the activation or inhibition of intracellular signaling pathways, bioactive factors such as cytokines and growth factors that are secreted from tumor cells and non-tumor cells in a paracrine or autocrine manner, play important roles in the formation of microenvironment that in turn facilitate tumor progression.

Non-tumor cells in tumor microenvironment

In addition to tumor cells, the surrounding non-tumor cells, such as fibroblasts and immune cells, are the major components of tumor microenvironment. These non-tumor cells are not bystanders but key players in tumor microenvironments.

Cancer-associated fibroblast (CAFs)

As the principal cellular component of connective tissues, fibroblasts are embedded in the fibrillar matrix of connective tissues. Fibroblasts within the tumor microenvironment are perpetually activated. Such activated fibroblasts have been termed cancer-associated fibroblasts (CAFs), peri-tumoral fibroblasts, and reactive stromal fibroblasts. Similar to the important roles in inflammation, fibroblasts in reactive stroma can promote tumor progression by providing supportive matrix and oncogenic signals that facilitate angiogenesis, tumor cell proliferation, and invasion.[23–25]

Two major subsets of CFAs are defined based on the expression of various markers.[25] One subset of fibroblasts express FSP1 (fibroblasts-specific protein-1) but not NG2 (neuron-glial antigen-2), αSMA (α-smooth-muscle actin), and PDGF (platelet-derived growth factor) β-receptor while the other subset of fibroblasts co-express NG2, αSMA and PDGF β-receptor but not FSP1. In addition to local fibroblasts or fibroblast precursors that have been considered as the major source of CAFs, bone-marrow derived mesenchymal precursor or stem cells can also be recruited into the tumor microenvironment and differentiated into fibroblasts.[26,27] Furthermore, CAFs can also be derived from epithelial cells or endothelial cells undergoing epithelial- or endothelial-mesenchymal transition, respectively.[28,29]

Immune cells

Among the large amount of immune cells presented in cancer tissues, macrophages (Tumor-associated macrophages, TAMs) are of particular importance.[30,31] TAMs have been extensively studied for their relationship with tumor cells and their multi-faceted functions in tumor microenvironments. Based on their pivotal roles in antigen presentation and lymphocyte activation, macrophages were assumed to play some roles in the host response against the growing tumor. Indeed, when

Table 2. Differences between two types of macrophages.

M1-type macrophage	**M2-type macrophage**
Inducing signals	
GM-CSF, IFN-γ, LPS, and other bacterial products,	M-CSF, IL-4, IL-13, IL-10, Corticosterloids, PGE, VitD3
Cytokine phenotype	
IL-1, TNF, IL-12, CXCL-9, CXCL-10. CXCL-11, NO, ROI	IL-1ra, decoy IL-1RII, IL-10, CCL-17, CCL18, CCL-22, Ployamine, Scavenger R, Mannose R
Functions	
Tumor suppression, Bactericidal activity, Inflammatory cytokines, Immuno-stimulation	Tumor promotion, Scavenging, Matrix remodeling, Tissue repair, Angiogenesis

GM-CSF: granulocyte-macrophage colony stimulating factor; M-CSF: Macrophage colony stimulating factor; PGE: prostaglandin E; VitD3: vitamin D3; NO: Nitric oxide; ROI: Reactive oxygen intermediates; NO: Nitric oxide; CXCL: CXC chemokine ligand; IL-1ra: IL-1 receptor antagonist; CCL: Chemokine (CC motif) ligand

appropriately activated *in vitro*, macrophages show some potential to inhibit tumor growth. However, numerous clinical studies revealed that infiltration of macrophages often correlated with tumor progression and poor outcome rather than tumor regression and good prognosis. It was later realized that TAMs are M2-type macrophages instead of M1-type macrophages. The differentiation of monocytes into different types of macrophages was induced by different signals. While bacterial products like LPS (Lipopolysaccharides) and Th1 cytokines like IFN-γ (Interferon-γ) can promote the M1 type polarization, cytokines rich in tumor microenvironment such as IL-10 (Interleukin-10) can not only inhibit M1 type polarization but also induce the differentiation of monocytes toward M2 type macrophages. Differences between two types of macrophages were summarized in Table 2.[32]

By producing various bioactive factors such as cytokines important to angiogenesis and matrix remodeling, M2-type macrophages can promote tumor growth, survival, invasion, and metastasis. In contrast to M1-type macrophages, TAMs can facilitate the suppression of adaptive immunity, one of major characters of tumor-permissive microenvironment different from non-tumor-permissive microenvironment. IL-10, IL-6 and TGF-β produced by TAMs can inhibit the maturation and activation of tumor-associated dendritic cells (TADCs), the major type of antigen-presenting cells (APCs) in tumor microenvironment. CCL18 from TAMs can attract the naïve T cells into TADC- and TAM-rich tumor microenvironment and induce its anergy. In addition, TAMs are unable to trigger Th1 polarized immune response but rather induce the conversion of conventional $CD4^+$ T cells into T regulatory (Treg) cells that can suppress T cell-mediated anti-tumor response.[33,34]

Other immune cells including T lymphocytes, TADC and Treg cells also present in the tumor microenvironment. However, as mentioned above, TADC are immature to function as APCs and T lymphocytes are in a state of anergy. Together with other factors such as the prevalence of immune-suppressive cytokines, abundant Treg cells in the tumor microenvironment play important roles in the remodeling of immune microenvironment.

Bioactive factors in tumor microenvironment

As morphogenesis is controlled by morphogens, tumor-permissive microenvironment is formulated by local bioactive soluble factors including cytokines, growth factors, and various metabolic intermediates.

Chemokines

A complex network of chemokines play important roles on the remodeling of tumor microenvironment by influencing immune cell infiltration, angiogenesis, tumor cell growth, survival, and migration.[35,36] Based on the position of the first two cysteines adjacent to the amino terminus, chemokines are classified into four highly conserved groups, CXC, CC, C and CX3C. More than 50 human chemokines have been discovered so far.

In contrast to infection-related inflammation where the tissue leukocytes are the major source of chemokine production, tumor cells in addition to leukocytes, CAFs, and endothelial cells can produce a huge amount of chemokines important for the formation of tumor-permissive microenvironment. The patterns of chemokines vary with different tumor types so that they can be used as markers for cancer detection and prognosis prediction.[37–39]

Target cells respond to chemokine gradients through the interaction of chemokines with their receptors. Tumor cells from different tissue origins express different profiles of chemokine receptors. Among the tens of chemokine receptors, CXCR4 is most commonly found on human and murine cancer cells and is generally a characteristic of tumor cells but not their normal counterpart.[40] CXCR4 is upregulated in tumor cells as an outcome of various oncogenic signals such as growth factor stimulation, oncogene activation or tumor suppression gene inactivation.[41–43] For instance, CXCR4 upregulation can be promoted by the mutation of VHL (von Hippel-Lindau) tumor suppressor gene, which regulates the intracellular level of the oncoprotein HIF-α (hypoxia-induced factor). As hypoxia and VHL mutations are poor prognostic signs and associated with advanced cancers, CXCR4 upregulation can stimulate the migration, invasion and metastasis of cancer cells and CXCR4 activation is associated with the metastatic capacity of various cancers.[35]

As the only ligand for CXCR4, CXCL12 is also involved in tumor cell growth and survival. CXCL12 can stimulate the proliferation and survival of CXCR4-expressing cancer cells under suboptimal conditions such as low serum concentrations. CXCL12 is supposed as the major cytokine involved in the establishment of tumor-cytokine network and growth of the metastatic tumor after the tumors arrive at a new location. Interestingly, CXCL12 plays a role in retaining tumor cells in the primary site rather than promote them to metastasize. Only when CXCR4 expression is increased or local level of proteinases such as MMPs is high enough to degrade CXCL12 to a certain extent, CXCL12-CXCR4 interaction might encourage sub-populations of tumor cells to leave the primary niche and disseminate to a new location.[35]

Together with CXCL12-CXCR4, many other chemokine-chemokine receptors constitute the complex chemokine network in tumor microenvironment. Given that chemokine network is critical to tumor progression, new anti-cancer drugs targeting chemokine network are being developed. However, there is still much to learn about chemokines and cancer. The comprehensive study on chemokines and receptors in primary tumors, metastatic lesions, and normal tissues will be crucial to further understanding of the cancer chemokine network, eventually facilitating the development of new effective therapeutic strategies for cancer.

Growth factors

Numerous growth factors play significant roles in angiogenesis and tumor growth in tumor microenvironment.

Transforming growth factor-β (TGF-β) is one of most important growth factors in tumor microenvironment. The effect of TGF-β on tumor progression is dynamic. Prior to initiation and early progression TGF-β acts on epithelial cells as a suppressor of tumorigenesis, whereas at later stages it is a tumor promoter. TGF-β signaling has multiple roles, ranging from inhibition of cell growth to enhancing cellular migration and epithelial-mesenchymal transition (EMT).[44]

Insulin-like growth factors (IGFs), one group of transforming growth factors that inhibits cell apoptosis, induces angiogenesis and at high concentrations, suppresses cell-mediated immunity, are enriched in tumor microenvironment.[45,46] There is increasing evidence linking high concentrations of IGFs with the high risk of various cancers such as breast cancer, prostate cancer, and colorectal cancer.

Other growth factors such as epidermal growth factor (EGF), platelet-derived growth factor (PDGF) and vascular endothelial growth factor (VEGF) are prevalent in tumor microenvironment. EGFs are important to tissue regeneration and tumor growth while PDGFs and VEGFs are predominant regulators of angiogenesis.[47–49]

MMPs and TIMPs (tissue inhibitors of metalloproteinases)

The functions of growth factors to activate their cognate receptors are often subjected to the regulation mediated by other soluble factors such as matrix metalloproteinases (MMPs). MMPs are a multigene family of zinc-dependent proteinases important to extracellular matrix (ECM) remodeling that can foster angiogenesis, tumor growth, and metastasis during tumor progression.[50] MMPs are also important to the activity regulation of numerous growth factors and cytokines such as TNF-α (tumor necrosis factor-α), CXCL12, EGF and TGF-β.[51–54] Many growth factors such as VEGF and basic fibroblast growth factor (bFGF) are stored in ECM and liberated after MMP-mediated ECM remodeling. Furthermore, proteolytic activation of latent TGF-β is essential to MMP-28-induced EMT.[55] MMPs are found at higher levels in many cancers and proposed as biomarkers for cancer diagnosis and prognosis prediction, especially longitudinal assessment of disease progression and therapeutic efficacy.

The activities of MMPs are regulated by their endogenous inhibitors such as TIMPs so that the extent of tissues remodeling is tightly controlled. Recent findings demonstrated that TIMPs in tumor microenvironment can regulate other important processes such as proliferation and apoptosis independent of metalloproteinase inhibition.[56] To date, only four TIMPs have been identified: TIMP-1, -2, -3 and -4. TIMPs expressions are decreased in tumor microenvironment at least partly due to the promoter-methylation mediated down-regulation of TIMPs in tumor cells.[57–59]

Other cytokines

There are many more other cytokines important for the remodeling of tumor microenvironment and tumor growth, such as IL-6, tumor necrosis factor-α (TNF-α). The production of IL-6 was upregulated in response to the treatment of carcinogen diethylnitrosamine (DEN), which can eventually induce hepatocellular carcinoma (HCC). Moreover, male mice which are usually much more susceptible to HCC than female mice had much higher levels of IL-6 and male mice deficient in IL-6 have similar incidence of HCC as female mice, strongly indicating the critical role of IL-6 in the development of HCC.[60] In addition to enhancing proliferation of tumor-initiating cells, IL-6 also protects premalignant intestinal epithelial cells from apoptosis, thus facilitating the development of colitis-associated colon cancer (CAC).[61]

TNF-α, the first active component discovered in the Coley toxins , is a multifunctional cytokine involved in many cellular functions such as apoptosis and survival by acting via two receptors. The dysregulation of TNF-α production has been implicated in a variety of human diseases including cancer. Based on the growth inhibitory function of TNF-α, several TNF-α related molecules are currently under detailed investigation as potential anti-cancer agents.

Intracellular signaling pathways

Bioactive soluble factors like growth factors function to regulate intercellular signaling pathways fundamental for cellular phenotypes. Many signaling pathways are aberrantly regulated in tumor cells or non-tumor cells in tumor microenvironment.

NF-κB (nuclear factor κ light chain polypeptide gene enhancer in B cells) pathway

NF-κB pathway has been used as the evidence to convince the link between chronic inflammation and carcinogenesis, since NF-κB plays important roles in both inflammation and cancer.[62,63] NF-κB is indispensible for Ras-mediated transformation and can function downstream of active Ras to promote the epigenetic silencing of tumor suppressors that would otherwise inhibit tumorigenesis.[64,65] Blocking NF-κB activity can suppress proliferation, induce apoptosis or sensitize tumor cells to various anti-cancer treatments.

NF-κB was first discovered via its interaction with the enhancer of genes encoding the immunoglobulin light chain. NF-κB is a transcription factor triggered largely in response to pro-inflammatory factors. Once activated, NF-κB can regulate the transcription of genes with NF-κB-binding sites (5'-GGGRNNYYCC-3', R: purine; Y: pyrimidine; N: any nucleotide). The target genes containing this cis-acting sequence are usually cytokines playing important roles in the remodeling of inflammatory tumor microenvironment, such as IL-6.

Inactive NF-κB is usually sequestered in the cytoplasm by a family of inhibitors, called I-κBs (inhibitors of κB), allowing the rapid response to a variety of extracellular stimuli since no new protein synthesis will be needed. NF-κB activation is initiated by a posttranslational protein modification cascade starting from the activation of IKK (I-κB kinase) which can phosphorylate two serine residues located in the I-κB regulatory domain. When phosphorylated on these serines, I-κB are subjected to ubiquitination and the subsequent proteasome-mediated protein degradation so that NF-κB will be liberated and translocated into the nucleus to regulate the expression of target genes.

NF-κB is constitutively active in tumors to keep tumor cells proliferating and protect cells from apoptosis. The molecular link between chronic inflammation and carcinogenesis has been revealed by several animal models with defects in NF-κB pathway.[61] Mice lacking IKKβ in their intestinal epithelial cells had a markedly reduced incidence of carcinogen-induced colon cancer compared with controls. One of the plausible reasons is the increased apoptosis of epithelial cells in conditional IKKβ-deficient mice. On the other hand, incidence of carcinogen-induced colon cancer was also reduced in mice in which IKKβ was specifically absent in the myeloid/macrophage lineage. Such a low tumor incidence was correlated with lower levels of inflammatory cytokines and lower proliferation of intestinal epithelial cells.[61,66] Similar results were also observed in HCC using multidrug resistance 2 (MDR2)-knockout mice which can spontaneously develop chronic hepatitis and HCC.[67] Therefore, NF-κB contributes to carcinogenesis by playing dual roles: preventing the cells with malignant potential from inflammation-driven apoptosis and stimulating the survival and proliferation of premalignant cells by promoting the transcription of inflammatory cytokines in non-tumor cells.

NF-κB is activated in tumor microenvironment because of mutations in genes encoding components in NF-κB signaling pathway in tumor cells or deregulation of cytokine network in tumor microenvironment. One of the major cytokines responsible for the activation of NF-κB is TNF-α which is produced by stromal cells and tumor-initiating or premalignant cells in response to inflammation or other damages such as ultraviolet irradiation.

STAT3 (signal transducer and activator of transcription 3) pathway

Another major pathway responsible for inflammation-induced carcinogenesis is the STAT3 pathway.[68,69] STAT3 belongs to the STAT protein family. In response to various stimuli such as cytokines and growth factors, STAT family proteins are phosphorylated by the receptor associated kinases and then form homo- or hetero-dimers to translocate into nucleus where they act as transcription factors. STAT family proteins especially STAT3 are playing crucial roles in selectively inducing and maintaining a procarcinogenic inflammatory microenvironment during tumor initiation and progression. In contrast to NF-κB pathway which is indispensible for both innate and T cell-mediated anti-tumor immunity, STAT3 can restrain anti-tumor immune response in tumor microenvironment in addition to promoting the oncogenic potential of tumor cells. The direct targets regulated by active STAT3 include oncogenes important to maintain malignant phenotypes such as Bcl-2 and Cox-2. In addition, STAT3 is also responsible for the transcription of numerous genes encoding cytokines, chemokines and growth factors that can in turn activate STAT3 in stromal cells. By doing so, a STAT3 feedforward loop is established between tumor cells and non-tumor cells in tumor microenvironment.[68]

In response to numerous bioactive factors including IL-6, IFNs and BMPs (Bone morphogenetic proteins), STAT3 is phosphorylated at tyrosine 705 and 727 by Janus kinases (JAKs). STAT3 can also be transactivated by receptor tyrosine kinases such as EGFRs as well as non-receptor tyrosine kinases such as c-src. The activity of STAT3 pathway is negatively regulated on multiple levels. Suppressors of cytokine signaling (SOCSs) can inhibit STAT3 phosphorylation by binding and inhibiting JAKs or competing with STAT3 for phosphotyrosine binding sites on cytokine receptors.[70] In addition, PIASs (protein inhibitors of activated STATs) can inhibit the transcriptional activity of STAT3 in the nucleus by binding to the DNA sequence that would otherwise be bound by STAT3.[71]

Although no natural mutations in STATs have been reported so far, STAT3 is constitutively active in tumor microenvironment to promote tumor growth. In addition to the increased production of cytokines in inflammatory tumor microenvironment, the epigenetic silencing of various inhibitors such as SOCSs and PIASs contribute to the persistent activation of STAT3 in the tumor microenvironment.

STAT3 interacts with NF-κB at multiple levels. The nuclear accumulation and activation of RelA, one major form of NF-κB, is promoted by p300-mediated acetylation, which requires the activity of STAT3.[72] On the other hand, the persistent activation of STAT3 in tumor cells, especially in the early stage of group I cancers, is dependent on NF-κB activation since many activators of STAT3 are subjected to the regulation of NF-κB. The most crucial STAT3 activator is IL-6, which is the target gene of NF-κB. The pro-proliferation and pro-survival effects of IL-6 on intestinal epithelial cells (IECs) are actually dependent on STAT3 since IEC-specific ablation has a profound impact on CAC development.[61] This

NF-κB-IL-6-STAT3 cascade is most likely important to the initiation of not only CAC but also many group I cancers. For example, in response to NF-κB activation, IL-6 derived from immune cells can activate STAT3 in hepatocytes, leading to the development of HCC.[60] Suppression of IL-6 dependent STAT3 activation can largely reduce the incidence of HCC.

Conclusions

Either chronic inflammation or genetic and epigenetic changes in cancer stem cells can be the first step in the initiation of cancer development. However, the interaction between cancer stem cells and non-tumor cells will anyway create an inflammatory microenvironment essential for the progression of tumors. A complex network of soluble bioactive factors formulates such a tumor-permissive inflammatory environment, which is featured by the suppression of cell-mediated immune response, pro-angiogenesis, and inhibition of apoptosis. Together with NF-κB, STAT3 is persistently activated in tumor microenvironment and plays pivotal roles in carcinogenesis-associated inflammation.

References

1. Reedy J. (1975) Galen on cancer and related diseases. *Clio Med* **10**(3):227–38.
2. Schafer M, Werner S. (2008) Cancer as an overhealing wound: An old hypothesis revisited. *Nat Rev Mol Cell Biol* **9**(8):628–38.
3. Balkwill F, Mantovani A. (2001) Inflammation and cancer: Back to Virchow? *Lancet* **357**(9255):539–45.
4. Coussens LM, Werb Z. (2002) Inflammation and cancer. *Nature* **420**(6917):860–7.
5. Ito M, Takata S, Tatsugami M *et al.* (2009) Clinical prevention of gastric cancer by *Helicobacter pylori* eradication therapy: A systematic review. *J Gastroentero* **44**(5):365–71.
6. Khan K, Curtis CR, Ekwueme DU *et al.* (2008) Preventing cervical cancer : overviews of the national breast and cervical cancer early detection program and 2 US immunization programs. *Cancer***113**(10 Suppl):3004–12.
7. Kao JH, Chen DS. (2002) Global control of hepatitis B virus infection. *Lancet Infect Dis* **2**(7):395–403.

8. Cha YI, DuBois RN. (2007) NSAIDs and cancer prevention: Targets downstream of COX-2. *Annu Rev Med* **58**:239–52.
9. Dvorak HF. (1986) Tumors: Wounds that do not heal. Similarities between tumor stroma generation and wound healing. *N Engl J Med* **315**(26):1650–9.
10. Rook GA, Hernandez-Pando R, Lightman SL. (1994) Hormones, peripherally activated prohormones and regulation of the Th1/Th2 balance. *Immunol Today* **15**(7):301–3.
11. Ketcham AS, Sindelar WF. (1975) Risk factors in breast cancer. *Prog Clin Cancer* **6**:99–114.
12. Sandhu JS. (2008) Prostate cancer and chronic prostatitis. *Curr Urol Rep* **9**(4):328–32.
13. Knudson AG. (2001) Two genetic hits (more or less) to cancer. *Nat Rev Cancer* **1**(2):157–62.
14. Beachy PA, Karhadkar SS, Berman DM. (2004) Tissue repair and stem cell renewal in carcinogenesis. *Nature* **432**(7015):324–31.
15. Meira LB, Bugni JM, Green SL *et al.* (2008) DNA damage induced by chronic inflammation contributes to colon carcinogenesis in mice. *J Clin Invest* **118**(7):2516–25.
16. Borrello MG, Alberti L, Fischer A *et al.* (2005) Induction of a proinflammatory program in normal human thyrocytes by the RET/PTC1 oncogene. *Proc Natl Acad Sci USA* **102**(41):14825–30.
17. Guerra C, Schuhmacher AJ, Canamero M *et al.* (2007) Chronic pancreatitis is essential for induction of pancreatic ductal adenocarcinoma by K-Ras oncogenes in adult mice. *Cancer Cell* **11**(3):291–302.
18. Sparmann A, Bar-Sagi D. (2004) Ras-induced interleukin-8 expression plays a critical role in tumor growth and angiogenesis. *Cancer Cell* **6**(5):447–58.
19. Sumimoto H, Imabayashi F, Iwata T *et al.* (2006) The BRAF-MAPK signaling pathway is essential for cancer-immune evasion in human melanoma cells. *J Exp Med* **203**(7):1651–6.
20. Shchors K, Shchors E, Rostker F *et al.* (2006) The Myc-dependent angiogenic switch in tumors is mediated by interleukin 1beta. *Genes Dev* **20**(18):2527–38.

21. Soucek L, Lawlor ER, Soto D *et al.* (2007) Mast cells are required for angiogenesis and macroscopic expansion of Myc-induced pancreatic islet tumors. *Nat Med* **13**(10):1211–8.
22. Mantovani A, Allavena P, Sica A *et al.* (2008) Cancer-related inflammation. *Nature* **454**(7203):436–44.
23. Angeli F, Koumakis G, Chen MC *et al.* (2009) Role of stromal fibroblasts in cancer: Promoting or impeding? *Tumour Biol* **30**(3):109–20.
24. Kalluri R, Zeisberg M. (2006) Fibroblasts in cancer. *Nat Rev Cancer* **6**(5):392–401.
25. Ostman A, Augsten M. (2009) Cancer-associated fibroblasts and tumor growth — bystanders turning into key players. *Curr Opin Genet Dev* **19**(1):67–73.
26. Haviv I, Polyak K, Qiu W *et al.* (2009) Origin of carcinoma associated fibroblasts. *Cell Cycle* **8**(4):589–95.
27. Ishii G, Sangai T, Oda T *et al.* (2003) Bone-marrow-derived myofibroblasts contribute to the cancer-induced stromal reaction. *Biochem Biophys Res Commun* **309**(1):232–40.
28. Kim KK, Kugler MC, Wolters PJ *et al.* (2006) Alveolar epithelial cell mesenchymal transition develops *in vivo* during pulmonary fibrosis and is regulated by the extracellular matrix. *Proc Natl Acad Sci USA* **103**(35):13180–5.
29. Zeisberg EM, Potenta S, Xie L *et al.* (2007) Discovery of endothelial to mesenchymal transition as a source for carcinoma-associated fibroblasts. *Cancer Res* **67**(21):10123–8.
30. Sica A, Bronte V. (2007) Altered macrophage differentiation and immune dysfunction in tumor development. *J Clin Invest* **117**(5):1155–66.
31. Martinez FO, Sica A, Mantovani A *et al.* (2008) Macrophage activation and polarization. *Front Biosci* **13**:453–61.
32. Sica A, Schioppa T, Mantovani A *et al.* (2006) Tumour-associated macrophages are a distinct M2 polarised population promoting tumour progression: Potential targets of anti-cancer therapy. *Eur J Cancer* **42**(6):717–27.
33. Wang HY, Wang RF. (2007) Regulatory T cells and cancer. *Curr Opin Immunol* **19**(2):217–23.
34. Nizar S, Copier J, Meyer B *et al.* (2009) T-regulatory cell modulation: The future of cancer immunotherapy? *Br J Cancer* **100**(11):1697–703.

35. Balkwill F. (2004) Cancer and the chemokine network. *Nat Rev Cancer* **4**(7):540–50.
36. Balkwill F. (2003) Chemokine biology in cancer. *Semin Immunol* **15**(1):49–55.
37. Struyf S, Schutyser E, Gouwy M *et al.* (2003) PARC/CCL18 is a plasma CC chemokine with increased levels in childhood acute lymphoblastic leukemia. *Am J Pathol* **163**(5):2065–75.
38. Moran CJ, Arenberg DA, Huang CC *et al.* (2002) RANTES expression is a predictor of survival in stage I lung adenocarcinoma. *Clin Cancer Res* **8**(12):3803–12.
39. Monti P, Leone BE, Marchesi F *et al.* (2003) The CC chemokine MCP-1/CCL2 in pancreatic cancer progression: Regulation of expression and potential mechanisms of antimalignant activity. *Cancer Res* **63**(21):7451–61.
40. Balkwill F. (2004) The significance of cancer cell expression of the chemokine receptor CXCR4. *Semin Cancer Biol* **14**(3):171–9.
41. Sengupta S, Schiff R, Katzenellenbogen BS. (2009) Post-transcriptional regulation of chemokine receptor CXCR4 by estrogen in HER2 overexpressing, estrogen receptor-positive breast cancer cells. *Breast Cancer Res Treat* **117**(2):243–51.
42. Mehta SA, Christopherson KW, Bhat-Nakshatri P *et al.* (2007) Negative regulation of chemokine receptor CXCR4 by tumor suppressor p53 in breast cancer cells: Implications of p53 mutation or isoform expression on breast cancer cell invasion. *Oncogene* **26**(23):3329–37.
43. Schioppa T, Uranchimeg B, Saccani A *et al.* (2003) Regulation of the chemokine receptor CXCR4 by hypoxia. *J Exp Med* **198**(9):1391–402.
44. Bierie B, Moses HL. (2006) TGF-beta and cancer. *Cytokine Growth Factor Rev* **17**(1–2):29–40.
45. Gualberto A, Pollak M. (2009) Emerging role of insulin-like growth factor receptor inhibitors in oncology: Early clinical trial results and future directions. *Oncogene* **28**(34):3009–21.
46. Belfiore A, Frasca F, Pandini G *et al.* (2009) Insulin receptor isoforms and insulin receptor/insulin-like growth factor receptor hybrids in physiology and disease. *Endocr Rev* **30**(6):586–623.
47. De Luca A, Carotenuto A, Rachiglio A *et al.* (2008) The role of the EGFR signaling in tumor microenvironment. *J Cell Physiol* **214**(3):559–67.
48. Ostman A, Heldin CH. (2007) PDGF receptors as targets in tumor treatment. *Adv Cancer Res* **97**:247–74.

49. Perona R. (2006) Cell signalling: Growth factors and tyrosine kinase receptors. *Clin Transl Oncol* **8**(2):77–82.
50. Roy R, Yang J, Moses MA. (2009) Matrix metalloproteinases as novel biomarkers and potential therapeutic targets in human cancer. *J Clin Oncol* **27**(31):5287–97.
51. Levesque JP, Hendy J, Takamatsu Y *et al.* (2003) Disruption of the CXCR4/CXCL12 chemotactic interaction during hematopoietic stem cell mobilization induced by GCSF or cyclophosphamide. *J Clin Invest* **111**(2):187–96.
52. Hurtado M, Lozano JJ, Castellanos E *et al.* (2007) Activation of the epidermal growth factor signalling pathway by tissue plasminogen activator in pancreas cancer cells. *Gut* **56**(9):1266–74.
53. Pai R, Soreghan B, Szabo IL *et al.* (2002) Prostaglandin E2 transactivates EGF receptor: A novel mechanism for promoting colon cancer growth and gastrointestinal hypertrophy. *Nat Med* **8**(3):289–93.
54. Guerrero J, Santibanez JF, Gonzalez A *et al.* (2004) EGF receptor transactivation by urokinase receptor stimulus through a mechanism involving Src and matrix metalloproteinases. *Exp Cell Res* **292**(1):201–8.
55. Illman SA, Lehti K, Keski-Oja J *et al.* (2006) Epilysin (MMP-28) induces TGF-beta mediated epithelial to mesenchymal transition in lung carcinoma cells. *J Cell Sci* **119**(Pt 18):3856–65.
56. Stetler-Stevenson WG. (2008) The tumor microenvironment: Regulation by MMP-independent effects of tissue inhibitor of metalloproteinases-2. *Cancer Metastasis Rev* **27**(1):57–66.
57. Dulaimi E, Ibanez de Caceres I, Uzzo RG *et al.* (2004) Promoter hypermethylation profile of kidney cancer. *Clin Cancer Res* **10**(12 Pt 1):3972–9.
58. Gu P, Xing X, Tanzer M *et al.* (2008) Frequent loss of TIMP-3 expression in progression of esophageal and gastric adenocarcinomas. *Neoplasia* **10**(6):563–72.
59. Pulukuri SM, Patibandla S, Patel J *et al.* (2007) Epigenetic inactivation of the tissue inhibitor of metalloproteinase-2 (TIMP-2) gene in human prostate tumors. *Oncogene* **26**(36):5229–37.
60. Naugler WE, Sakurai T, Kim S *et al.* (2007) Gender disparity in liver cancer due to sex differences in MyD88-dependent IL-6 production. *Science* **317**(5834):121–4.

61. Grivennikov S, Karin E, Terzic J *et al.* (2009) IL-6 and Stat3 are required for survival of intestinal epithelial cells and development of colitis-associated cancer. *Cancer Cell* **15**(2):103–13.
62. Karin M, Cao Y, Greten FR *et al.* (2002) NF-kappaB in cancer: From innocent bystander to major culprit. *Nat Rev Cancer* **2**(4):301–10.
63. Karin M, Greten FR. (2005) NF-kappaB: Linking inflammation and immunity to cancer development and progression. *Nat Rev Immunol* **5**(10):749–59.
64. Karin M. (2006) Nuclear factor-kappaB in cancer development and progression. *Nature* **441**(7092):431–6.
65. Liu X, Wang X, Zhang J *et al.* (2010) Warburg effect revisited: An epigenetic link between glycolysis and gastric carcinogenesis. *Oncogene* **29**(3):442–50.
66. Greten FR, Eckmann L, Greten TF *et al.* (2004) IKKbeta links inflammation and tumorigenesis in a mouse model of colitis-associated cancer. *Cell* **118**(3):285–96.
67. Pikarsky E, Porat RM, Stein I *et al.* (2004) NF-kappaB functions as a tumour promoter in inflammation-associated cancer. *Nature* **431**(7007):461–6.
68. Yu H, Pardoll D, Jove R. (2009) STATs in cancer inflammation and immunity: A leading role for STAT3. *Nat Rev Cancer* **9**(11):798–809.
69. Hodge DR, Hurt EM, Farrar WL. (2005) The role of IL-6 and STAT3 in inflammation and cancer. *Eur J Cancer* **41**(16):2502–12.
70. Croker BA, Kiu H, Nicholson SE. (2008) SOCS regulation of the JAK/STAT signalling pathway. *Semin Cell Dev Biol* **19**(4):414–22.
71. Shuai K, Liu B. (2005) Regulation of gene-activation pathways by PIAS proteins in the immune system. *Nat Rev Immunol* **5**(8):593–605.
72. Lee H, Herrmann A, Deng JH *et al.* (2009) Persistently activated Stat3 maintains constitutive NF-kappaB activity in tumors. *Cancer Cell* **15**(4):283–93.

Section II

Models of Chronic Inflammation–Induced Cancers and Their Treatments

Chapter 5

Advances in the Treatment of *Helicobacter pylori* Infection and Gastric Cancer

Guy D. Eslick*

The Whiteley-Martin Research Centre, Discipline of Surgery, The University of Sydney, Sydney Medical School Nepean, Nepean Hospital, Australia

Helicobacter pylori infection treatment is a dynamic process dependent on antibiotic resistance. Triple therapy remains the first line approach to patients. Sequential therapy may hold the key to recalcitrant patients however, further data is required. Novel alternative therapies are in the early days and still require further investigation. Treatment of gastric cancer patients is currently sub-optimal and advances in molecular and targeted agents shows promise, although trial data is still in progress. On a population level the treatment of *H. pylori* is not a feasible option for the prevention of gastric cancer. Future studies should take a multidisciplinary approach to treating gastric cancer patients to provide the most favorable outcomes for patients.

Introduction

This chapter will review some of the historical aspects and the latest developments in the treatment of *Helicobacter pylori* infection and gastric cancer separately and then discuss what effect eliminating *H. pylori* infection might have on the progression to gastric cancer. Before the discovery of *H. pylori* in 1982 and the publication of Barry Marshall and Robin Warren's

* E-mail: eslickg@med.usyd.edu.au

letters in the *Lancet*,[1,2] the link between *H. pylori* infection and gastric cancer was unknown. This pivotal medical discovery has provided opportunities to cure a number of gastric conditions including gastritis, peptic ulcer disease, MALToma, and adenocarcinoma.[3,4] Currently, the indications for the treatment of *H. pylori* infection does vary depending on the condition (Box 1).[5–7]

Box 1. Indications for *H. pylori* treatment.

- Peptic ulcer disease
- Gastric MALT lymphoma
- Post endoscopic resection of early stage gastric cancer
- Uninvestigated dyspepsia
- Atrophic gastritis
- Non-ulcer dyspepsia
- Gastroesophageal reflux disease (GERD)
- Individuals using non-steroidal drugs (NSAIDs)
- Unexplained iron deficiency anemia
- Populations at higher risk of gastric cancer
- Patients with a first degree relative with gastric cancer
- Unexplained idiopathic thrombocytopenic purpura
- Early gastric cancer

The International Agency for Research on Cancer (IARC) published a report on biological agents and their potential to cause cancer,[8] this included Schistosomes, liver flukes and *Helicobacter pylori*. The evaluation determined that there was sufficient evidence to classify *H. pylori* as a definite class 1 carcinogen to humans however, there was inadequate evidence to classify the organism as a carcinogen to animals. The conflicting studies based around this association have led some to question if a causal link really exists or if confounding factors have not been adequately controlled for in these studies.[9] Several meta-analyses have been conducted which appear to have produced consistent data to support a relationship between *H. pylori* and the development of gastric cancer

Table 1. Findings from *H. pylori* and gastric cancer meta-analyses.

Meta-analysis	Number of studies	Odds ratio	Confidence interval
Huang *et al.*[10]	19	1.92	1.32–2.78
Danesh[11]	10	2.50	1.90–3.40
Eslick *et al.*[12]	42	2.04	1.69–2.45
Xue *et al.*[13]	11	2.56	1.85–3.55
HCCG[14]	12	2.36	1.98–2.81
Huang *et al.*[15,§]	16	2.28	1.71–3.05
Wang *et al.*[16,*]	19	3.38	2.15–5.33

§ cagA; * early gastric cancer.

(Table 1).[10–16] These findings have paved the way for future public health interventions that would include the possibility of treating *H. pylori* infection to prevent the development of gastric cancer, but there remains much debate as to the true benefit of undertaking this monumental task.[17,18]

The majority of these meta-analyses have looked at the overall relationship between *H. pylori* and gastric cancer, but there have been some that specifically aimed to assess other aspects of this relationship. For example, Huang and colleagues[15] specifically aimed to determine the role of cagA seropositivity in the development of gastric cancer, while a meta-analysis by Wang and colleagues determined the role of *H. pylori* in the development of early gastric cancer.[16] Because *H. pylori* infection is treatable the belief that eradicating this organism from peoples stomach will significantly reduce the incidence of gastric cancer.

Treatment of *Helicobacter pylori* infection

There a several options in treating *H. pylori* infection. These fit into the following groups:

- Standard triple therapy
- Quadruple therapy
- Sequential therapy
- Alternative therapy

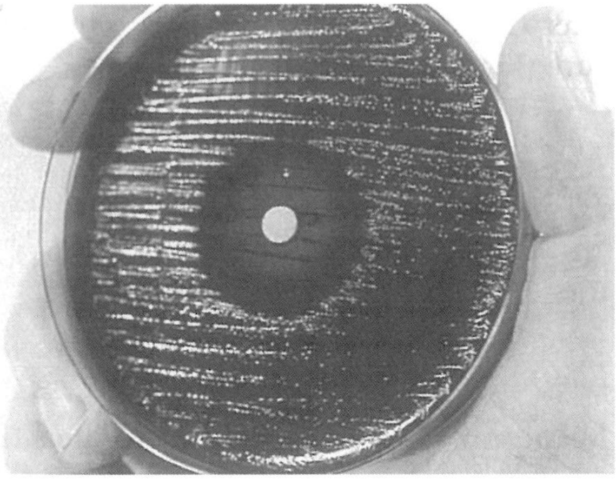

Figure 1. Three-day-old culture of *H. pylori* inhibited by colloidal bismuth subcitrate ("DeNol"). The disc contains 50 μg of bismuth subcitrate (*with permission*, from Marshall BJ, *et al. Helicobacter pylori* in peptic ulceration and gastritis, p. 161 (1991). Blackwell Scientific Publishing, Boston).[19]

Therapies for the treatment of *H. pylori* have come along way since the days of "DeNol" (colloidal bismuth subcitrate), which was used extensively during the early *H. pylori* treatment era.[19] Historically, bismuth salts had been used to a great extent in gastroenterology.[20] Bismuth subcitrate inhibited the growth of *H. pylori* (Figure 1), and the major reason for its use related to the response shown among those with duodenal ulcers even before the discovery of *H. pylori*.[21]

In 1983, the first bismuth/antibiotic combination was used to treat *H. pylori* and consisted of "DeNol" and amoxicillin which eradicated the organism.[22] It was noted that the failure rate of this combination was high with between 20%–50% of patients not responding and remaining infected. In 1986–87, an Australian group developed the first triple therapy, which consisted of tripotassium dicitratobismuthate combined with ten days of tindazole (1 g/day) with or without either amoxicillin, erythromycin, or tetracycline (each 250 mg/4 times/day for 4 weeks).[23] This was the impetus for a multitude of clinical trials over the next two decades comparing various combinations of antibiotics and proton pump inhibitors for the optimal treatment of *H. pylori* infection.

For more than a decade the initial treatment option for *H. pylori* has been triple therapy which generally consists of a proton pump inhibitor (PPI), amoxicillin (1 g), and clarithromycin (500 mg) all twice per day, for up to 14 days.[24] However, there has been a growing number of reports suggesting that cure rates using this triple therapy have dropped below 80%.[25] Solutions to improving this situation have included prolonging the treatment period or by changing the dose of the proton pump inhibitor. These factors obviously affect the compliance of the specific therapy for *H. pylori*, along with side effects of the treatments (Figure 2). For triple therapy, amoxicillin is one of the most widely used antibiotics, but resistance appears to be uncommon, while rates of resistance for clarithromycin are generally between 5–20%.[26] Levofloxacin has been proposed as an alternative to clarithromycin for those cases with clarithromycin-resistant strains. Increasing the duration of treatment has not resulted in substantial improvement in cure rates and in many Western countries triple therapy cure rates have fallen to unacceptable levels.

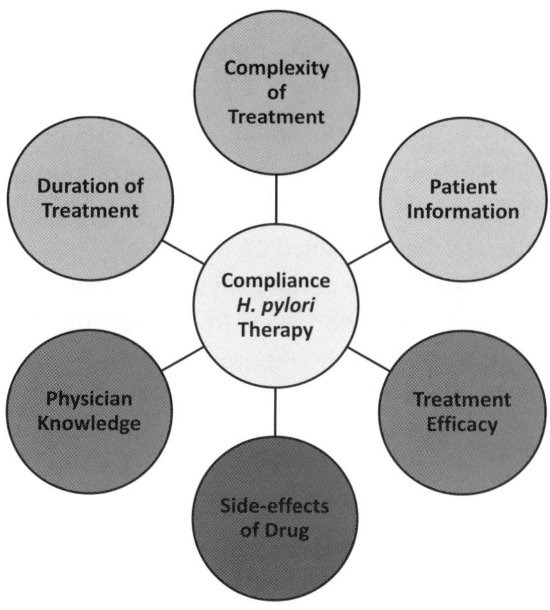

Figure 2. Factors affecting compliance of *H. pylori* therapy (adapted from O'Conner *et al.*[27]).

The increasing number of treatment failures occurring with triple therapy lead to the development of quadruple therapy, which consisted of bismuth, tetracycline, metronidazole and a proton pump inhibitor. Resistance to metranidazole has been a major issue for the quadruple therapy regimes with over one-third of strains resistant.[27] Furthermore, studies have suggested that metronidazole resistance not only reduces the efficacy of triple therapy but that it leads to secondary clarithromycin resistance, which results in duel resistance increasing the chances of treatment failure.[28]

A recently developed alternative has been receiving a lot of attention and this is known as sequential therapy. It consists of two five day periods where a combination of a duel therapy and subsequently a triple therapy are used during each period. The first five day duel treatment aims to significantly decrease the bacterial load, while the second five day triple therapy kills the remaining organisms.[29] Two pooled analyses report that cure rates using sequential therapy are greater than 90%.[30,31] However, it must be note that the majority of studies all come from Italy and as such are not representative of other populations.[32] In fact some other countries have much lower cure rates, for example, a study from Korea had a cure rate of 78%.[33]

The complexity of the treatments in terms of number of drugs taken, number of times taken each day, will have a determining effect on adherence and thus cure rate among individuals, these factors must always be taken into consideration and adapted on a patient by patient basis. Indeed sequential therapy involves a complicated timetable of drugs and one study reported that it might be easier to provide the same four drugs together for 8–10 days, which should provide similar cure rates.[34]

Guidelines for the treatment of *H. pylori*

Worldwide there are a number of guidelines that have been formulated to provide a consensus on the optimal therapy for *H. pylori* infection. I will discuss the three main guidelines used around the world with these being the American College of Gastroenterology, Maastricht III, and the Second Asia-Pacific guidelines.[5,7,35] A brief outline of these guidelines are shown in Table 2. These guidelines are similar with some minor differences

Table 2. Comparison of *H. pylori* treatment guidelines.

Criteria	ACG[5]	Maastricht III[35]	Asia-Pacific[7]
Testing	Active gastric or duodenal ulcer, gastric MALT, early gastric cancer, endoscopic resection of early gastric cancer, or uninvestigated dyspepsia	Active gastric or duodenal ulcer, gastric MALT, early gastric cancer, uninvestigated dyspepsia, gastric cancer first degree relative, atrophic gastritis, unexplained iron deficiency anemia, or chronic idiopathic thrombocytopenic purpura.	Active gastric or duodenal ulcer, gastric MALT, early gastric cancer, uninvestigated dyspepsia, gastric cancer first degree relative, atrophic gastritis, unexplained iron deficiency anemia, or chronic idiopathic thrombocytopenic purpura, post gastric cancer resection, NSAID users, patients on low-dose aspirin, GERD, individuals at high risk of gastric cancer, Patients' wishes.
Treatment strategy	Age < 55 years and no alarm symptoms*	Age <45 years and no alarm symptoms*	Not specified
Duration of therapy	10–14 days	7 days	7 days

* Alarm symptoms: dysphagia, weight loss, evidence of gastrointestinal bleeding, and persistent vomiting.

between them. It should be noted that while the American and Maastricht guidelines did set age cut-offs for test and treat strategies, the Asia-Pacific guidelines did not specify this because of the diversity of the Asian populations and due to the increased risk of gastric cancer among these populations, in particular among younger age groups.

In terms of the duration of treatment stated in each guideline is dependent on the type of therapy undertaken, with the Maastricht III recommending longer treatment periods (10–14 days), while the American and Asia-Pacific guidelines recommended shorter 7 day treatment periods due to the increasing risk of clarithromycin resistance. All guidelines stated that further research is required to determine optimal therapies in terms of dose, duration, and improving adherence. The Asia-Pacific guidelines also highlighted the importance of genetic polymorphisms (CYP2C19) and cigarette smoking in affecting *H. pylori* eradication rates.

Based on current knowledge, first-line treatment should be triple therapy assuming that there is no high level of clarithromycin resistance (Figure 3). Additional therapy should not be undertaken unless the presence of *H. pylori* is confirmed. More data is needed on sequential therapies in different populations before this will take over from triple therapy as the first-line option for treating *H. pylori* infection.

Alternative therapies for *H. pylori* infection

There are a number of alternative therapies that have been assessed for treating *H. pylori* infection. These alternative therapies include: traditional Chinese medicine, phytoceuticals, probiotics, and other alternative options. Currently, there have been a number of clinical trials assessing various traditional Chinese medicines, which have included *in vitro* studies of herbs such as *Radix scutellariae*, *Lonicera*, *Radix Isatidis Seu Baphicacanthi*, *Coptis chinensis Franch* and *Fructus Aurantii Immaturus* which appear to have potential inhibitory effects on *H. pylori*. A recent systematic review of 16 trials using traditional Chinese medicine with a proton pump inhibitor or bismuth subcitrate.[36] There was a large amount of heterogeneity among the trials. The eradication rates between the two groups was 72% vs 78% for traditional Chinese medicine and triple therapy, respectively. Therefore, traditional Chinese medicine may not be as effective as triple therapy, however, the quality of the studies was poor and thus further studies that meet CONSORT guidelines would be required to provide a more appropriate recommendation on the potential use of traditional Chinese medicine for the treatment of *H. pylori* infection.

The use of probiotics has also been of recent interest with a few systematic reviews and meta-analyses published.[37–39] Probiotics are live microorganisms which when administered in adequate amounts confer a health benefit on the host. The most commonly used microorganisms

(a)

Triple therapy

7-14 days

Amoxicillin: 1 g twice/day
Clarithromycin: 500 mg twice/day
Proton Pump Inhibitor: 20-40 mg twice/day

↓

Quadruple therapy

10-14 days

Bismuth: 120 mg four times/day
Tetracycline: 500 mg four times/day
Metronidazole: 250 mg four times/day
Proton Pump Inhibitor: 20-40 mg twice/day

↓

Sequential therapy

Days 1-5

Amoxicillin: 1 g twice/day
Proton Pump Inhibitor: 20-40 mg twice/day

Days 6-10

Tindazole: 500 mg twice/day
Clarithromycin: 500 mg twice/day
Proton Pump Inhibitor: 20-40 mg twice/day

(b)

Triple therapy

7-14 days

Amoxicillin: 1 g twice/day
Metronidazole: 500 mg twice/day
Proton Pump Inhibitor: 20-40 mg twice/day

Figure 3. (a) First-line treatment options for *H. pylori* infection. (b) Second-line treatment option for previous triple therapy using clarithromycin for *H. pylori* infection.

include: lactic acid-producing bacteria such as *Lactobacillus* spp, *Bifidobacterium*, and *Bacillus*. A recent meta-analysis assessed the effect of fermented milk-based probiotic preparations on *H. pylori* eradication and identified ten randomized controlled trials consisting of 953 patients (498 treatment group vs 465 control group).[38] Fermented milk-based probiotics improved *H. pylori* eradication rates by only 10%, with mixed results in terms of the impact on adverse effects.

Probiotics may work on *H. pylori* via a number of mechanisms including:

- Growth inhibition of *H. pylori* via urease inhibition
- Blocking *H. pylori* by adherence of the probiotic to gastric cells
- Restoration of gastric mucosal permeability
- Modification of the immune response (e.g. reduce IL-8)

Probiotics appear to offer excellent anti-inflammatory properties with several studies showing improvement of *H. pylori* gastritis and a decrease in *H. pylori* density.[39] Moreover, the use of probiotics in conjunction with standard *H. pylori* therapies greatly reduces *H. pylori* therapy-associated side effects (23% vs 46%, $p = 0.04$).[39] However, no study thus far has demonstrated eradication of *H. pylori* infection using a probiotic treatment. Further research is ongoing and larger well designed studies are required to establish the usefulness of probiotics in treating *H. pylori* infection in humans.

Phytoceuticals such as Korean red ginseng, green tea, red wine, flavonoids, broccoli sprouts, and garlic have been shown to inhibit *H. pylori* colonization, reduce gastric inflammation and repress precancerous changes.[40] The potential mechanisms by which some of these events occur predominantly include:

- Inhibiting cytokine and chemokine release
- Inhibiting nuclear factor-kappa B DNA

Studies have shown the Korean red ginseng has a substantial protective effect in reducing *H. pylori* cytotoxicity and DNA mutagenesis.[41,42] Additional research has revealed that *Panax* ginseng can inhibit *H. pylori* mitogen-activated protein kinase (MAPK).[43] It has been suggested that long-term use of red ginseng might offer significant protection from gastric inflammation due to *H. pylori* infection.

Green tea has long been purported to offer a number of health benefits to those who consume it on a regular basis. Green tea has been shown to inhibit the urease enzyme which is essential for *H. pylori* to colonise the human stomach, thus reducing the potential for bacterial colonization.[44] Other mechanisms include an anti-adhesive effect via a pectin-type acidic polysaccharide in the green tea. Furthermore, green tea may reduce urea and therefore affect vacuolation via the vacA cytotoxin. The polyphenols in green tea may also prevent *H. pylori*-associated gastroduodenal diseases. Extensive studies are required in this interesting area of research.

Other agents with antibacterial activity have been reported to offer benefit against *H. pylori* infection. One of these agents is Manuka honey which is from New Zealand. This particular type of honey is believed to have very potent antibacterial properties. A small study consisted of 12 *H. pylori* positive (by CLO test) patients with six treated with manuka honey four times per day for 2 weeks and six treated with honey and omeprazole (20 mg twice/day) for 2 weeks.[45] All 12 patients remained positive after the trial as determined by ^{14}C urea breath tests. Further studies over longer periods (3 months treatment) and with larger sample sizes are required.

Treatment of gastric cancer

Gastric cancer remains one of the most recalcitrant cancers to treat and while more new chemotherapeutic agents are becoming available the median survival times have not improved substantially over the last two decades. Metastatic gastric cancer remains an incurable disease, with a relative 5-year survival of 7%–27%.[46] However, the development of new targeted therapies may offer promise with results from ongoing trials to determine their clinical role in the treatment of gastric cancer.

It has been observed that patients in phase II clinical trials involving chemotherapy for gastric cancer have up to 60% response to treatment, however, due to the development of drug resistance within a few months

Table 3. Single agent use in gastric cancer (advanced).

Agents	Response rate (%)
Mitomycin C	30
Doxorubicin	17
Epirubicin	19
Cisplatin	19
BCNU	18
5-Flurouracil	21
Etopside	21
Hydroxurea	19
UFT	27
Capectiabina	19
S-1	45
Paclitaxel	17–23
Docetaxel	17–29
CPT-11	18

the median survival is approximately eight months.[46] Moreover, the toxic effects of the chemotherapy have had many clinicians ask whether the treatment benefit is acceptable compared with the quality of life. Older treatment options usually involved a single agent (Table 3), while more current therapies usually consist of a combination of chemotherapeutic agents.

There have been a few meta-analyses that have aimed to determine the efficacy of various approaches to chemotherapy for gastric cancer.[47,48] One of these meta-analyses assessed 14 randomised controlled trials using intravenous chemotherapy after gastrectomy and it was reported that it was better than surgery alone, even though two patients did died from chemotherapy toxicity (OR = 0.56, 95% CI: 0.40–0.79).[47]

Because the spread of gastric cancer often involves the intraperitoneal cavity, the use of intraperitoneal chemotherapy among patients having a curative resection was assessed among 11 trials.[48] The overall pooled estimate was (OR = 0.51, 95% CI: 0.40–0.65) suggesting this might be of benefit for patients. However, further studies are still required using a rigorous design and using large numbers of patients.

A recent meta-analysis of 20 randomized clinical trials conducted over the course of 25 years determined the impact of radiotherapy (pre-operative, post-operative and/or intra-operative) on 3- and 5-years survival for patients with resectable gastric cancer.[49] Studies using radiotherapy in the treatment of gastric cancer have produced conflicting results. The quality of the studies included was low and there was no heterogeneity and no publication bias. There was a 5-year survival benefit from preoperative radiotherapy (OR = 1.26, 95% CI: 1.08–1.48).

In 2006, the Medical Research Council Adjuvant Gastric Infusional Chemotherapy (MAGIC) Trial comparing perioperative chemotherapy versus surgery alone for resectable gastroesophaeal cancer was reported in the New England Journal of Medicine.[50] The study consisted of patients randomized to chemotherapy with epirubicin, cisplatin, and infused fluorouracil (ECF) plus surgery compared to surgery alone. Five-year survival was 36% in the chemotherapy group compared with 23% in the surgery-only group. There were a number of important issues associated with this trial. Patients were given three cycles of ECF before and after surgery, however, more than half the patients in both groups did not complete all six cycles of chemotherapy (58.4 perioperative chemotherapy vs 50.5 perioperative chemotherapy and surgery. In total, 503 patients were randomized between 1994 and 2002, a trial period twice what was initially expected. The main aim of the study was to determine a survival difference between the two treatment arms, with a 90% statistical power to detect a 15% survival difference at 5 years. One hundred patients were older than 70 years and 125 patients had gastroesophageal junction or lower esophageal cancers. Other issues included the fact that 31% of patients did not have their tumor size documented before randomization. At surgery, there were more patients with advanced disease based on tumor stage and nodal status in the surgery group compared with the perioperative chemotherapy group.

A year later another paper was published by a group from Japan comparing patients with stage II or III gastric cancer who had a D2 gastrectomy followed by adjuvant therapy with oral fluropyrimidine (S-1) or just surgery alone.[51] At 3-year overall survival the surgery and chemotherapy group had a 10% higher survival rate compared with the surgery alone group (80.1% vs 70.1%, $p = 0.003$). It should be noted that the approach to gastric cancer patients in Japan is more aggressive than those taken in Western countries, especially with the D2 gastrectomy and this may account for the findings in this study.

In a recent comparison of two phase I and II trials (Intergroup 0116 and Dutch Gastric Cancer Group Trail (DGCT)) found that after D1 surgery the addition of postoperative chemotherapy improved survival and decreased local recurrence of gastric cancer.[52] Local recurrence after 2-years was higher in the surgery only (DGCT) group (17% vs 5%, $p = 0.001$). There were less local recurrences for those undergoing the D2 resection compared to the D1 resection. Figure 4 shows the overall survival analyses: (A) Local recurrence: chemoradiotherapy (CRT) versus surgery only. Hazard ratio (HR), 3.23; $p = 0.0015$. (B) Overall survival: CRT versus surgery only. HR, 1.14; $p = 0.51$. (C) Local recurrence: CRT D1 versus surgery only D1. HR, 11.10; $p = 0.001$. (D) Overall survival: CRT D1 versus surgery only D1. HR, 1.46; $p = 0.18$. (E) Local recurrence: CRT D2 versus surgery only D2. HR, 1.10; $p = 0.84$. (F) Overall survival: CRT D2 versus surgery only D2. HR, 1.05; $p = 0.88$.

In addition a recent meta-analysis of 17 randomized controlled trials consisting of 3838 patients with a median follow-up time of seven years determined that the use of postoperative adjuvant chemotherapy using regimes based on flurouracil provided reduced risk of death when compared to surgery alone.[53] Surgery alone had a higher number of deaths (57%) than among the chemotherapy group (52%). The use of chemotherapy increased 5-year survival by 5.7%. There were a number of limitations to this meta-analysis which included using studies from more than 30 years ago, underpowered trials, trials with poor design, mixed chemotherapeutic agents, different surgical approaches, differing duration of treatments, various levels of treatment completion, and incomplete resection.[53] Some feel that these limitations along with the heterogeneity of gastric cancers in terms of the biology, therapy or both did not make postoperative adjuvant chemotherapy a standard option for Western patients with gastric cancer.[53] More specifically directed and well designed trials are required to determine if trials would be more

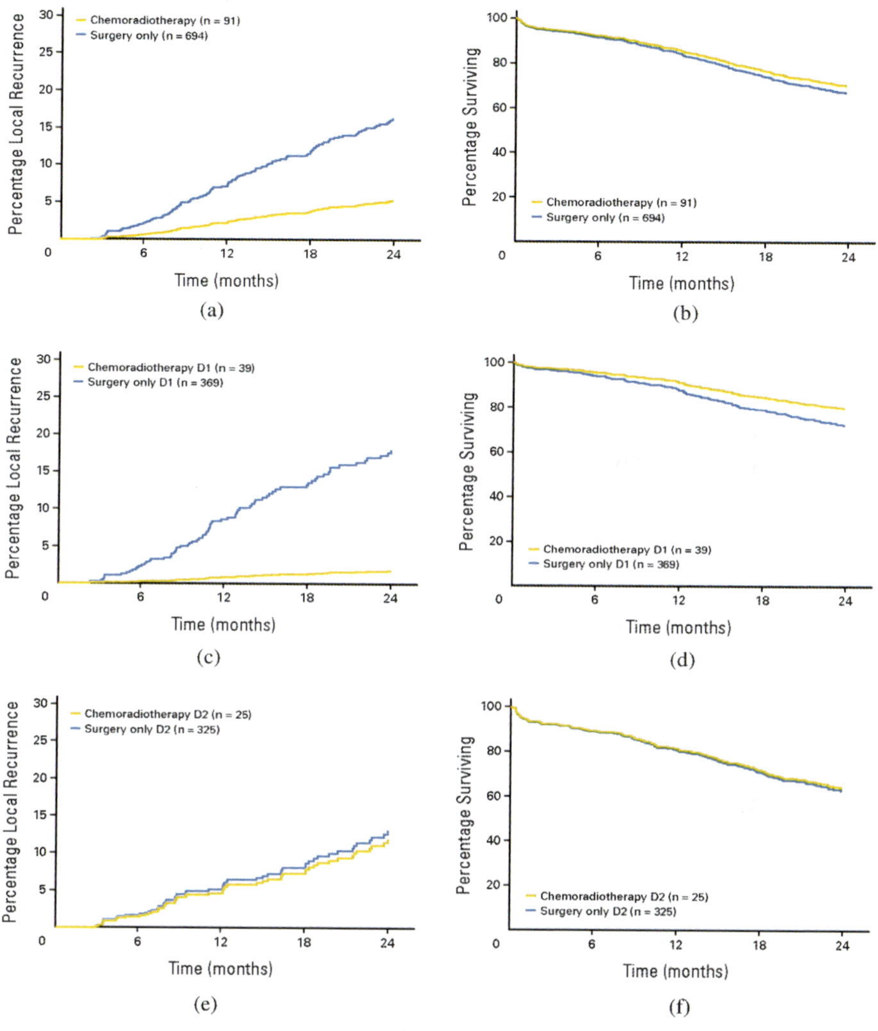

Figure 4. Multivariate analyses of local recurrence and overall survival. From: Dikken JL, Jansen EP, Cats A, *et al.* Impact of the extent of surgery and postoperative chemoradiotherapy on recurrence patterns in gastric cancer. *J Clin Oncol* 2010;28:2430–2436.[52] (*with permission*)

successful on subsets of patients (e.g., those with *ERBB2*-positive tumors) using a more targeted approach based on molecular and biomarker strategies. This appears to be the future direction of therapy options for gastric cancer.

Future directions in gastric cancer treatment

Currently, it is well recognized that therapies for advanced gastric cancer do not have any prognostic impact on patient survival. It is envisaged that with the development of targeted and molecular therapies that patient outcomes might improve and that overall survival could extend beyond the current average of ten-months.[54] Future strategies will revolve around the following drugs:

- Epidermal growth factor receptor (EGFR) inhibitors
- Anti-angiogenic agents
- Multitryrosine kinase inhibitors
- Cell cycle inhibitors
- Apoptosis promoters
- Matrix metalloproteinase inhibitors

There are a number of clinical trials currently underway using targeted therapies (Table 4).

It is beyond the scope of this article to discuss the variety of mechanisms and pathways used to induce a cellular effect on cancer cells (Figure 5). However, excellent sources include the following published papers.[54,55]

Prevention of gastric cancer by treating *H. pylori* infection

The potential to reduce morbidity and mortality associated with gastric cancer by treating *H. pylori* infection has enormous public health implications. Currently, there are six published trials that have aimed to determine if *H. pylori* treatment reduces gastric cancer. The results of these trials have recently been reported in a meta-analysis (Table 5).[56]

None of the studies produced a statistically significant result, however, overall there was a significant finding, suggesting that treatment for *H. pylori* infection does reduce gastric cancer incidence. It is important to note the small sample sizes in these trials and obviously large multicentre trials might assist in confirming these results. However, due to the logistical, financial and methodological problems associated with undertaking such studies,

Table 4. Current clinical trials for gastric cancer.

Target	Agent	Description	Status
Angiogenesis	Bevacizumab	Humanized monoclonal antibody anti-VEGF	Phase III
	Sunitinib	Small molecule targeting VEGFRs, PDGFR-β, and c-Kit	Phase I–II
	Sorafenib	Small molecule targeting RAF, VEGFRs, PDGFR-β	Phase I–II
EGFR/HER-2	Cetuximab	Chimeric, human-murine immunoglobulin anti-EGFR	Phase III
	Matuzumab	Humanized monoclonal antibody anti-EGFR	Phase I
	Panitumumab	Fully human monoclonal antibody anti-EGFR	Phase II
	Gefitinib	Tyrosine kinase inhibitor of EGFR	Phase II
	Erlotinib	Tyrosine kinase inhibitor of EGFR	Phase II
	Trastuzumab	Monoclonal antibody anti-HER-2	Phase III
	Lapatinib	Small-molecule dual inhibitor of EGFR and HER-2	Phase III
Cell cycle	Flavopiridol	Pan cyclin-dependent kinases inhibitor	Phase I–II
Matrix metalloproteinase	Marimastat	Matrix metalloproteinases inhibitor	Phase III
Proteasome	Bortezomib	Small molecule proteasome inhibitor	Phase II
Gastrin 17	G17DT	Immunogen	Phase II

From: Morabito A, Carillio G, Longo R. Systemic treatment of gastric cancer. *Crit Rev Oncol Hematol* 2009;70:216–234.[55] (*with permission*)

these trials would not be advisable. Moreover, the fact that few people who have *Helicobacter pylori* infection go on to develop gastric cancer would make a more focused approach not only practical but economical. Identification of those individuals at high risk would provide a more optimal approach to treating such patients and should be the focus of future research. Recently, de Vaies *et al.*[57] suggested that treatment of *H. pylori* infection does not prevent the development of gastric cancer even after long term

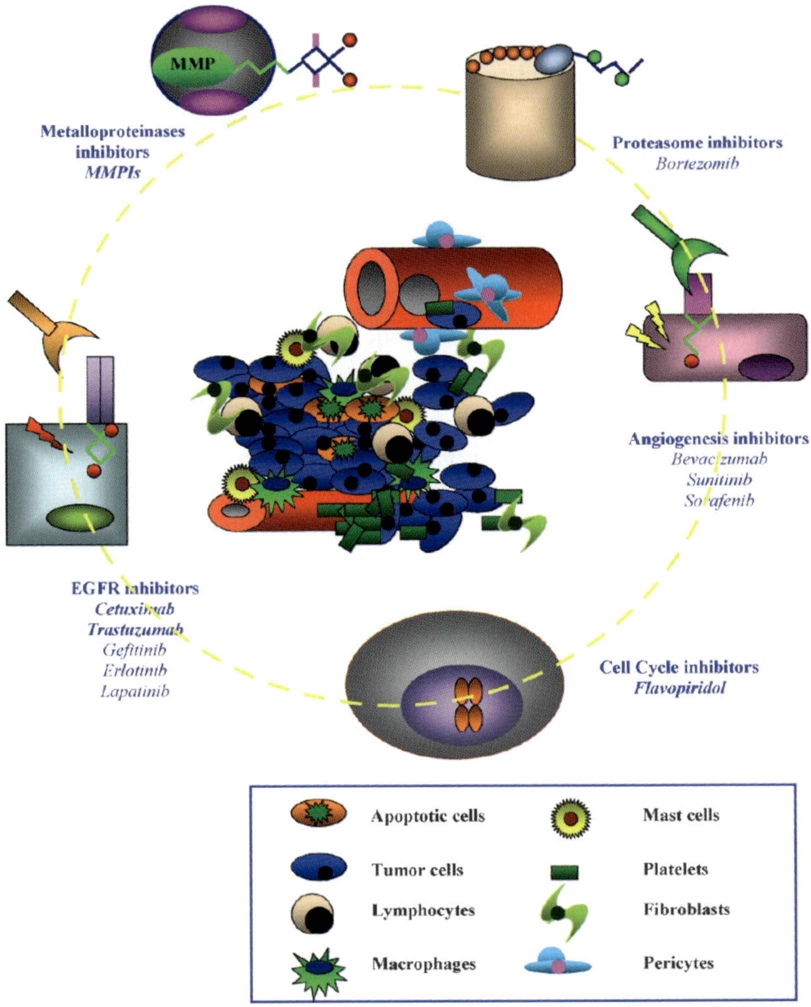

Figure 5. Tumor microenvironment and target-based agents. From: Morabito A, Carillio G, Longo R. Systemic treatment of gastric cancer. *Crit Rev Oncol Hematol* 2009;70:216–234.[55] (*with permission*)

follow-up.[57] There have also been conflicting opinions regarding this approach to reduce gastric cancer rates, even in areas of high risk.[58–62]

Guidelines have been proposed for those individuals at intermediate or high risk for the development of gastric cancer (Figure 6)[63].

Table 5. Findings from six trials using *H. pylori* therapy for gastric cancer.

Author, year	Relative risk (95% confidence interval)	Treatment group events (n/n)	Control group events (n/n)
Correa *et al.* 2000	1.48 (0.25–8.83)	3/491	2/485
Leung *et al.* 2004	0.66 (0.19–2.31)	4/295	6/292
Wwong *et al.* 2004	0.63 (0.25–1.63)	7/817	11/813
Satio *et al.* 2005	0.55 (0.09–3.27)	2/379	3/313
You *et al.* 2006	0.70 (0.39–1.26)	19/1130	27/1128
Zhou 2008	0.29 (0.06–1.36)	2/276	7/276
Overall	0.65 (0.43–0.98)	37/3388	56/3307

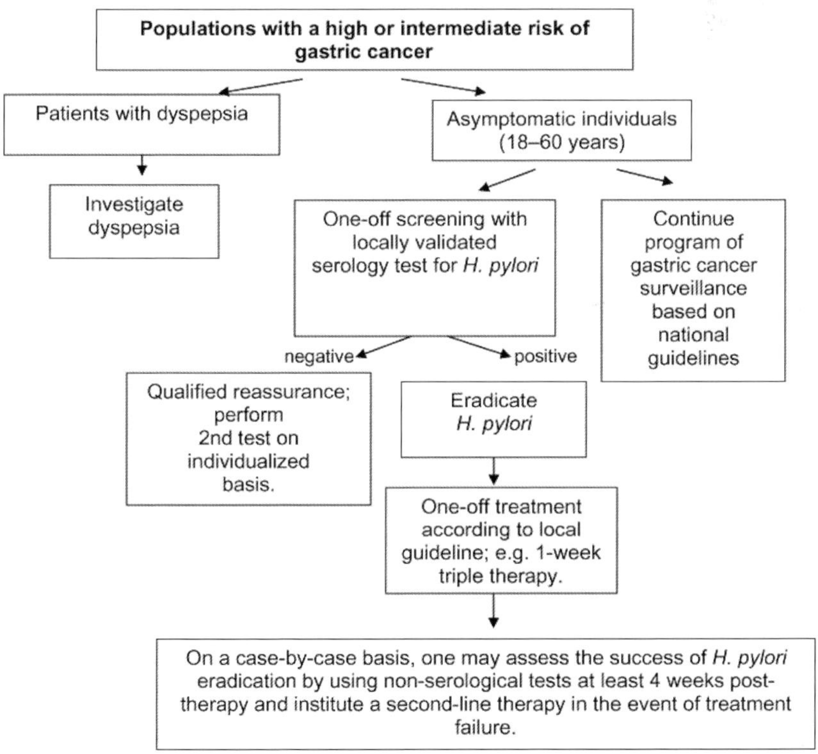

Figure 6. Strategy of *H. pylori* screening and eradication in populations at high or intermediate risk for gastric cancer. From: Fock KM, Talley NJ, Moayyedi P *et al.* Asia-Pacific consensus guidelines on gastric cancer prevention. *J Gastroenterol Hepatol* 2008;23:351–365. (*with permission*)

Conclusions

The burden produced by *Helicobacter pylori* infection in terms of morbidity and mortality is unimaginable. It is a cause of benign and malignant gastric disease, with a select group of the organism's afflictions curable using antibiotics. Antibiotic treatments have advanced over the last quarter of a century and with the difficulties associated with the development of antibiotic resistance this will continue to be an essential element in the progress and ultimate success of therapy for this infection. Currently, there are numerous complementary and alternative therapies being assessed to determine what role they may play in the treatment of this ubiquitous infection. Pooled estimates from six trials suggest that treatment of *H. pylori* infection would reduce the incidence of gastric cancer, however, the logistics and methodological issues associated with conducting future trials which would confirm these data are impractical.

Gastric cancer treatments have not improved survival in over 40 years, and it is hoped that newer molecular and targeted therapies may provide an increase in survival for these patients. Although much research and numerous high quality trials will be required to determine the potential of these therapies, current trials may offer new hope in the fight against gastric cancer.

Acknowledgments

This work was supported by a generous bequest of Nita Whiteley to the Discipline of Surgery at The University of Sydney, Australia.

Dedication

I would like to thank my good friend and colleague, Professor Harry H-X. Xia for all his support, friendship, and inspiration over the many years I have been fortunate to know him. He is an outstanding researcher and his work on *Helicobacter pylori* infection has provided numerous key insights into this amazing infection of the gastrointestinal system.

References

1. Marshall BJ. (1983) Unidentified curved bacilli on gastric epithelium in active chronic gastritis. *Lancet* **i**:1273–5.
2. Warren RJ. (1983) Unidentified curved bacilli on gastric epithelium in active chronic gastritis. *Lancet* **i**:1273.
3. Lee Y-C, Liou J-M, Wu M-S *et al.* (2008) Eradication of *Helicobacter pylori* to prevent gastroduodenal diseases: Hitting more than one bird with the same stone. *Ther Advan Gastroenterol* **1**:111–20.
4. McColl KE. (2010) Clinical Practice: *Helicobacter pylori* infection. *N Engl J Med* **362**:1597–604.
5. Chey WD, Wong BCY. (2007) American College of Gastroenterology guideline on the management of *Helicobacter pylori* infection. *Am J Gastroenterol* **102**:1808–25.
6. Kim N, Kim JJ, Choe YH *et al.* (2009) Diagnosis and treatment for *Helicobacter pylori* inection in Korea. *Korean J Gastroenterol* **54**:269–78.
7. Fock KM, Katelaris P, Sugano K *et al.* (2009) Second Asia-Pacific consensus guidelines for *Helicobacter pylori* infection. *J Gastroenterol Hepatol* **24**:1587–600.
8. International Agency for Research on Cancer. Schistosomes, liver flukes and *Helicobacter pylori*. IARC Monographs on the Evaluation of Carcinogenic risks to Humans, No. 61. IARC, Lyon; 1994.
9. Gonzalez CA, Lopez-Carrillo L. (2010) *Helicobacter pylori*, nutrition and smoking interactions: Their impact ain gastric carcinogenesis. *Scand J Gastroenterol* **45**:6–14.
10. Huang J-Q, Sridhar S, Chen Y *et al.* (1998) Meta-analysis of the relationship between *Helicobacter pylori* seropositivity and gastric cancer. *Gastroenterology* **114**:1169–79.
11. Danesh J. (1999) *Helicobacter pylori* infection and gastric cancer: systematic review of the epidemiological studies. *Aliment Pharmacol Ther* **13**:851–6.
12. Eslick GD, Lim LL-Y, Byles JE *et al.* (1999) Association between *Helicobacter pylori* infection and gastric carcinoma: A meta-analysis. *Am J Gastroenterol* **94**:2373–9.
13. Xue F-B, Xu Y-Y, Wan Y *et al.* (2001) Association of *H. pylori* infection with gastric cancinoma: A meta-analysis. *World J Gastroenterol* **7**:801–4.

14. *Helicobacter* and Cancer Collaborative Group. (2001) Gastric cancer and *Helicobacter pylori*: A combined analysis of 12 case controls studies nested within prospective cohorts. *Gut* **49**:347–53.
15. Huang J-Q, Zheng GF, Sumanac K *et al.* (2003) Meta-analysis of the relationship between *cagA* seropositivity and gastric cancer. *Gastroenterology* **125**:1636–44.
16. Wang C, Yuan Y, Hunt RH. (2007) The association between *Helicobacter pylori* infection and early gastric cancer: A meta-analysis. *Am J Gastroenterol* **102**:1789–98.
17. Parsonnet J, Forman D. (2004) *Helicobacter pylori* infection and gastric cancer — For want of more outcomes. *JAMA* **291**:244–5.
18. Lee Y-C, Lin J-T, Chen TH-H *et al.* (2008) Is eradication of *Helicobacter pylori* the feasible way to prevent gastric cancer? New evidence and progress, but still a long way to go. *J Formos Med Assoc* **107**:591–9.
19. Marshall BJ, McCallum RW, Guerrant RL. (1991) Treatment of *Helicobacter pylori*. In, *Helicobacter pylori in peptic ulceration and gastritis.* Blackwell Scientific Publishing, Boston, USA.
20. Ogle JW. (1864) Effervescing bismuth water. *Br Med J* **i**:249–50.
21. Martin DF, May SJ, Tweedle DE *et al.* (1980) Difference in the relapse rates of duodenal ulcer healing with cimetidine or tripotassium dicitratobismuthate. *Lancet* **i**:7–10.
22. Goodwin CS, Armstrong JA, Marshall BJ. (1986) *Campylobacter pyloridis*, gastritis, and peptic ulceration. *J Clin Pathol* **39**:353–65.
23. Borody TJ, Carrick J, Hazell SL. (1987) Symptoms improve after the eradication of gastric *Campylobacter pyloridis*. *Med J Aust* **146**:450–1.
24. O'Conner A, Gisbert J, O'Morain C. (2009) Treatment of *Helicobacter pylori* infection. *Helicobacter* **14**(Suppl 1):46–51.
25. Xia HX, Daw MA, Beattie S *et al.* (1993) Prevalence of metronidazole-resistant *Helicobacter pylori* in dyspeptic patients. *Irish J Med Sci* **162**:91–4.
26. Xia HX, Buckley M, Keane CT *et al.* (1996) Clarithromycin resistance in *Helicobacter pylori*: Prevalence in untreated dyspeptic patients and stability *in vitro*. *J Antimicro Chemotherapy* **37**:473–81.
27. Buckley MJ, Xia HX, Hyde DM *et al.* (1997) Metronidazole resistance reduces efficacy of triple therapy and leads to secondary clarithromycin resistance. *Dig Dis Sci* **42**:2111–5.

28. O'Conner JP, Teneike I, O'Morain C. (2009) Improving compliance with *Helicobacter pylori* eradication therapy: When and how? *Ther Advan Gastroenterol* **2**:273–9.
29. Varia D, Zullo A, Hassan C *et al.* (2009) Sequential therapy for *Helicobacter pylori* eradication: the time is now! *Ther Advan Gastroenterol* **2**:317–22.
30. Gatta L, Vakil N, Leandro G *et al.* (2009) Sequential therapy or triple therapy for *Helicobacter pylori* infection: Systematic review and meta-analysis of randomized controlled trials in adults and children. *Am J Gastroenterol* **104**:3069–79.
31. Gisbert JP, Calvet X, O'Conner A *et al.* (2010) Sequential therapy for *Helicobacter pylori* eradication: A critical review. *J Clin Gastroenterol* **44**:313–25.
32. Moayyedi P, Malfertheiner P. (2009) Sequential therapy for eradication of *Helicobacter pylori*: A new guiding light or a false dawn? *Am J Gastroenterol* **104**:3081–3.
33. Choi WH, Park DI, Oh SJ *et al.* (2008) Effectiveness of 10-day sequential therapy for *Helicobacter pylori* eradication in Korea. *Korean J Gastroenterol* **51**:280–4.
34. Wu D, Hsu P, Wu J *et al.* (2008) Randomized controlled comparison of sequential and quadruple (concomitant) therapies for *H. pylori* infection. Gastroenterology **134**: A-24.
35. Malfertheiner P, Megraud F, O'Morain C *et al.* (2007) Current concepts in the management of *Helicobacter pylori* infection: The Maastricht III consensus report. *Gut* **56**:772–81.
36. Lin J, Huang W-H. (2009) A systematic review of treating *Helicobacter pylori* infection with traditional Chinese medicine. *World J Gastroenterol* **15**:4715–9.
37. Lionetti E, Indiro F, Pavone L *et al.* (2010) Role of probiotics in pediatric patients with *Helicobacter pylori* infection: A comprehensive review of the literature. *Helicobacter* **15**:79–87.
38. Sachdeva A, Nagpal J. (2009) Effect of fermented milk-based probiotic preparations on *Helicobacter pylori* eradication: A systematic review and meta-analysis of randomined-controlled trials. *Eur J Gastroenterol Hepatol* **21**:45–53.
39. Lesbros-Pantoflickova D, Corthesy-Theulaz, Blum AL. (2007) *Helicobacter pylori* and probiotics. *J Nutrition* **137**:812S-8S.

40. Kim DK, Lee JA, Kim YB *et al.* (2007) A randomized controlled trial assessing Korea red ginseng treatment of *Helicobacter pylori*–associated chronic gastritis. *Korean J Med* **72**:20–8.
41. Park S, Yeo M, Jin JH *et al.* (2005) Rescue of *Helicobacter pylori*-induced cytotoxicity by red ginseng. *Dig Dis Sci* **50**:1218–27.
42. Lee JH, Shim JS, Lee JS *et al.* (2006) Pectin-like acidic polysaccharide from *Panax* ginseng with selective antiadhesive activity against pathogenic bacteria. *Carbohydr Res* **341**:1154–63.
43. Matsubara S, Shibata H, Ishikawa F *et al.* (2003) Suppression of *Helicobacter pylori* — induced gastritis by green tea extract in Mongolian gerbils. *Biochem Biophys Res Commun* **310**:715–9.
44. Lee S-Y, Shin YW, Hahm K-B. (2008) Phytoceuticals: Mighty but ignored weapons against *Helicobacter pylori* infection. *J Dig Dis* **9**:129–39.
45. McGovern DP, Abbas SZ, Vivian G *et al.* (1999) Manuka honey against *Helicobacter pylori*. *J Royal Soc Med* **92**:439.
46. Rosati G, Ferrara D, Manzione L. (2009) New perspectives in the treatment of advanced metastatic gastric cancer. *World J Gastroenterol* **15**:2689–92.
47. Hu J-H, Chen H-X, Zhou Z-G *et al.* (2002) Intravenous chemotherapy for resected gastric cancer: Meta-analysis of randomized controlled trials. *World J Gastroenterol* **8**:1023–8.
48. Xu D-Z, Zhan Y-Q, Sun X-W *et al.* (2004) Meta-analysis of intraperitoneal chemotherapy for gastric cancer. *World J Gastroenterol* **10**:2727–30.
49. Valentini V, Cellini F, Minsky BD *et al.* (2009) Survival after radiotherapy in gastric cancer: Systematic review and meta-analysis. *Radiother Oncol* **92**:176–83.
50. Cunningham D, Allum WH, Stenning SP *et al.* (2006) Perioperative chemotherapy versus surgery alone for resectable gastroesophageal cancer. *N Engl J Med* **355**:11–20.
51. Sakuramoto S, Sasako M, Yamaguchi T *et al.* (2007) Adjuvant chemotherapy for gastric cancer with S-1, an oral fluoropyrimidine. *N Engl J Med* **357**:1810–20.
52. Dikken JL, Jansen EP, Cats A *et al.* (2010) Impact of the extent of surgery and postoperative chemoradiotherapy on recurrence patterns in gastric cancer. *J Clin Oncol* **28**:2430–6.
53. The Gastric Group. (2010) Benefit of adjuvant chemotherapy for resectable gastric cancer. *JAMA* **303**:1729–37.

54. Wagner AD, Moehler M. (2009) Development of targeted therapies in advanced gastric cancer: Promising exploratory steps in a new era. *Curr Opin Oncol* **21**:381–5.
55. Morabito A, Carillio G, Longo R. Systemic treatment of gastric cancer. *Crit Rev Oncol Hematol* 2009;**70**:216–34.
56. Fuccio L, Mauirizo R, Eusebi LH *et al.* (2009) Meta-analysis: Can *Helicobacter pylori* eradication treatment reduce the risk for gastric cancer. *Ann Intern Med* **151**:121–8.
57. De Varies AC, Kuipers EJ, Rauws EA. (2009) *Helicobacter pylori* eradication and gastric cancer: When is the horse out of the barn? *Aam J Gastroenterol* **104**:1342–5.
58. Lee Y-C, Lin J-T, Chen TH *et al.* (2008) Is eradication of *Helicobacter pylori* the feasible way to prevent gastric cancer? New evidence and progress, but still a long way to go. *J Formos Med A ssoc* **107**:591–9.
59. Herrera V, Parsonnet J. (2009) *Helicobacter pylori* and gastric adenocarcinoma. *Clin Microbiol Infect* **15**:971–6.
60. Peek RM. (2008) Prevention of gastric cancer: When is treatment of *Helicobacter pylori* warranted? *Ther Advan Gastroenterol* **1**:19–31.
61. Malfertheiner P, Bornchein J, Selgrad M. (2010) Role of *Helicobacter pylori* infection in gastric cancer pathogenesis: A chance for prevention. *J Dig Dis* **11**:2–11.
62. De Varies AC, Kuipers EJ. (2007) *Helicobacter pylori* eradication for the prevention of gastric cancer. *Aliment Pharmacol Ther* **26**(Suppl 2):25–35.
63. Fock KM, Talley NJ, Moayyedi P *et al.* (2008) Asia-Pacific consensus guidelines on gastric cancer prevention. *J Gastroenterol Hepatol* **23**:351–65.

Chapter 6

Inflammatory Bowel Disease and Colorectal Cancer and Their Treatment

Crispin Corte and Rupert WL Leong*

Gastroenterology and Liver Services, Sydney Local Health Network, Sydney, Australia

Colorectal cancer is one of the most devastating complications of chronic colitis in the setting of inflammatory bowel disease (IBD).[1] Current strategies in the reduction or management of colitis-associated colorectal cancer are chemoprophylaxis, colonoscopy surveillance of at-risk individuals and proctocolectomy is a potentially curative treatment for those with precancerous dysplasia or early cancer. Maintaining colitis in remission may reduce colorectal carcinogenesis in IBD. 5-aminosalicylic acid compounds may have additional chemoprophylactic effects and ursodeoxycholic acid reduces colorectal carcinogenesis in the setting of primary sclerosing cholangitis. Anti-tumour necrosis factor agents and thiopurine analogues may not only treat colitis but also have chemoprophylactic benefits. New endoscopic imaging techniques, such as chromoendoscopy, may improve the yield of identifying flat dysplasia during surveillance colonoscopy. This chapter summarises the epidemiology of dysplasia in IBD, its classification, and outlines the current endoscopic surveillance strategies, treatment algorithm and dysplasia chemoprophylaxis.

Introduction

Colorectal cancer (CRC) in patients with IBD accounts for only 1% of CRC cases. However, patients with chronic colitis carry a significantly

* Corresponding author. Email: rupertleong@hotmail.com

elevated risk of developing colorectal neoplasia. The development of CRC in the context of IBD is a grave complication and accounts for up to one sixth of deaths from ulcerative colitis.[2,3] Screening for colitis-associated CRC is based on the premise that early detection of premalignant lesions is possible, and that therapy of these lesions is associated with a decrease in their associated morbidity and mortality.

Epidemiology

Since it was first recognised in 1925[4] the literature surrounding CRC in IBD has shown substantial variation in its incidence. This is thought to be due to referral centre bias, heterogeneity in study design and possibly environmental or geographical factors.[5] Furthermore, changes to the surveillance and management of dysplasia including the improvement of endoscopic technologies in the earlier identification of pre-cancerous dysplasia have undoubtedly affected both the reported rates and outcomes of dysplasia and CRC. Initial data suggested a difference in risk of CRC between those with UC and CD, but it is generally accepted that the risks are approximately equivalent stratifying for the extent of colonic involvement.[6–9] A metanalysis of 116 studies including 54,478 patients derived an overall prevalence of CRC in any UC patient to be 3.7%. The incidence was reported as 3 cases per 1,000 person years duration (pyd).[10] When stratified for disease duration, the incidence increased from 2 to 7 to 12/1000 pyd for the first, second and third decades respectively (corresponding to cumulative probabilities of 2%, 8% and 18%). Similar findings have been recently described amongst a large Korean multicentre study[11] indicating that the cumulative incidence of CRC in IBD patients in low prevalence countries is equivalent to that in western countries. Owing to the previously held perception that CRC in IBD was less likely in Asian populations, screening and chemoprophylaxis have been underutilised, and as a result CRC may become an emerging problem in this geographical region.

Subsequent studies, especially utilising population-based data, have reported lower incidences. A single centre experience from England spanning almost 6,000 patient-years of follow-up reported a CRC incidence of only 2.5%, 7.6% and 10.8% at 20, 30 and 40 years respectively.[12] Data from Olmsted County in the USA following 692 IBD patients over 60 years did not demonstrate an overall increase in the incidence of CRC.[6] A large Swedish study of 7,607 IBD patients over 198,227 person years demonstrated a low incidence of CRC at 1%, 1.5% and 2.7% at 10, 20 and 30 years after diagnosis. Incidence of CRC in IBD and the associated mortality appear to be declining in recent years.[13] Ongoing reductions in the incidence of CRC in longstanding IBD may continue to be seen with regular surveillance colonoscopy, improvements in imaging and adenoma detection, and aggressive use of maintenance therapies through their chemoprotective effects.

Pathological characteristics

Colorectal dysplasia is defined as unequivocal neoplastic epithelium without invasion beyond the basement membrane in which is originates.[14] Dysplasia is characterised by atypical nuclear morphology, cytoplasmic abnormalities suggesting impaired differentiation and clonality, and altered growth patterns due to uncontrolled cellular proliferation. (Figure 1) Intraepithelial dysplasia (superficial to the lamina propria) is the premalignant lesion in IBD associated CRC, and is classified as low grade (LGD) or high grade (HGD) according to histopathological features. The differentiation of LGD from HGD is based on the degree and extent of nuclear stratification, haphazardness and loss of nuclear polarity, nuclear atypia, nucleoli size, nuclear clumping and presence of atypical mitotic figures. LGD needs to be differentiated from reactive changes due to inflammation. The presence of neoplastic invasion is diagnostic of CRC. For the most part, IBD-associated CRC is histologically similar to sporadic CRC, although it exhibits several different pathobiological features. CRC in IBD, like its sporadic counterpart, is most commonly adenocarcinoma. However, poorly differentiated, mucinous and anaplastic carcinomas, are overrepresented in the IBD population. Dysplasia in IBD is typically multifocal, and variously described as flat, indistinct, ulcerated, plaque-like, nodular, velvety, stricturing, or mass-like, whereas sporadic dysplasia is more classically unifocal and associated with discrete polyp formation.[9] Lesions arise from areas of the colon currently or previously inflamed, but may be in areas of microscopic inflammation

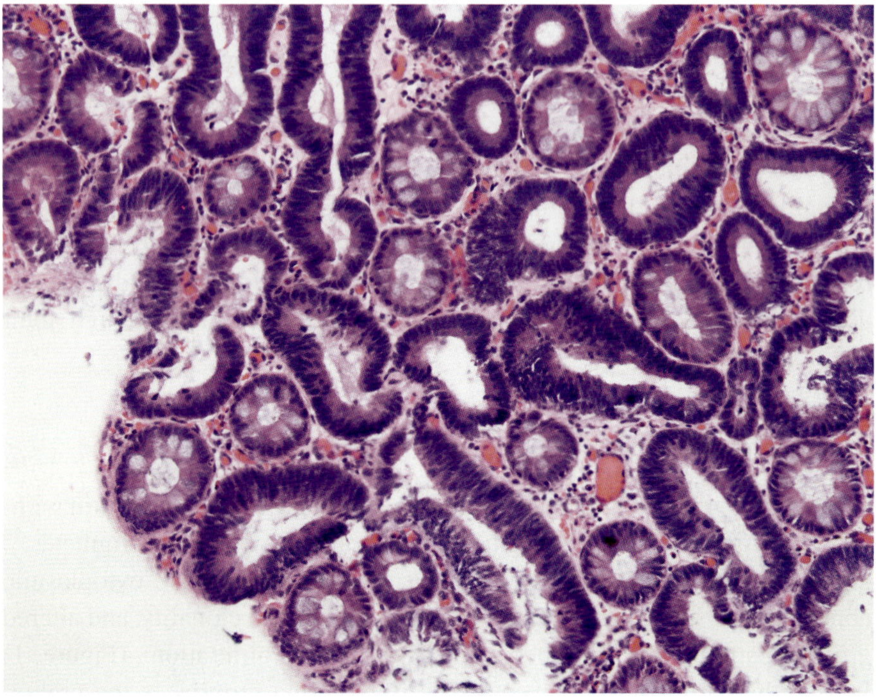

Figure 1. Low grade dysplasia (H&E stain) demonstrating epithelial nuclear crowding.

rather than macroscopic involvement.[15] Being associated with chronic inflammation, colitis-associated dysplasia is most commonly located in the distal colon. The mean age at onset is lower in IBD than for sporadic CRC, and synchronous tumours are more common in IBD, occurring in up to 12%.[16]

Chronic inflammation underlies the carcinogenesis pathways, and the exact molecular pathways are still being researched.[17] Genomic instability arises prior to the development of dysplasia and is precipitated by oxidative stress from reactive oxygen and nitrogen species from the colitis.[18] Loss of p53 occurs as an early event IBD related CRC with loss of APC as a late event — the opposite of what is normally seen in sporadic CRC. Similarly, the methylation molecular phenotypes associated with microsatellite instability differ to those of sporadic CRC.[19] Dysplasia can progress rapidly from LGD to HGD to CRC.[20] Low grade tubuloglandular adenocarcinoma may not evolve through HGD at all, arising instead from LGD.[21] Sporadic CRC is classically thought to undergo a stepwise progression towards frankly invasive adenocarcinoma.

Risk of dysplasia

Inflammation and tumorigenesis are inexorably linked[17] and the evolution of dysplasia in the colon of a patient with IBD is thought to reflect cumulative inflammatory insults. The threshold to develop dysplasia may be raised or lowered through associated risk factors such as the presence of primary sclerosing cholangitis (PSC) or an inherited predisposition toward CRC.

Much of the data on prevalence of CRC in IBD reflects the relationship between duration of disease and CRC risk.[6,10,12,22] The risk of developing CRC increases markedly after ten years of disease duration in pancolitis, (and 15–20 years in left sided disease), and surveillance is recommended from eight to ten years (and 15 years onwards in left sided disease) based upon these findings.

Whilst some data has indicated that the age of onset may be an independent predictor for development of CRC,[7] adjusting for disease duration appears to ameliorate this effect.[23] Calculations regarding commencement of surveillance are therefore based upon disease duration not patient age.

Greater extent of disease also provides an increase in cumulative inflammatory insults corresponding to the increased risk of CRC[13,23] in those with extensive colitis or pancolitis. A German study[24] demonstrated a relationship between backwash ileitis and CRC, but this has not been confirmed with subsequent reports.[25]

Disease activity has some bearing on the development of dysplasia. The historical difficulty with demonstrating this[26,27] may reflect the increased likelihood of patients with more severe disease to receive medical or surgical therapies, and poor correlation between clinical and histological assessment of disease activity.[28] A case control study of 68 patients demonstrated an increased risk of dysplasia associated with greater disease activity based on endoscopic and histological activity scores.[25] Colonic strictures,[25,29,30] a foreshortened colon[25] and pseudopolyps[25,31] represent healing of severe inflammation. These endoscopic features have been shown to be associated with a higher rate of CRC in IBD.

The risk of developing IBD related CRC in the presence of PSC is increased. A metanalysis performed by Soetikno *et al*[32] confirmed this risk to be in excess of four times the background rate seen in IBD patients. Whilst treating with moderate dose ursodeoxycholic acid goes some way to ameliorating this risk (see the section below on chemoprevention), the risk remains elevated following orthotopic liver transplantation[33] and ongoing yearly surveillance is recommended.[34]

As with sporadic CRC, family history of CRC is associated with a greater risk of developing dysplasia. For patients with IBD and a first degree relative with CRC the risk is at least two times baseline.[35–37] This is approximately the expected increase for non-IBD affected patients in a similar situation.

Colitis CRC surveillance guidelines

There is no direct evidence that surveillance colonoscopy prolongs survival in patients with extensive colitis.[38] However there is evidence that patients undergoing surveillance have their CRC detected at an earlier stage, and have corresponding improved outcomes.[38] Table 1 lists the five factors identified by the American Gastroenterology Association (AGA)[34] to influence the success of surveillance colonoscopy. Guidelines for colitis surveillance, therefore, focus on the timing of commencement of surveillance, the interval between surveillance colonoscopies, and the technical aspects of surveillance colonoscopy.

1. *Timing of commencement of surveillance*

Guidelines on the commencement of surveillance differ slightly. Expert consensus is that commencement of screening at between eight and ten years following the onset of symptoms in the absence of PSC is adequate.

Table 1. Factors influencing success of colonoscopic surveillance.

Factors influencing success of colonoscopic surveillance
Endoscopic recognition of dysplasia
Endoscopic resectability and completeness of resection
Adequacy of mucosal sampling
Interfering anatomic factors: strictures, pseudopolyps
Patient acceptance/compliance

The AGA technical review on this topic recommends that 'all patients [with ulcerative colitis], regardless of the extent of disease at initial diagnosis, should undergo a screening colonoscopy a maximum of 8 years after onset of symptoms, with multiple biopsy specimens obtained throughout the entire colon, to assess the true microscopic extent of inflammation.' As a high risk group; patients with PSC should begin surveillance colonoscopy at the time of this diagnosis if they are not already undergoing regular surveillance. These recommendations apply to patients with Crohn's disease involving at least one third of the colon.

2. *Surveillance interval*

Guidelines recommend surveillance colonoscopy every one to two years following screening colonoscopy. Following two negative surveillance colonoscopies the interval period between colonoscopies can be increased to three yearly, until colitis has been present for 20 years. At this point the frequency of surveillance colonoscopy should increase to every two years.

These guidelines have been significantly updated in the recent AGA technical review.[34] High risk patients (likely to benefit from yearly screening) and low risk patients (unlikely to develop dysplasia) are recommended different intervals between surveillance colonoscopies. In addition to the lack of data comparing screening strategies and surveillance intervals amongst different risk groups, it is unlikely that randomised controlled trials in this area will be performed. Guidelines therefore are based on expert opinion.

Therefore, interval screening for patients with chronic colitis who have undergone a negative screening colonoscopy should be determined according to the following three risk groups:

1. *High risk patients*: with PSC, ongoing active inflammation, previous history of dysplasia or strictures, or a strong family history of CRC should undergo yearly surveillance colonoscopy
2. *Intermediate risk patients*: with post-inflammatory polyps, a family history of CRC late in life and other risk factors, should undergo surveillance every three years
3. *Low risk patients*: with quiescent disease and no other risk factors, should undergo surveillance colonoscopy every five years

These surveillance intervals are based on the assumption that the examinations are successful, conducted on well prepared uninflamed colons, carried out by physicians trained in the detection of dysplasia, and performed using contemporary techniques for visualisation of dysplasia and mucosal sampling.

3. *Techniques in surveillance for CRC*

Prevention of CRC relies on the early and adequate detection of dysplasia. Detection of dysplasia in turn can be examined in terms of the efficacy of endoscopic visualisation of dysplasia and the adequacy of mucosal sampling. These two differing notions reflect a recent paradigm shift in the techniques used in endoscopic surveillance for CRC in IBD.

Until recently colonic dysplasia was thought to be endoscopically difficult-to-visualise. Therefore, random biopsies of the colonic mucosa were considered the only method of conducting a widespread survey of the colonic mucosa. Mucosal sampling by this method is thought at best to sample only one percent of colonic mucosa.[39] The recommendations[34,40–42] are to obtain biopsy specimens from two to four quadrants in each 10 cm segment of colon, with each segment submitted for pathology in a separate pot. The colon should be well prepared, and in order to minimise histological confusion between inflammation and dysplasia, colitis should be in remission wherever possible. Sensitivities for detecting dysplasia by this method were calculated to be 90% when 33 biopsies are taken and are improved to 95% when 64 biopsies are taken.[43] The scope for missed dysplasia with this method is considerable and interval cancers (CRC developing within the period between surveillance colonoscopies) occur when this approach has been employed.[44,45]

There is now considerable evidence that a large proportion of dysplasia is endoscopically visible.[46] Large prospective studies comparing targeted biopsies of colonic mucosa with abnormal endoscopic features with random biopsies have demonstrated higher dysplasia detection rates with the targeted approach. The dysplasia miss rates of targeted biopsies are likely to be lower than the random biopsy approach.

With the knowledge that early lesions in CRC development are endoscopically visible and that targeted biopsies are superior to random biopsies; considerable interest has been given to developing techniques for improving visualisation of dysplasia at the time of colonoscopy to enhance the sensitivity of targeted mucosal sampling. The techniques studied included dye-spray chromoendoscopy, narrow band imaging (NBI), and confocal endomicroscopy.

Dye-spray chromoendoscopy

Dye-spray chromoendoscopy is the most intensively studied technique for enhancing visualisation of colonic dysplasia. Chromoendoscopy improves visualisation of discrete colonic lesions, and is also used to improve evaluation of pit pattern allowing differentiation between benign and dysplastic lesions.[30] Two dyes have been studied for this purpose. Methylene blue is a vital stain that is absorbed by normal colonic mucosa, but less so by inflamed or dysplastic tissue. Indigocarmine is not taken up by colonic mucosa, but pools in pits and folds enhancing visibility of mucosal architecture and improving visualisation of dysplastic lesions. These dyes are sprayed topically onto the mucosal surface followed by careful endoscopic examination for any irregularities of interest. Indigo carmine is more expensive than methylene blue, however both are readily available in many countries. Earlier use of chromoendoscopy in this setting was with indigo carmine, although the technique has since been well validated using methylene blue.

Prospective studies comparing the sensitivity of chromoendoscopically targeted biopsies to those obtained by random sampling using conventional white-light colonoscopy[47–50] have demonstrated superiority of the targeted biopsy approach. In addition, the assessment of the extent and activity of disease is improved by chromoendoscopy, especially when combined with magnifying colonoscopy.[47,49] The use of a magnifying colonoscope in conjunction with chromoendoscopy further improves the sensitivity of targeted biopsies,[49] but this has not been further evaluated, and is a more time consuming technique, requiring specific instruments not available to many endoscopists at this stage.

Adoption of this technique is widespread in Europe, but has been delayed in the USA (perhaps because of the lack of local data until 2008).[34] Lack of adoption of this technique may also be due to earlier concerns regarding cost, and increased duration of the procedure. Indigo carmine is more expensive than methylene blue and dye spray catheters are relatively cheap. There has been concern that methylene blue may induce DNA damage and potentially promote carcinogenesis. However, there is little supportive evidence to support this and the enhanced dysplasia detection is likely to outweigh this theoretical risk.[50] The additional time taken to perform chromoendoscopy needs to be weighed against the time taken to perform random biopsies, and the benefit of increased dysplasia detection. Studies have demonstrated the time difference to be statistically insignificant.[46]

Chromoendoscopy relies on excellent bowel preparation and endoscopic cleansing. After intubating the caecum, application of 0.1% methylene blue or 0.1% indigo carmine is performed in one colonic segment at a time. Excess pools of the dye are suctioned and spasmolytic agents may improve visualisation. Careful inspection on withdrawal of the colonoscope is then undertaken and any identified lesion is biopsied or removed using polypectomy or endoscopic mucosal resection. Significant lesions require endoscopic tattooing, especially those that require biopsies of the surrounding flat area suspicious of dysplasia arising from flat mucosa. The procedure is repeated for the subsequent segments of colon. Chromoendoscopy for this indication is now recommended in the guidelines of the British Society of Gastroenterology[40] and also the Crohn's and Colitis Foundation of America.[42] The recent AGA technical review on this topic refers to high definition white light colonoscopy with random mucosal sampling as a reasonable method of surveillance, whilst describing chromoendoscopically targeted biopsies as an acceptable alternative for endoscopists who have experience with this technique.[34]

Narrow band imaging

NBI utilises optically filtered light of specified wavelengths to improve the visualisation of vessels and subtle fine structures. One study has examined the use of NBI to increase yield of surveillance colonoscopy. NBI increased the detection of mucosal lesions compared with conventional white light, but the frequency of dysplasia detected by targeted biopsies with these methods was not significantly different.[51] The sensitivity of NBI in its current form is not superior to white light alone, and it has not been directly compared to dye spray chromoendoscopy and further research in the use of this technique is required.

Fluorescence imaging

This method involves the topical (or the less effective systemic) administration of 5-amino-levulaenic acid hours prior to the examination, and requires blue light to demonstrate the differential fluorescence between dysplastic versus normal mucosa.[52] Autofluorescence imaging (AFI) obviates the use of exogenously applied fluorophores and detects differential fluorescent properties of endogenous fluorophores in dysplastic versus normal colonic mucosa.[53] Combined tri-modal imaging using high-resolution endoscopy, AFI and narrow-band imaging in the detection of neoplasia during UC surveillance showed that AFI lacked specificity in differentiating dysplasia from inflammation.[54]

Confocal endomicroscopy

Whilst histological analysis of biopsies (targeted or random) remains the gold standard for diagnosis of intraepithelial neoplasia, optical biopsy using confocal endomicroscopy (CEM) is gaining support. CEM uses focal laser illumination in combination with a detector to analyse reflected light. The light returning to the detector is 'pinhole limited' in order to reject light that is out of focus and the results in very high resolution and magnified imaging of the gastrointestinal mucosa down to subcellular structures. This technique has been validated in colorectal neoplasia and intraepithelial neoplasia.[55,56] Combining chromoendoscopy with CEM increased the yield of dysplasia detection five-fold compared to conventional white light colonoscopy, with a sensitivity of 95% when compared to histopathology as gold standard. This combination increases the sensitivity of identifying flat lesions using chromoendoscopy whereas CEM increased the specificity of finding dysplasia and reduced the need to take biopsies of non-dysplastic lesions.

Management of dysplasia

In order to appropriately manage colonic intraepithelial dysplasia in the setting of chronic colitis, further classification of the lesion is required. Management is further decided according to the histological features, morphological features, location and distribution of the lesion.

1. *Endoscopic management of dysplasia*

The most widely used histological classification of dysplasia is the Vienna classification that identifies five categories (Table 2).[57] Molecular markers such as Ki-67, AMACR (alpha-methylacyl-CoA racemase) and sialyl-Tn antigen may assist in differentiating dysplastic from regenerative or inflammatory epithelium.[34,58] Despite these advances, and increased awareness of this issue, inter-observer variability regarding biopsy specimens is high[59,60] and the identification of dysplasia and its grading should be confirmed by a second experienced pathologist.[14]

1.1. *Visualised lesions*

Endoscopic visualised dysplastic lesions have been termed 'dysplasia-associated lesion or mass' (DALM).[34] DALMs have been categorised into 'adenoma like' and 'non-adenoma like' based on their morphology

Table 2. Vienna classification of dysplasia in IBD.

Vienna Classification of Dysplasia in IBD
1. Negative for neoplasia/dysplasia
2. Indefinite for neoplasia/dysplasia
3. Non invasive low grade neoplasia (low grade adenoma/dysplasia)
4. Non invasive high grade neoplasia
4.1 High grade adenoma/dysplasia
4.2 Non invasive carcinoma (in situ)
4.3 Suspicious of invasive carcinoma
5. Invasive neoplasia
5.1 Intramucosal adenocarcinoma
5.2 Submucosal carcinoma or beyond

(reflecting the appearance of sporadic polyps or arising as irregular masses respectively). A more practical classification is whether the lesions are endoscopically resectable or unresectable. Endoscopically-resectable lesions may be managed by endoscopic removal (polypectomy or endoscopic mucosal resection) whereas unresectable lesions usually require proctocolectomy. The location and number of dysplastic lesions are also of relevance. Lesions appearing outside of colitis affected areas are more likely to be sporadic; and completely managed by simple polypectomies. Whilst unifocal dysplasia is reportedly more common than multifocal dysplasia,[46] it is not clear to what extent this is due to sampling error.

Adenoma like DALMs arising outside an area affected by colitis are likely to be sporadic adenomas. Treating these lesions as such (with polypectomy and surveillance) is advised providing that there is no evidence of surrounding inflammation or dysplasia, and there is no flat (invisible) dysplasia elsewhere in the colon.[61–63] Non-adenoma like DALMs (endoscopically unresectable lesions) have a high risk (38–83%) of containing invasive carcinoma, and should be managed with colectomy. Even if biopsies are consistent with lower grade neoplasia, the risk of synchronous lesions is high, and colectomy should be advised in this circumstance.

There is a recent paradigm shift in the treatment of adenoma-like DALMs arising within areas of colon affected by colitis. If the lesion is endoscopically resectable, and biopsies are taken from the surrounding mucosa to exclude surrounding flat dysplasia, it is now felt that these lesions can be adequately treated by polypectomy and surveillance. Following endoscopic resection, recurrence of polypoid lesions is not different between those with chronic colitis thought to have DALM or sporadic adenomas, and is between 10 and 60% at up to four years.[62,66]

1.2. *Flat lesions*

Flat or invisible lesions are those detected by random mucosal sampling or by chromoendoscopy. Flat-HGD is synchronous with CRC in 42%–67% of cases and colectomy is therefore recommended.[22,44,64] However, the management of flat-LGD is controversial. The data examining concurrent LGD and CRC lacks distinction between visible and flat lesions, which can be managed differently. The risk of LGD progressing to more advanced lesions range from 0–3% over 10 years to 35–54% over 5 years.[30] There are no trials comparing increased surveillance to colectomy, and the observational data regarding patients who undergo increased surveillance are conflicting. In a recent meta-analysis the reported incidence of HGD/CRC at colectomy for patients with LGD detected by random biopsy was 22%.[65] The management of unifocal LGD, and the decision for close surveillance versus colectomy should be individualised. However, multi-focal LGD requires colectomy due the presumption that the dysplasia is arising from a large field defect caused by the chronic colitis. Figure 2 summarises this proposed management algorithm.

2. *Chemoprophylaxis*

As with sporadic CRC, there is some evidence that pharmacologic therapy has a preventative effect on the development of CRC (in addition to the effect of disease control on the development of CRC).

2.1. *5-Aminosalicylatic acid*

The majority of evidence for chemoprevention of CRC in IBD centres around 5-ASA agents. There has never been, and is unlikely to be a

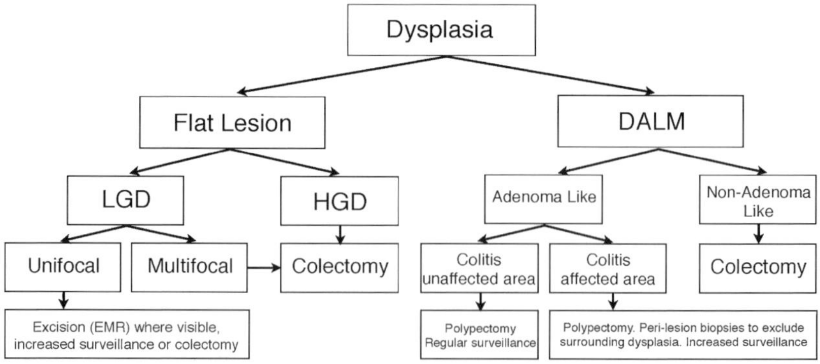

Figure 2. Management algorithm of colitis-associated dysplasia.

LGD = low grade dysplasia; HGD = high grade dysplasia, DALM = dysplasia-associated lesion or mass

large prospective trial addressing this issue but the widespread use of these agents amongst those with chronic colitis, and their low side effect profile make them an attractive prospect. Nine of the 17 published studies on this topic were included in a systematic review and meta-analysis.[67] A significant reduction in the development of CRC or dysplasia is seen with regular use of at least 1.2 grams per day of mesalamine or equivalent.

2.2. *Ursodeoxycholic acid*

Patients who have both PSC and UC represent one of the highest risk groups for developing CRC. Administration of ursodeoxycholic acid (UDCA) at doses used in PSC (8–15mg/kg/d) has been associated with significant reduction in the risk of developing advanced neoplasia.[68]

2.3. *Thiopurine analogues*

The thiopurine analogues azathioprine and mercaptopurine help maintain remission in IBD and were found to induce a three-fold decrease in the incidence of advanced colorectal neoplasia in chronic colitis.[69]

2.4. *Other agents*

Animal models confirm TNF alpha as an important mediator in the initiation and progression of carcinogenesis associated with chronic colonic inflammation.[70] Comparative cohort studies suggest a lower incidence of colonic neoplasia in patients treated with anti-TNF agents.[71,72] There is insufficient evidence to recommend their use for chemoprevention at this stage. Corticosteroid use has not been shown consistently to have a chemoprotective effect. Given the side effects of this class of agents, there is no evidence to recommend their long term use. There is little evidence to support the use of folate, calcium or multivitamin supplements in the prevention of dysplasia for patients with chronic colitis. There is little evidence to support the use of folate, calcium or multivitamin supplements in the prevention of dysplasia for patients with chronic colitis. One case control study suggested that long term (greater than five years) statin use is related to a considerable risk reduction in the development of CRC.[73] Further prospective studies are required before these drugs are recommended for chemoprophylaxis.

Conclusions

Prevention of colitis-associated carcinogenesis is recommended in high-risk individuals especially given the safety profiles of 5-aminosalicylates and ursodeoxycholic acid, the latter in those with concurrent PSC. Improving the control of colitis may underlie the efficacy of chemoprophylactic agents. The new paradigm in the management of IBD includes the aim towards the endpoint of mucosal healing. This may in the long term translate to a decline in colorectal dysplasia and change the natural history of IBD. Surveillance colonoscopies, especially employing new endoscopic technologies, may further improve the identification of early lesions prior to the development of incurable CRC. The identification of molecular and genomic biomarkers may further help improve the selection of patients most at risk of developing colorectal cancer.

References

1. Leong RW, Koo JH. (2009) Colorectal cancer in inflammatory bowel disease. *J Gastroenterol Hepatol* **24**(4):503–5.
2. Gyde S, Prior P, Dew NJ *et al.* (1982) Mortality in ulcerative colitis. *Gastroenterology* **83**:36–43.
3. Hendriksen C, Kreiner S, Binder V. (1985) Long term prognosis in ulcerative colitis-based on results from a regional patient group from the county of Copenhagen. *Gut* **26**:158–63.
4. Crohn B, Rosenberg H. (1925) The sigmoidoscopic picture of chronic ulcerative colitis (non- specific). *Am J Med Sci* **170**:220–8.
5. Zisman TL, Rubin DT. (2008) Colorectal cancer and dysplasia in inflammatory bowel disease. *World Journal of Gastroenterology* **14**(17):2662–9.
6. Jess T, Loftus E, Fernando S *et al.* (2006) 1046 risk of intestinal cancer in inflammatory bowel disease: A population-based study from olmsted county, minnesota. *Gastroenterology* **130**:1039–46.
7. Ekbom A, Helmick C, Zack M *et al.* (1990) *Lancet* **336** (8711):357–9.

8. Gillen C, Walmsley R, Prior P *et al.* (1994) Ulcerative colitis and Crohn's disease: A comparison of the colorectal cancer risk in extensive colitis. *Gut* **35**:1590–2.
9. Choi PM, Zelig MP. (1994) Similarity of colorectal cancer in Crohn's disease and ulcerative colitis: Implications for carcinogenesis and prevention. *Gut* **35**:950–4.
10. Eaden J, Abrams K, Mayberry J. (2001) The risk of colorectal cancer in ulcerative colitis: A meta-analysis. *Gut* **48**:526–35.
11. Kim BJ, Yan SK, Kim JS. (2009) Trends of ulcerative colitis-associated colorectal cancer in Korea: A KASID study. *Journal of Gastroenterology and Hepatology* **24**:667–71.
12. Rutter M, Saunders B, Wilkinson K. (2006) Thirty-year analysis of a colonoscopic surveillance program or neoplasia in ulcerative colitis. *Gastroenterology* **130**:1030–8.
13. Soderlund S, Brandt L, Lapidus A. (2009) Decreasing time-trends of colorectal cancer in a large cohort of patients with inflammatory bowel disease. *Gastroenterology* **136**:1561–7.
14. Riddell RH, Goldman H, Ransohoff DF *et al.* (1983) Dysplasia in inflammatory bowel disease: Standardized classification with provisional clinical applications. *Hum Pathol* **14**(11):931–68.
15. Mathy C, Schneider K, Chen YY *et al.* (2003) Gross versus microscopic pancolitis and the occurrence of neoplasia in ulcerative colitis. *Inflamm Bowel Dis* **9**(6):351–5.
16. Itzkowitz SH. (1997) Inflammatory bowel disease and cancer. *Gastroenterol Clin North Am* **26**(1):129–39.
17. Terzic J, Grivennikov S, Karin E *et al.* (2010) Inflammation and colon cancer. *Gastroenterology* **138**:2101–14.
18. Chen R, Rabinovitch PS, Crispin DA *et al.* (2005) The initiation of colon cancer in a chronic inflammatory setting. *Carcinogenesis* **26**(9):1513–9.
19. Schulmann K, Mori Y, Croog V *et al.* (2005) Molecular phenotype of inflammatory bowel disease — associated neoplasms with microsatellite instability. *Gastroenterology* **129**(1):74–85.
20. Itzkowitz SH. (2006) Molecular biology of dysplasia and cancer in inflammatory bowel disease. *Gastroenterology Clinics of North America* **35**(3):553–71.
21. Levi GS, Harpaz N. (2006) Intestinal low-grade tubuloglandular adenocarcinoma in inflammatory bowel disease. *Am J Surg Pathol* **30**:1022–9.

22. Bernstein C, Shanahan F, Weinstein W. (1994) Are we telling patients the truth about surveillance colonoscopy in ulcerative colitis? *Lancet* **343**:71–4.
23. Ekbom A, Helmick C, Zack M *et al.* (1990) Ulcerative colitis and colorectal cancer. A population-based study. *N Engl J Med* **323**(18):1228–33.
24. Heuschen U, Hinz U, Allemeye E. (2001) Backwash ileitis is strongly associated with colorectal carcinoma in ulcerative colitis. *Gastroenterology* **120**:841–847.
25. Rutter MD, Saunders BP, Wilkinson KH *et al.* (2004) Cancer surveillance in longstanding ulcerative colitis: Endoscopic appearances help predict cancer risk. *Gut* **53**:1813–6.
26. Eaden J, Abrams K, Ekbom A. (2000) Colorectal cancer prevention in ulcerative colitis: A case control study. *Aliment Pharmacol Ther* **14**:145–53.
27. Pinczowski D, Ekbom A, Baron J *et al.* (1994) Risk factors for colorectal cancer in patients with ulcerative colitis: A case-control study. *Gastroenterology* **107**:117–20.
28. Gomes P, du Boulay C, Smith C *et al.* (1986) Relationship between disease activity indices and colonoscopic findings in patients with colonic inflammatory bowel disease. *Gut* **27**:92–5.
29. Reiser JR, Waye JD, Janowitz HD *et al.* (1994) Adenocarcinoma in strictures of ulcerative colitis without antecedent dysplasia by colonoscopy. *Am J Gastroenterol* **89**:119–22.
30. Rutter M, Bernstein C, Matsumoto T *et al.* (2004) Endoscopic appearance of dysplasia in ulcerative colitis and the role of staining. *Endoscopy* **36**:1109–14.
31. Velayos F, Loftus E, Jess T *et al.* (2006) Predictive and protective factors associated with colorectal cancer in ulcerative colitis: A case-control Study. *Gastroenterology* **130**:1941–9.
32. Soetikno R, Lin O, Heidenreich P *et al.* (2002) Increased risk of colorectal neoplasia in patients with primary sclerosing cholangitis and ulcerative colitis: A meta-analysis. *Gastrointestinal Endoscopy* **56**:48–54.
33. Vera A, Gunson B, Ussatoff V *et al.* (2003) Colorectal cancer in patients with inflammatory bowel disease after liver transplantation for primary sclerosing cholangitis **75**:1983–8.
34. Farraye F, Odze R, Eaden J *et al.* (2010) AGA technical review on the diagnosis and management of colorectal neoplasia in inflammatory bowel disease. *Gastroenterology* **138**:746–74.

35. Nuako K, Ahlquist D, Mahoney D *et al.* (1998) Familial predisposition for colorectal cancer in chronic ulcerative colitis: A case-control study. *Gastroenterology* **115**:1079–83.
36. Askling J, Dickman P, Karlen P *et al.* (2001) Family history as a risk factor for colorectal cancer in inflammatory bowel disease. *Gastroenterology* **120**:1356–62.
37. Askling J, Dickman P W, Karlén P *et al.* (2001) Colorectal cancer rates among first-degree relatives of patients with inflammatory bowel disease: A population-based cohort study. *Lancet* **357**(9252):262–6.
38. Mpofu C, Watson AJ, Rhodes JM. (2004) Strategies for detecting colon cancer and/or dysplasia in patients with inflammatory bowel disease. *Cochrane Database Syst Rev* **2004**(2):CD000279.
39. Rosenstock E, Farmer R, Petras R *et al.* (1985) Surveillance for colonic carcinoma in ulcerative colitis. *Gastroenterology* **89**:1342–6.
40. Eaden J, Mayberry J. (2002) Guidelines for screening and surveillance of asymptomatic colorectal cancer in patients with inflammatory bowel disease. *Gut* **51**(Suppl 5):V10–V12.
41. Kornbluth A, Sachar D. (2004) Ulcerative colitis practice guidelines in adults (update): American college of gastroenterology, practice parameters committee. *Am J Gastroenterol* **99**:1371–85.
42. Itzkowitz SH, Present DH. (2005) Consensus conference: Colorectal cancer screening and surveillance in inflammatory bowel disease. *Inflamm Bowel Dis* **11**:314–21.
43. Rubin CE, Haggitt RC, Burmer GC *et al.* (1992) DNA aneuploidy in colonic biopsies predicts future development of dysplasia in ulcerative colitis. *Gastroenterology* **103**:1611–20.
44. Connell WR, Lennard-Jones JE, Williams CB *et al.* (1994) Factors affecting the outcome of endoscopic surveillance for cancer in ulcerative colitis. *Gastroenterology* **107**:934–44.
45. Lim CH, Dixon MF, Vail A *et al.* (2003) Ten year follow up of ulcerative colitis patients with and without low grade dysplasia. *Gut* **52**:1127–32.
46. Rutter MD, Saunders BP, Wilkinson KH *et al.* (2004) Most dysplasia in ulcerative colitis is visible at colonoscopy. *Gastrointest Endosc* **60**:334–9.
47. Kiesslich R, Fritsch J, Holtmann M *et al.* (2003) Methylene blue-aided chromoendoscopy for the detection of intraepithelial neoplasia and colon cancer in ulcerative colitis. *Gastroenterology* **124**:880–8.

48. Rutter MD, Saunders BP, Schofield G *et al.* (2004) Pancolonic indigo carmine dye spraying for the detection of dysplasia in ulcerative colitis. *Gut* **53**:256–60.
49. Hurlstone DP, Sanders DS, Lobo AJ *et al.* (2005) Indigo carmine assisted high-magnification chromoscopic colonoscopy for the detection and characterisation of intraepithelial neoplasia in ulcerative colitis: A prospective evaluation. *Endoscopy* **37**:1186–92.
50. Marion JF, Waye JD, Present DH *et al.* (2008) Chromoendoscopy targeted biopsies are superior to standard colonoscopic surveillance for detecting dysplasia in inflammatory bowel disease patients: A prospective endoscopic trial. *Am J Gastroenterol* **103**:2342–9.
51. Dekker E, van den Broek FJ, Reitsma JB *et al.* (2007) Narrow-band imaging compared with conventional colonoscopy for the detection of dysplasia in patients with longstanding ulcerative colitis. *Endoscopy* **39**:216–21.
52. Messmann H, Endlicher E, Freunek G *et al.* (2003) Fluorescence endoscopy for the detection of low and high grade dysplasia in ulcerative colitis using systemic or local 5-aminolaevulinic acid sensitization. *Gut* **52**:1003–7.
53. Matsumoto T, Moriyama T, Yao T *et al.* (2007) Autofluorescence imaging colonoscopy for the diagnosis of dysplasia in ulcerative colitis. *Inflammatory Bowel Disease* **13**(5): 640–1.
54. van den Broek FJ, Fockens P, van Eeden S *et al.* (2008) Endoscopic trimodal imaging for surveillance in ulcerative colitis: Randomised comparison of high-resolution endoscopy and autofluorescence imaging for neoplasia detection; and evaluation of narrow-band imaging for classification of lesions. *Gut* **57**(8):1083–9.
55. Kiesslich R, Burg J, Vieth M *et al.* (2004) Confocal laser endoscopy for diagnosing intraepithelial neoplasias and colorectal cancer *in vivo*. *Gastroenterology* **127**:706–13.
56. Kiesslich R, Goetz M, Lammersdorf K *et al.* (2007) Chromoscopyguided endomicroscopy increases the diagnostic yield of intraepithelial neoplasia in ulcerative colitis. *Gastroenterology* **132**:874–82.
57. Schlemper RJ, Riddell RH, Kato Y *et al.* (2000) The Vienna classification of gastrointestinal epithelial neoplasia. *Gut* **47**:251–5.
58. Wong NA, Mayer NJ, MacKell S *et al.* (2000) Immunohistochemical assessment of Ki67 and p53 expression assists the diagnosis and grading of ulcerative colitis-related dysplasia. *Histopathology* **37**:108–14.

59. Odze RD, Goldblum J, Noffsinger A *et al.* (2002) Interobserver variability in the diagnosis of ulcerative colitis-associated dysplasia by telepathology. *Mod Pathol* **15**:379–86.
60. Eaden J, Abrams K, McKay H *et al.* (2001) Inter-observer variation between general and specialist gastrointestinal pathologists when grading dysplasia in ulcerative colitis. *J Pathol* **194**:152–7.
61. Friedman S, Odze RD, Farraye FA. (2003) Management of neoplastic polyps in inflammatory bowel disease. *Inflamm Bowel Dis* **9**:260–6.
62. Engelsgjerd M, Farraye FA, Odze RD. (1999) Polypectomy may be adequate treatment for adenoma-like dysplastic lesions in chronic ulcerative colitis. *Gastroenterology* **117**:1288–94.
63. Vieth M, Behrens H, Stolte M. (2006) Sporadic adenoma in ulcerative colitis: Endoscopic resection is an adequate treatment. *Gut* **55**:1151–5.
64. Hata K, Watanabe T, Kazama S *et al.* (2003) Earlier surveillance colonoscopy programme improves survival in patients with ulcerative colitis associated colorectal cancer: Results of a 23-year surveillance programme in the Japanese population. *Br J Cancer* **89**:1232–6.
65. Thomas T, Abrams KA, Robinson RJ *et al.* (2007) Meta-analysis: Cancer risk of low-grade dysplasia in chronic ulcerative colitis. *Aliment Pharmacol Ther* **25**:657–68.
66. Hurlstone DP, Sanders DS, Atkinson R *et al.* (2007) Endoscopic mucosal resection for flat neoplasia in chronic ulcerative colitis: Can we change the endoscopic management paradigm? *Gut* **56**:838–46.
67. Velayos FS, Terdiman JP, Walsh JM. (2005) Effect of 5-aminosalicylate use on colorectal cancer and dysplasia risk: A systematic review and metaanalysis of observational studies. *Am J Gastroenterol* **100**:1345–53.
68. Pardi DS, Loftus EV Jr, Kremers WK *et al.* (2003) Ursodeoxycholic acid as a chemopreventive agent in patients with ulcerative colitis and primary sclerosing cholangitis. *Gastroenterology* **124**: 889–93.
69. Beaugerie L, Seksik P, Carrat F. (2009) Thiopurine therapy is associated with a three-fold decrease in the incidence of advanced colorectal neoplasia in IBD patients with longstanding extensive colitis: The CESAME prospective data. *J Crohn's Colitis* **2009**:3S5–6.
70. Popivanova BK, Kitamura K, Wu Y *et al.* (2008) Blocking TNF-alpha in mice reduces colorectal carcinogenesis associated with chronic colitis. *J Clin Invest* **118**:560–70.

71. Fidder H, Schnitzler F, Ferrante M *et al.* (2009) Long-term safety of infliximab for the treatment of inflammatory bowel disease: A single-centre cohort study. *Gut* **58**:477–8.
72. Biancone L, Orlando A, Kohn A *et al.* (2006) Infliximab and newly diagnosed neoplasia in Crohn's disease: A multicentre matched pair study. *Gut* **55**:228–33.
73. Poynter JN, Gruber SB, Higgins PD *et al.* (2005) Statins and the risk of colorectal cancer. *N Engl J Med* **352**:2184–92.

Chapter 7

Hepatitis B and Hepatocellular Carcinoma and Their Treatment

Chi-Jen Chu,[1,3,*] Teh-Ia Huo[1,2] and Shou-Dong Lee[1,3]

[1]*Division of Gastroenterology, Department of Medicine, Taipei Veterans General Hospital, Taipei, Taiwan*
[2]*Institute of Pharmacology,*
[3]*Faculty of Medicine,*
National Yang-Ming University, Taipei, Taiwan

Chronic hepatitis B virus (HBV) infection is a major cause of liver-associated morbidity and mortality worldwide. An increased knowledge of hepatitis B virology, immunology and natural history has identified active HBV replication as the key driver of immune-mediated liver injury and disease progression. In the past two decades, the clinical use of interferon and oral antiviral agents has improved long-term prognosis of chronic hepatitis B patients. To achieve a better treatment response, important issues regarding the treatment candidacy, end points of therapy and predictors of sustained virological response remain to be investigated. Currently, emergence of drug resistance is the major drawback of oral antiviral therapy. In the future, the use of new antiviral agents with greater potency and a high genetic barrier to resistance, as well as on-treatment monitoring of virological response, may result in improved outcomes in HBV therapy. Hepatocellular carcinoma (HCC) is a common liver cancer worldwide and is highly prevalent in Asia. Surgical treatment of HCC includes partial hepatectomy and liver transplantation. Liver transplantation is indicated in patients fulfilling the Milan criteria. The Milan criteria have been challenged with less restrictive

* Corresponding author. E-mail: cjchu@vghtpe.gov.tw

criteria, the UCSF criteria which did not significantly increase the post-transplant tumor recurrence rate. For patients who had unresectable lesions, loco-regional therapy included transarterial chemoembolization, percutaneous acetic or ethanol acid injection, or radiofrequency ablation is recommended depending on the size and number of tumor nodules. Sorafenib, an oral form multi-targeted kinase inhibitor, can prolong the overall survival of patients with advanced HCC.

Introduction

Despite the universal vaccination of neonates and infants during the last two decades, chronic hepatitis B virus (HBV) infection remains a significant public health problem worldwide. An estimated 400 million people worldwide have chronic HBV infection and more than 500,000 people die every year because of complications from HBV-related chronic liver disease including the development of hepatocellular carcinoma (HCC).[1] The therapeutic management of chronic hepatitis B (CHB) has improved substantially over the past decade, and continuing development of more effective anti-HBV agents might improve long-term prognosis in patients with chronic HBV infection. In this chapter, the new advances in the indications and end points for CHB treatment and the characteristics of available therapeutic options will be reviewed. Besides, current status regarding the prognosis of HCC and treatment modalities will be discussed.

Natural history of chronic HBV infection

The natural history of chronic HBV infection involves a complex interplay between the virus and the host's immune system (Figure 1). It includes four phases of varying duration distinguished by the presence in the serum of HBeAg or its antibody (anti-HBe) and serum concentrations of HBV DNA and alanine aminotransferases (ALT).[2,3] Chronic HBV infection, which is common after neonatal or childhood infection, usually starts with an HBeAg-positive immune-tolerant phase, characterized by high viremia, normal serum ALT, and few histological changes. These patients gradually progress to the HBeAg seroconversion phase (HBeAg-positive CHB),

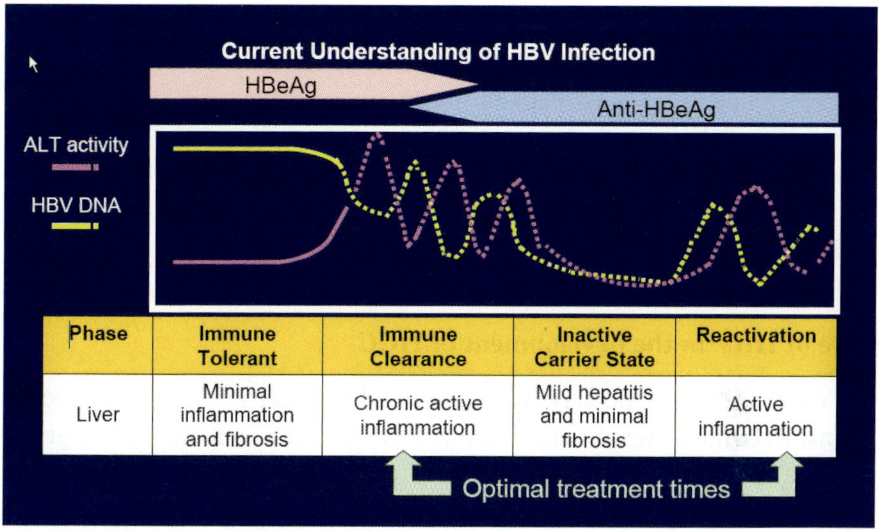

Figure 1. Natural history of chronic HBV infection.

which is characterized initially by positive HBeAg, high serum HBV DNA concentrations, increased ALT level, and active necroinflammation and/or fibrosis.[4,5] The annual probability of HBeAg seroconversion depends on the age of infection, ethnicity, and HBV genotypes (lower with genotype C than B).[6–9] If spontaneous HBeAg seroconversion occurs, patients progress to the HBeAg-negative phase, which is classified as either an inactive chronic HBV carrier state, characterized by low levels of viral replication, normal ALT, and few histological lesions,[2,3] or as HBeAg-negative CHB, characterized by higher viral replication, increased ALT, and active liver necroinflammation and fibrosis.[10,11] HBeAg-negative CHB may develop immediately after the HBeAg seroconversion phase or after several years of an inactive chronic carrier state. It is associated with the emergence of HBV strains that replicate but do not express HBeAg, and is more likely to run a fluctuating course, leading to cirrhosis and decompensation. In general, chronic HBV infection is characterized by its dynamic natural course, which includes apparent periodic activation of the host immune system against the infected hepatocytes to eradicate the virus, but this activation usually causes disease exacerbations and leads to the accumulation of fibrosis and development of cirrhosis.[2,3] Approximately 15–20% of patients with chronic hepatitis B develop cirrhosis within 5 years,[12] whereas 15% of patients with compensated cirrhosis and more than 60% of those with decompensated cirrhosis die within 5 years.[13,14] Moreover, all patients with chronic HBV infection are at increased risk of HCC, although the risk increases substantially in patients with long-term high viremia and cirrhosis.[15,16]

Role of HBV in the development of HCC

HBV likely causes hepatocarcinogenesis by direct and indirect mechanisms. Laboratory results showed that HBV could be integrated into genes that are responsible for the control of cell proliferation, differentiation, and viability.[17,18] Of all the HBV genes, the HBx gene has generated the most interest in HBV-related hepatocarcinogenesis, and is the most commonly integrated gene. More than 95% of patients with HBV-related cirrhosis and dysplasia are positive for HBx, and HBx is expressed in 70% of patients with HBV related HCC. The exact mechanism by which HBx can induce HCC development remains to be fully elucidated. HBx is known to be a transcription activator through its interaction with a wide range of both viral and host regulatory elements.[19] These include the major histocompatibility complex, epidermal growth factor receptor, c-myc, c-jun, c-fos, TP53, AP-1, NF-κB and SP1, among others.[20,21] Through its effect on these regulator elements, HBx can interfere with the hepatocyte DNA repair system and the controlling elements of cellular proliferation.[22] In addition, HBx can bind with p53, with subsequent inhibition of p53-mediated apoptosis.[23] Through the other pathway, HBV can incite chronic injury to the hepatocytes, with continuous necroinflammation and regeneration activity and a resultant increase in hepatocyte turnover. The net effect of this is the accumulation of potential critical mutations in the hepatocyte genome, with subsequent malignant transformation and clonal expansion, leading to HCC.

To date, several viral factors are associated with the increased risk of HCC development. The most important and perhaps most clinically relevant is the level of serum HBV DNA. Large cohort studies have shown that higher levels of HBV DNA were associated with an increased risk of

HCC.[24,25] A cut-off level of >2,000 IU/mL was shown to be a strong predictor of HCC, although even lower HBV DNA levels still indicated a risk of HCC development.[24,26] Although HBeAg positivity had previously been considered as a risk factor, it has not been shown to be an independent predictor of HCC in subsequent studies, and its effect is likely dependent on both the underlying HBV DNA levels and the HBV genotypes.[27] In addition to HBV DNA level, genotype C has been shown to be an independent predictor related to HCC development.[24,28] The core promoter variants of HBV (A1762T and G1764A) have also been shown to be associated with the development of HCC[29,30] but the underlying mechanisms remain to be investigated.

Treatment candidacy

Every patient with chronic HBV infection is potentially infectious and at risk of liver complications and is ideally a candidate for therapy. However, current medications rarely achieve viral eradication in patients with chronic HBV infection and therefore only patients who are at risk for progression to advanced liver disease should be considered for treatment. According to the most recent guidelines,[31–35] treatment is recommended to all patients with either HBeAg-positive or HBeAg-negative CHB who have serum HBV DNA >20,000 IU/mL and alanine aminotransferase (ALT) higher than two times the upper limit of normal (>2 ×ULN) for at least 3 months. In such cases, liver biopsy is considered to be optional, as it may offer prognostic information but it is not expected to affect the decision to treat. On the other hand, treatment is also recommended for HBV carriers with ALT between 1–2 ×ULN and serum HBV DNA between 2,000–20,000 IU/mL who have at least moderate necroinflammatory activity and/or significant fibrosis. A lower threshold of HBV DNA (2,000 IU/mL) for initiation of antiviral therapy should be considered for patients with compensated cirrhosis. For patients with decompensated liver cirrhosis, oral antiviral therapy was indicated when serum HBV DNA could be detected by polymerase chain reaction (PCR) assay. It should be mentioned here that currently available treatment guidelines are based on specific criteria and require certain cut-off points, which may sometimes be arbitrary and not applicable to all patients.

Therapeutic strategies for specific group of patients should be considered on an individual basis based on improving long-term outcomes.

Definition of treatment response

Irrespective of the type of treatment, the therapeutic response can be classified as (1) biochemical, based on aminotransferases (mainly ALT) concentrations, (2) virological, based on serum HBV DNA concentrations and HBeAg seroconversion to anti-HBe, which represents an important therapeutic goal in HBeAg-positive chronic HBV infection, and (3) histological, based on hepatic histological changes.[31] Response is defined as complete in cases with biochemical and virological responses accompanied by clearance of HBsAg. Biochemical and virological responses can be estimated during therapy (on-therapy response) or after cessation of therapy (sustained off -therapy response).[31]

Interferon (IFN)-based therapy

IFN therapy, in the form of either standard IFN α-2b[36] or long-acting pegylated IFN (Peg-IFN) α-2a,[37] is approved for the treatment of chronic hepatitis B. IFNs are known to have direct antiviral and immunomodulatory effects which can be used for HBV suppression. The response rates in HBeAg-positive patients after 4–6 months of short-acting IFN were about 30–40%, with a risk difference of 23–25% against untreated controls.[36] A duration of 48 weeks of Peg-IFN therapy yields a sustained HBeAg seroconversion rate of 29–32% when assessed 24 weeks after completion of therapy.[38,39] Patients with genotype A (vs D) or B (vs C) infection tend to have a better response to IFN-based regimen.[38,40] HBeAg seroconversion response is sustained in more than 80% of patients, and can be followed by HBsAg loss.[41–43] Additional predictors of response include elevated levels of baseline ALT, lower HBV DNA levels, and lower quantitative HBeAg levels at baseline or after 24 weeks of treatment.[44,45] Long-term follow-up studies suggest IFN-based therapy has long-term benefits by promoting cumulative HBeAg seroconversion, increasing HBsAg loss, reducing development of cirrhosis and HCC, and extending survival, especially in responders.[41–43] Patients with HBeAg-negative CHB respond to IFN therapy but often relapse after treatment completion.[46,47] The combined response to Peg-IFN α-2a therapy (ALT normalization plus HBV DNA <2 $\times$ 10^4 copies/mL) in HBeAg-negative patients is 36% at 6 months post treatment.[48,49]

The advantages of interferon-based therapy are the finite treatment duration and no reported to select drug-resistant strain. However, IFN-based therapy is associated with more common adverse events, including influenza-like symptoms, fatigue, anorexia, weight loss, hair loss, thyroid dysfunction, emotional instability, and bone marrow suppression. Patients under IFN-based therapy might need symptomatic treatment to alleviate adverse effects, and some require dose modification or discontinuation of therapy. Despite this, most patients are able to complete 48 weeks of Peg-IFN treatment with tolerable side effects.[38,39,48]

Oral antiviral agents and end points of therapy

Five nucleoside or nucleotide analogs are currently available as approved therapy for CHB, each with variable rates of efficacy and incidence of drug resistance. These oral antiviral agents have fast and potent inhibitory effects on HBV polymerase and reverse transcriptase activity, and are safe and effective for HBV DNA suppression, ALT normalization, and histological improvement. Table 1 summarizes the efficacy of various oral antiviral agents in HBeAg-positive CHB patients based on 1-year treatment duration.[50–54] Entecavir, tenofovir and telbivudine are more potent antiviral agents as compared with lamivudine or adefovir. However, higher antiviral potency does not result in an increasing HBeAg seroconversion rate — which was seen at a rate of around 20% after 1 year of treatment and HBsAg loss is very rare.[50–54] Higher baseline ALT (>5 $\times$ ULN) was associated with higher HBeAg seroconversion in patients treated by lamivudine, indicating stronger endogenous immune response is important for successful antiviral therapy. If HBeAg seroconversion was not achieved after one-year treatment, antiviral agents can be continued but the benefits of long-term therapy should be weighed against the risk of selection of drug-resistance mutants.[31–35] Therefore, carefully monitoring HBV DNA levels during therapy and early switching antiviral regimens were highly recommended especially when low genetic barrier

Table 1. Responses to approved oral antiviral agents among treatment-naïve patients with HBeAg-positive CHB based on one-year treatment duration.

	Lamivudine 100 mg qd	Adefovir 10 mg qd	Entecavir 0.5 mg qd	Telbivudine 600 mg qd	Tenofovir 300 mg qd
Undetectable HBV DNA by PCR	40%–44%	21%	67%	60%	76%
HBeAg loss	17%–32%	24%	22%	26%	NA
HBeAg seroconversion	16%–21%	12%	21%	22%	21%
HBsAg loss	1%	0%	2%	0%	3.2%
ALT normalization	41%–75%	48%	68%	77%	68%
Histologic improvement	49%–56%	53%	72%	65%	74%
Durability of response	50%–80%	~ 90%	69%	~ 80%	NA

NA: not answered

antiviral agents such as lamivudine or telbivudine were used. In general, oral antiviral agents should be continued beyond the point of HBeAg seroconversion until at least 6 months after the appearance of anti-HBe to solidify the durability of response.[31–35] If possible, a preferred approach would be to continue therapy beyond the point of HBeAg seroconversion and for an additional 12 months once HBV DNA became undetectable by PCR assay. Following discontinuation of therapy, patients must be monitored closely for evidence of reactivation of HBV infection or disease progression.

The response to approved oral antiviral agents in HBeAg-negative CHB patients based on 1-year treatment duration is summarized in Table 2.[53–57] The majority of patients can achieve undetectable HBV DNA by PCR assay at the end-of-treatment. However, the durability of response was very poor (<10%). Therefore, long-term antiviral therapy was recommended in cases of HBeAg-negative CHB and HBsAg loss would be an ultimate goal. Results of a large randomized controlled trial in patients with advanced fibrosis or cirrhosis showed the benefits

Table 2. Responses to approved oral antiviral agents among treatment-naïve patients with HBeAg-negative CHB based on one-year treatment duration.

	Lamivudine 100 mg qd	**Adefovir 10 mg qd**	**Entecavir 0.5 mg qd**	**Telbivudine 600 mg qd**	**Tenofovir 300 mg qd**
Undetectable HBV DNA by PCR	60%–73%	51%	90%	88%	93%
ALT normalization	60%–79%	72%	78%	74%	76%
Histologic improvement	60%–66%	64%	70%	67%	72%
Durability of response	< 10%	~ 5%	3%	NA	NA

NA: not answered.

of long-term lamivudine therapy for 3 years can reduce disease progression and HCC development.[58] Unfortunately, the beneficial effects could be negated in patients with lamivudine resistance. Published results suggested that sustained off-therapy responses might be achieved in a proportion for HBeAg-negative CHB patients treated with some oral antiviral agents for years.[59,60] However, the optimal duration of therapy in the setting of HBeAg-negative CHB is uncertain and more studies are needed before firm conclusions can be drawn.

Antiviral resistance

The main limitation of long-term therapies with antiviral agents is the progressively increasing rates of viral resistance due to selection of treatment-resistant HBV mutant strains.[61,62] The emergence of genotypic viral resistance is usually followed by the subsequent development of virological breakthrough or secondary antiviral treatment failure, which is defined as reappearance or >1 $\log_{10}$ IU/mL increase of serum HBV DNA. Virological breakthroughs are usually followed by biochemical breakthroughs, which eventually worsen liver histology and may even result in decompensation and death, particularly in patients with pre-existing cirrhosis. Viral resistance may develop under any anti-HBV oral agent, but the rate of resistance differs markedly among the different agents (Table 3).[63–70] Long-term lamivudine monotherapy results in rather high rates of resistance due to emergence of HBV strains with mutation within the YMDD motif (rtM204V/I with or without rtL180M). Lamivudine resistance rates usually exceed 15–20% at year 1 and 60–65% at year 4.[63–64] Resistance to entecavir in nucleoside naive CHB patients seems to be rare, since it has been detected in <1.5% of naive patients treated with entecavir monotherapy for up to five years.[67] The above phenomenon was attributed to entecavir resistance which requires selection of two lamivudine-resistant mutations (rtM204V/I and rtL180M) and at least one additional substitution (rtI169, rtT184, rtS202, or rtM250).

Besides antiviral drug alone, several baseline patient and viral indices have been associated with the emergence of drug resistance. It has been reported that male sex, older age, high body mass index, high HBV DNA concentration, high histological scores, and presence of core promoter mutations are associated with risk of lamivudine resistance. Another factor associated with the emergence of drug resistance is the persistence of viral replication during antiviral treatment. Clinical data from lamivudine[71] and telbivudine[53] studies suggested that the rate of emergence of drug-resistant HBV was directly proportional to the HBV DNA concentration at week 24 after treatment. Based on these, nucleos(t)ide analogues that cause rapid viral suppression with a high genetic barrier to resistance should be the treatment of choice.[31–35] Early assessment of viral load reduction at week 24 of treatment to aid decision-making should be mandatory, especially for patients who are receiving nucleoside analogues with a low genetic barrier such as lamivudine or telbuivudine. It might be possible to predict the response and development of resistance as early as 4 weeks of treatment, although more data are needed to confirm this. To achieve a better clinical response in patients with drug resistance, the addition of another nucleoside analogue from a different group without cross resistance should be given as early as possible, preferably at the time when genotypic resistance emerges. If antiviral resistance was confirmed, switching or add-on therapy without cross-resistance should be instituted (Table 3).[31–35] Switching to IFN-based therapy could be an option for selected patients.[72]

Table 3. Characteristics of oral antiviral agents, cumulative resistant rates and options of rescue therapy.

	Lamivudine 100 mg qd	**Adefovir 10 mg qd**	**Entecavir 0.5 mg qd**	**Telbivudine 600 mg qd**	**Tenofovir 300 mg qd**
Antiviral potency	++	+	+++	+++	+++
Genetic barrier of resistance	+	++	+++	+	?
Selection of resistant strain	+++	++	+	++	+
Drug resistance for HBeAg (+) CHB					
Year 1	11%–14%	0%	0%	5%	0%
Year 2	40%		0%	25%	0% (to week 72)
Year 5	69%	20%	1.2%		
Drug resistance for HBeAg (–) CHB					
Year 1	6%–27%	0%	0%	2%	0%
Year 2	26%–54%	3%	0%	11%	0% (to week 72)
Year 5	65%	29%	1.2%		
Rescue therapy when antiviral resistance	1. Add adefovir or tenofovir 2. Switch to Truvada	1. Add lamivudine 2. Switch to or add entecavir 3. Switch to Truvada	1. Switch to tenofovir or Truvada	1. Add adefovir or tenofovir 2. Switch to Truvada	

+++ = high, ++ = intermediate, + = low
Truvada: combination pill with emtricitabine 200 mg and tenofovir 300 mg

Clinical features of HCC

HCC is a common liver cancer worldwide and is highly prevalent in Asia. With the exception of Japan, where hepatitis C virus (HCV) is the predominantly cause of HCC, most countries in Asia are endemic for HBV infection. Chronic HBV or HCV infections are probably the most important causes for the development of HCC. The HBx gene can secret hepatitis B X protein, which can induce malignant transformation, whereas HCV can secret oncoproteins such as core protein and non-structural 5A protein.[73] In addition, these two viruses share a common mechanism to induce HCC. Chronic HBV or HCV infection can induce cirrhosis, a precancerous state with high genomic instability, through persistent inflammation and repair of liver tissue. Other causes of cirrhosis, such as primary biliary cirrhosis, hemochromatosis, autoimmune hepatitis, can also induce the formation of HCC.

About 70–80% of patients with HCC also have coexisting liver cirrhosis at the time of diagnosis. Therefore, the selection of treatment modality for HCC is dependent on several factors: the extent of tumor involvement, the severity of cirrhosis and the performance of the patient. The prognosis of HCC is highly variable and closely linked with cancer stage and treatment, with an average 5-year survival rate of 10–40%. Patients with HCC often have a poor prognosis because HCC usually does not have distinct clinical presentations until the tumor is at an advanced stage. Therefore, periodical surveillance for high-risk patients, such as patients with HBV or HCV infection, is necessary to prolong the survival.

Surgical treatment

Surgical resection of HCC is usually the standard curative treatment for HCC. This procedure involves partial resection of the liver in an attempt to totally remove the tumor. However, surgical resection cannot be performed when there are multiple tumors in liver and complete tumor resection is considered not possible, or patients have severe cirrhosis and hepatic decompensation may develop after resection. The criteria of surgical resection for patients with HCC include (1) patients with tumor involving no more than 3 Healey's segments, (2) Child-Turcotte-Pugh

(CTP) class A with less than 25% retention of indocyanine green 15 minutes after injection, and (3) no main portal vein trunk involvement or distant metastasis. However, patients undergoing curative surgical resection often develop tumor recurrence after surgery. Tumor recurrence within 2 years of surgery is considered to be due to the existence of small HCC foci that are not detected before the operation, whereas tumor recurrence after 2 years is linked with continuing viral inflammation that may induce new HCC formation.[74] Risk factors for post-resection tumor recurrence include large tumors, vascular invasion and high serum alpha-fetoprotein levels. Post-operative adjuvant chemotherapy may be beneficial for preventing tumor recurrence in selected high-risk patients. Persistent viral replication may also contribute to post-resection tumor recurrence. In this regard, interferon therapy may reduce the incidence of tumor recurrence through suppressing viral replication in patients with HCV-related small HCC undergoing surgical resection.[75]

Liver transplantation is another treatment option especially for patients with advanced cirrhosis, but patients on the waiting list of transplantation far outnumber the potential cadaveric or living liver donors. In addition, tumor recurrence is not uncommon even after transplantation, therefore strict criteria for liver transplantation have been proposed for transplant candidates. Patients indicated for liver transplantation should fulfill the Milan criteria (a single tumor up to 5 cm in diameter or up to three lesions, none larger than 3 cm).[76] The Milan criteria have been challenged with less restrictive criteria, the University of California at San Francisco (UCSF) criteria (single HCC up to 6.5 cm in diameter or with up to three HCCs, none larger than 4.5 cm, with a cumulative diameter up to 8 cm).[77] The UCSF criteria have been employed in many transplant centers without significantly increasing the post-transplant tumor recurrence rate or compromising long-term survival.

Medical treatment

The majority of HCC patients also have cirrhosis. Surgical resection is less likely to perform in these patients because the risk of post-operative liver decompensation is high. For patients who had unresectable lesions, loco-regional therapy included transarterial chemoembolization (TACE), percutaneous acetic or ethanol acid injection (PAI, PEI), or radiofrequency ablation (RFA) was performed depending on the size and number of tumor nodules.

TACE has been used to treat liver cancers to several decades. Early results were discouraging because of high incidence of liver failure after repeated TACE procedure. Recent studies showed that TACE is beneficial for selected HCC patients. TACE can only be safely performed in patients with compensated cirrhosis. The advantage of TACE is that it can target multiple liver tumors during one treatment session. Post-embolization syndrome, including abdominal pain, anorexia, fever, infection, liver failure and renal failure may occur. Radio-embolization using Yttrium-90 microsphere has been used in the TACE procedure to induce tumor necrosis through the effect of local irradiation. A phase II study showed that Yttrium-90 microsphere therapy in patients with HCC complicated by portal vein thrombosis is effective and appears to have a favorable toxicity.[78]

PEI technique was first initiated by the Japanese researchers in the 1980s when the real-time ultrasound guidance became possible. The injected pure ethanol induces local tumor necrosis through the mechanisms of protein denaturation, cell dehydration and thrombosis of tumor vessels. HCC is often a hypervascular structure and is well encapsulated by a tumor capsule that can limit the spread of ethanol within the tumor nodule, which is usually soft in consistency. These features make PEI one of the most commonly used methods of percutaneous ablation therapy. PEI has the advantages of being safer, less expensive, and easy to perform. In addition, PEI allows selective treatment of HCC without damaging the adjacent unaffected liver parenchyma. Side effects are minimal. Patients with tumor nodules less than 3 cm and no more than 3 nodules are more suitable for PEI.[79] Small (<3 cm) HCC nodule treated by PEI may have a complete response rate of 80% or higher, whereas the response rate may significantly decrease with increasing size of tumor nodule. Comparison of PEI and surgical resection in patients with small HCC indicated that PEI therapy might be as effective as surgical resection.

Acetic acid, at a concentration of 15–50%, induces profound tumor necrosis through a similar mechanism as ethanol. It has a strong ability to penetrate and dissolve lipids and collagen tissue that are present in intra-tumoral septa and capsule. Generally the PAI technique has similar treatment efficacy and safety profiles as PEI.[80]

RFA was first applied for human HCC in 1993. The radiofrequency energy emitted from the needle tip induces ionic agitation and frictional heat. RFA has become one of the highly efficient local ablative therapies for HCC due to its excellent necrotizing effect.[81] A major breakthrough of RFA over PAI or PEI is that RFA can be used to treat medium- or large-sized HCC up to 8 cm in diameter.[82] The effect of RFA for small HCC was reported to be comparable to patients undergoing surgical resection.[83] While RFA is generally considered a safe procedure, the complication rate of RFA could be higher than that previously assumed in published studies. RFA has some other limitations in addition to the potentially high complication rate. When the location of tumor nodule is close to the major blood vessels, the radiofrequency energy will be carried away by the blood flow (the "heat sink" phenomenon) and result in a sub-optimal treatment response.

By combining different anti-tumor mechanisms in combination therapy, the treatment response may be enhanced and could be extended to treat medium (3–5 cm) or large-sized (>5 cm) HCC. Examples of combination therapy include TACE and PEI, TACE and PAI and RFA after TACE. Combination therapy frequently induces a higher rate of complete tumor necrosis. Overall, RFA may be considered the first choice. PEI or PAI is preferred for nodules at risk for RFA, and selective TACE is preferred for nodules not recognizable at ultrasound examination or for multiple nodules.

Systemic chemotherapy has a limited effect in treating advanced HCC. Single-agent doxorubicin produces a response rate of 10–15% without significant survival benefit; combination chemotherapy also provided unimpressive results. With recent advances in the knowledge of carcinogenesis pathway, there has been encouraging development in the targeted therapy of advanced HCC. Among the newly identified targets, targeting the anti-angiogenic pathway and the Raf/mitogen-activated protein kinase pathways have been shown to play an important role in anti-cancer treatment. Sorafenib, a multi-targeted kinase inhibitor, has been demonstrated to prolong the overall survival of patients with advanced HCC in the phase III clinical trial.[84] Currently, sorafenib is the only approved targeted therapy for patients with advanced HCC and well-compensated cirrhosis. For far-advanced HCC patients, including those with Child class C cirrhosis, main portal vein thrombosis and evidence of distant metastasis, only the best supportive care is given and no aggressive treatment is recommended.

Summary of HCC therapy

The clinical scenarios of HCC at presentation may vary widely. The size and number of tumor nodules and the severity of coexisting cirrhosis are the two major factors to affect the survival. The choice of optimal therapy for patients with HCC depends on the experience and facility of the referral center. Although a long-term survival in patients with unresectable HCC is possible in selected patients, the overall outcome remains unsatisfactory especially among those with poor prognostic predictors. Surgical resection remains the first choice of treatment. Liver transplantation has the advantages of treating both HCC and cirrhosis at the same time. Various forms of loco-regional therapies can be used to treat patients who are not indicated for surgical treatment. In clinical practice, combination therapy or multi-modality treatment is often used to treat patients at difference cancer stages. Targeted therapy should be considered for advanced stage patients who have well-compensated liver disease but are not suitable for any aggressive forms of treatment.

References

1. Lee WM. (1997) Hepatitis B virus infection. *N Engl J Med* **337**:1733–45.
2. Lok AS, Heathcote EJ, Hoofnagle JH. (2001) Management of hepatitis B: 2000—summary of a workshop. *Gastroenterology* **120**:1828–53.
3. Fattovich G. (2003) Natural history and prognosis of hepatitis B. *Semin Liver Dis* **23**:47–58.
4. Hoofnagle JH, Dusheiko GM, Seeff LB *et al.* (1981) Seroconversion from hepatitis B e antigen to antibody in chronic type B hepatitis. *Ann Intern Med* **94**:744–8.
5. Fattovich G, Rugge M, Brollo L *et al.* (1986) Clinical, virologic and histologic outcome following seroconversion from HBeAg to anti-HBe in chronic hepatitis type B. *Hepatology* **6**:167–72.

6. Lok AS, Lai CL, Wu PC *et al.* (1987) Spontaneous hepatitis B e antigen to antibody seroconversion and reversion in Chinese patients with chronic hepatitis B virus infection. *Gastroenterology* **92**:1839–43.
7. Chu CJ, Hussain M, Lok AS. (2002) Hepatitis B virus genotype B is associated with earlier HBeAg seroconversion compared with hepatitis B virus genotype C. *Gastroenterology* **122**:1756–62.
8. Yuen MF, Sablon E, Yuan HJ *et al.* (2003) Significance of hepatitis B genotype in acute exacerbation, HBeAg seroconversion, cirrhosis-related complications, and hepatocellular carcinoma. *Hepatology* **37**:562–7.
9. Chu CJ, Keeffe EB, Han SH *et al.* (2003) Hepatitis B virus genotypes in the United States: results of a nationwide study. *Gastroenterology* **125**:444–51.
10. Brunetto MR, Giarin M, Oliveri F *et al.* (1991) Wild type and e antigen-minus hepatitis B virus in course of chronic hepatitis. *Proc Natl Acad Sci USA* **88**:4186–90.
11. Hadziyannis SJ, Vassilopoulos D. (2001) Hepatitis B e antigen-negative chronic hepatitis B. *Hepatology* **34**:617–24.
12. Liaw YF, Tai DI, Chu CM *et al.* (1988) The development of cirrhosis in patients with chronic type B hepatitis: A prospective study. *Hepatology* **8**:493–6.
13. Realdi G, Fattovich G, Hadziyannis S *et al.* (1994) Survival and prognostic factors in 366 patients with compensated cirrhosis type B: A multicenter study. *J Hepatol* **21**:656–66.
14. de Jongh FE, Janssen HL, de Man RA *et al.* (1992) Survival and prognostic indicators in HBsAg-positive cirrhosis of the liver. *Gastroenterology* **103**:1630–5.
15. Beasley RP. (1988) The major etiology of hepatocellular carcinoma. *Cancer* **61**:1942–56.
16. Yu MW, Yeh SH, Chen PJ *et al.* (2005) Hepatitis B virus genotype and DNA level and hepatocellular carcinoma: A prospective study in men. *J Natl Cancer Inst* **97**:265–72.
17. Kremsdorf D, Soussan P, Paterlini-Brechot P *et al.* (2006) Hepatitis B virus-related hepatocellular carcinoma: Paradigms for viral-related human carcinogenesis. *Oncogene* **25**:3823–33.
18. Bonilla Guerrero R, Roberts LR. (2005) The role of hepatitis B virus integrations in the pathogenesis of human hepatocellular carcinoma. *J Hepatol* **42**:760–77.

19. Rossner MT. (1992) Review: Hepatitis B virus X-gene product: a promiscuous transcriptional activator. *J Med Virol* **36**:101–17.
20. Su F, Schneider RJ. (1996) Hepatitis B virus HBx protein activates transcription factor NF-kappa B by acting on multiple cytoplasmic inhibitors of rel-related proteins. *J Virol* **70**:4558–66.
21. Yeh CT. (2000) Hepatitis B virus X protein: Searching for a role in hepatocarcinogenesis. *J Gastroenterol Hepatol* **15**:339–41.
22. Becker SA, Lee TH, Butel JS *et al.* (1998) Hepatitis B virus X protein interferes with cellular DNA repair. *J Virol* **72**:266–72.
23. Takada S, Kaneniwa N, Tsuchida N *et al.* (1997) Cytoplasmic retention of the p53 tumor suppressor gene product is observed in the hepatitis B virus X gene-transfected cells. *Oncogene* **15**:1895–901.
24. Chen CJ, Yang HI, Su J *et al.* (2006) Risk of hepatocellular carcinoma across a biological gradient of serum hepatitis B virus DNA level. *JAMA* **295**:65–73.
25. Chen G, Lin W, Shen F *et al.* (2006) Past HBV viral load as predictor of mortality and morbidity from HCC and chronic liver disease in a prospective study. *Am J Gastroenterol* **101**:1797–803.
26. Fung J, Yuen MF, Yuen JC *et al.* (2007) Low serum HBV DNA levels and development of hepatocellular carcinoma in patients with chronic hepatitis B: A case–control study. *Aliment Pharmacol Ther* **26**:377–82.
27. Yang HI, Lu SN, Liaw YF *et al.* (2002) Hepatitis B e antigen and the risk of hepatocellular carcinoma. *N Engl J Med* **347**:168–74.
28. Chan HL, Hui AY, Wong ML *et al.* (2004) Genotype C hepatitis B virus infection is associated with an increased risk of hepatocellular carcinoma. *Gut* **53**:1494–8.
29. Chou YC, Yu MW, Wu CF *et al.* (2008) Temporal relationship between hepatitis B virus enhancer II/basal core promoter sequence variation and risk of hepatocellular carcinoma. *Gut* **57**:91–7.
30. Kao JH, Chen PJ, Lai MY *et al.* (2003) Basal core promotor mutations of hepatitis B virus increase the risk of hepatocellular carcinoma. *Gastroenterology* **124**:327–34.
31. Lok AS, McMahon BJ. (2007) Chronic hepatitis B. *Hepatology* **45**:507–39.
32. Keeffe EB, Dieterich DT, Han SH *et al.* (2008) A treatment algorithm for the management of chronic hepatitis B virus infection in the United States: 2008 update. *Clin Gastroenterol Hepatol* **6**:1315–41.

33. Liaw YF, Leung N, Kao JH *et al.* (2008) Asian-Pacific consensus statement on the management of chronic hepatitis B: A 2008 update. *Hepatol Int* **2**:263–83.
34. European Association for the Study of the Liver. (2009) EASL clinical practice guidelines: Management of chronic hepatitis B. *J Hepatol* **50**:227–42.
35. Lok AS, McMahon BJ. (2009) Chronic hepatitis B: Update 2009. *Hepatology* **50**:661–2.
36. Craxi A, Di Bona D, Camma C. (2003) Interferon-alpha for HBeAg-positive chronic hepatitis B. *J Hepatol* **39** (suppl 1):99–105.
37. Cooksley WGF, Piratvisuth T, Lee SD *et al.* (2003) Peginterferon alpha 2a (40kDa): An advance in the treatment of hepatitis B e antigen positive chronic hepatitis B. *J Viral Hepat* **10**:298–305.
38. Janssen HLA, van Zonneveld M, Senturk H *et al.* (2005) Pegylated interferon alfa-2b alone or in combination with lamivudine for HBeAg-positive chronic hepatitis B: A randomised trial. *Lancet* **365**:123–9.
39. Lau GK, Piratvisuth T, Luo KX *et al.* (2005) Peginterferon Alfa-2a, lamivudine, and the combination for HBeAg-positive chronic hepatitis B. *N Engl J Med* **352**:2682–95.
40. Kao JH. (2007) Role of viral factors in the natural course and therapy of chronic hepatitis B. *Hepatol Int* **1**:415–30.
41. Lin SM, Yu ML, Lee CM *et al.* (2007) Interferon therapy in HBeAg positive chronic hepatitis reduces cirrhosis and hepatocellular carcinoma. *J Hepatol* **46**:45–52.
42. Niederau C, Heintges T, Lange S *et al.* (1996) Long-term follow-up of HBeAg-positive patients treated with interferon alfa for chronic hepatitis B. *N Engl J Med* **334**:1422–7.
43. van Zonneveld M, Honkoop P, Hansen BE *et al.* (2004) Long-term follow-up of alpha-interferon treatment of patients with chronic hepatitis B. *Hepatology* **39**:804–10.
44. Fried MW, Piratvisuth T, Lau GK *et al.* (2008) HBeAg and hepatitis B virus DNA as outcome predictors during therapy with peginterferon alfa-2a for HBeAg-positive chronic hepatitis B. *Hepatology* **47**:428–34.
45. Piratvisuth T, Lau G, Chao YC *et al.* (2008) Sustained response to peginterferon alfa-2a (40 kD) with or without lamivudine in Asian patients with HBeAg-positive and HBeAg-negative chronic hepatitis B. *Hepatol Int* **2**:102–10.

46. Brunetto MR, Oliveri F, Coco B *et al.* (2002) Outcome of anti-HBe positive chronic hepatitis B in alpha-interferon treated and untreated patients: A long term cohort study. *J Hepatol* **36**:263–70.
47. Papatheodoridis GV, Dimou E, Dimakopoulos K *et al.* (2005) Outcome of hepatitis B e antigen-negative chronic hepatitis B on long-term nucleos(t)ide analog therapy starting with lamivudine. *Hepatology* **42**:121–9.
48. Marcellin P, Lau GKK, Bonino F *et al.* (2004) Peginterferon alfa-2a alone, lamivudine alone and the two in combination in patients with HBeAg negative chronic hepatitis B. *N Engl J Med* **35**:1206–17.
49. Bonino F, Marcellin P, Lau GK *et al.* (2007) Predicting response to peginterferon alpha-2a, lamivudine and the two combined for HBeAg-negative chronic hepatitis B. *Gut* **56**:699–705.
50. Lai C, Chien R, Leung N *et al.* (1998) A one-year trial of lamivudine for chronic hepatitis B. Asia Hepatitis Lamivudine Study Group. *N Engl J Med* **339**:61–8.
51. Marcellin P, Chang T, Lim SG *et al.* (2003) Adefovir dipivoxil for the treatment of hepatitis B e antigen-positive chronic hepatitis B. *N Engl J Med* **348**:808–16.
52. Chang TT, Gish RG, de Man R *et al.* (2006) A comparison of entecavir and lamivudine for HBeAg-positive chronic hepatitis B. *N Engl J Med* **354**:1001–10.
53. Lai CL, Gane E, Liaw YF *et al.* (2007) Telbivudine versus lamivudine in patients with chronic hepatitis B. *N Engl J Med* **357**:2576–88.
54. Marcellin P, Heathcote EJ, Buti M *et al.* (2008) Tenofovir disoproxil fumarate versus adefovir dipivoxil for chronic hepatitis B. *N Engl J Med* **359**:2442–55.
55. Tassopoulos NC, Volpes R, Pastore G *et al.* (1999) Efficacy of lamivudine in patients with hepatitis B e antigen-negative/hepatitis B virus DNA-positive (precore mutant) chronic hepatitis B. Lamivudine Precore Mutant Study Group. *Hepatology* **29**:889–96.
56. Hadziyannis SJ, Tassopoulos NC, Heathcote EJ *et al.* (2003) Adefovir dipivoxil for the treatment of hepatitis B e antigen-negative chronic hepatitis B. *N Engl J Med* **348**:800–7.
57. Lai CL, Shouval D, Lok AS *et al.* (2006) Entecavir versus lamivudine for patients with HBeAg-negative chronic hepatitis B. *N Engl J Med* **354**:1011–20.

58. Liaw YF, Sung JJY, Chow WC *et al.* (2004) Lamivudine for patients with chronic hepatitis B and advanced liver disease. *N Engl J Med* **351**:1521–31.
59. Fung SK, Wong F, Hussain M *et al.* (2004) Sustained response after a 2-year course of lamivudine treatment of hepatitis B e antigen-negative chronic hepatitis B. *J Viral Hepat* **11**:432–8.
60. Hadziyannis S, Sevastianos V, I. R. (2009) Outcome of HBeAg-negative chronic hepatitis B (CHB) 5 years after discontinuation of long term adefovir dipivoxil (ADV) treatment [Abstract 18]. *J Hepatol* **50** (suppl 1):S9.
61. Zoulim F. (2004) Mechanism of viral persistence and resistance to nucleoside and nucleotide analogs in chronic hepatitis B virus infection. *Antiviral Res* **64**:1–15.
62. Shaw T, Bartholomeusz A, Locarnini S. (2006) HBV drug resistance: Mechanisms, detection and interpretation. *J Hepatol* **44**:593–606.
63. Chang TT, Lai CL, Chien RN *et al.* (2004) Four years of lamivudine treatment in Chinese patients with chronic hepatitis B. *J Gastroenterol Hepatol* **19**:1276–82.
64. Lok AS, Lai CL, Leung N *et al.* (2003) Long-term safety of lamivudine treatment in patients with chronic hepatitis B. *Gastroenterology* **125**:1714–22.
65. Marcellin P, Chang TT, Lim SG *et al.* (2008) Long-term efficacy and safety of adefovir dipivoxil for the treatment of hepatitis B e antigen-positive chronic hepatitis B. *Hepatology* **48**:750–8.
66. Hadziyannis S, Tassopoulos N, Heathcote E *et al.* (2006) Long-term therapy With adefovir dipivoxil for HBeAg-negative chronic hepatitis B for up to 5 years. *Gastroenterology* **131**:1743–51.
67. Tenney DJ, Rose RE, Baldick CJ *et al.* (2009) Long-term monitoring shows hepatitis B virus resistance to entecavir in nucleoside-naive patients is rare through 5 years of therapy. *Hepatology* **49**:1503–14.
68. Liaw YF, Gane E, Leung N *et al.* (2009) 2-Year GLOBE trial results: Telbivudine is superior to lamivudine in patients with chronic hepatitis B. *Gastroenterology* **136**:486–95.
69. Amini-Bavil-Olyaee S, Herbers U, Sheldon J *et al.* (2009) The rtA194T polymerase mutation impacts viral replication and susceptibility to tenofovir in hepatitis B e antigen-positive and hepatitis B e antigen-negative hepatitis B virus strains. *Hepatology* **49**:1158–65.
70. Snow-Lampart A, Chappell BJ, Curtis M *et al.* (2008) Week 96 resistance surveillance for HBeAg positive and negative subjects with chronic HBV

infection randomized to receive tenofovir DF 300 mg qd [Abstract]. *Hepatology* **48**(suppl):745A.

71. Yuen MF, Sablon E, Hui CK *et al.* (2001) Factors associated with hepatitis B virus DNA breakthrough in patients receiving prolonged lamivudine therapy. *Hepatology* **34**:785–91.
72. Flink HJ, Hansen BE, Heathcote EJ *et al.* (2006) Successful treatment with peginterferon α-2b of HBeAg-positive HBV non-responders to standard interferon or lamivudine. *Am J Gastroenterol* **101**:2523–9.
73. Anzola M. (2004) Hepatocellular carcinoma: Role of hepatitis B and hepatitis C viruses proteins in hepatocarcinogenesis. *J Viral Hepat* **11**:383–93.
74. Cucchetti A, Piscaglia F, Caturelli E *et al.* (2009) Comparison of recurrence of hepatocellular carcinoma after resection in patients with cirrhosis to its occurrence in a surveilled cirrhotic population. *Ann Surg Oncol* **16**:413–22.
75. Kubo S, Nishiguchi S, Hirohashi K *et al.* (2001) Effects of long-term postoperative interferon-alpha therapy on intrahepatic recurrence after resection of hepatitis C virus-related hepatocellular carcinoma: A randomized, controlled trial. *Ann Intern Med* **134**:963–7.
76. Mazzaferro V, Regalia E, Doci R *et al.* (1996) Liver transplantation for the treatment of small hepatocellular carcinomas in patients with cirrhosis. *N Engl J Med* **334**:693–9.
77. Yao FY, Ferrell L, Bass NM *et al.* (2001) Liver transplantation for hepatocellular carcinoma: Expansion of the tumor size limits does not adversely impact survival. *Hepatology* **33**:1394–403.
78. Kulik LM, Carr BI, Mulcahy MF *et al.* (2008) Safety and efficacy of 90Y radiotherapy for hepatocellular carcinoma with and without portal vein thrombosis. *Hepatology* **47**:71–81.
79. Ng KK, Lam CM, Poon RT *et al.* (2003) Thermal ablative therapy for malignant liver tumors: A critical appraisal. *J Gastroenterol Hepatol* **18**:616–29.
80. Huo TI, Huang YH, Wu JC *et al.* (2002) Survival benefit of cirrhotic patients with hepatocellular carcinoma treated by percutaneous ethanol injection as a salvage therapy. *Scand J Gastroenterol* **37**:350–5.
81. Lencioni RA, Allgaier HP, Cioni D *et al.* (2003) Small hepatocellular carcinoma in cirrhosis: Randomized comparison of radio-frequency thermal ablation versus percutaneous ethanol injection. *Radiology* **228**:235–40.

82. Livraghi T, Goldberg SN, Lazzaroni S *et al.* (2000) Hepatocellular carcinoma: Radio-frequency ablation of medium and large lesions. *Radiology* **214**:761–8.
83. Vivarelli M, Guglielmi A, Ruzzenente A *et al.* (2004) Surgical resection versus percutaneous radiofrequency ablation in the treatment of hepatocellular carcinoma on cirrhotic liver. *Ann Surg* **240**:102–7.
84. Llovet JM, Ricci S, Mazzaferro V *et al.* (2008) Sorafenib in advanced hepatocellular carcinoma. *N Engl J Med* **359**:378–90.

Chapter 8

Hepatitis C and Hepatocellular Carcinoma: Implications for Pathogenesis and Treatment

Geoffrey C. Farrell*

Australian National University Medical School, The Canberra Hospital, ACT, Australia

Infection with hepatitis C virus (HCV) is the second commonest cause of hepatocellular carcinoma (HCC) worldwide, the number one cause in Japan and a major reason for increasing HCC incidence in North America and Australia. HCV is an RNA virus whose genome does not enter the host nucleus to damage DNA directly. In chronic HCV infection, viral persistence is related to suppression of host innate immunity and dampening of the adaptive immune response. Conversely, immunosuppression facilitates viral replication and progression of chronic hepatitis C (CHC). In cell culture and transgenic mice, HCV proteins, such as core, NS3 and NS5A produce multiple effects on transcriptional regulation of gene expression and cell signaling of potential relevance to inflammatory recruitment, cell death and proliferation of hepatocytes. This has led many authors to conclude that HCV has direct hepatocarcinogenic properties, but there are potential flaws in this interpretation related to the experimental systems used. Instead, clinicopathological correlations indicate that the HCV pathway to liver cancer proceeds via chronic liver inflammation (CHC) and cirrhosis, and this takes decades to unfold. Other host determinants of HCC risk in HCV-infected patients include older age, male gender, genetic factors/ethnicity, previous heavy alcohol intake, hepatitis B virus (HBV) infection, obesity, type 2 diabetes and cigarette smoking. While interactions between viral proteins, alcohol and hepatic lipid metabolism or

* E-mail: geoff.farrell@anu.edu.au

insulin receptor signaling are evident experimentally, these co-morbid environmental factors are likely to operate principally by worsening the inflammatory activity and rate of fibrotic progression of CHC to cirrhosis. Conversely, effective antiviral therapy abolishes liver inflammation and injury when sustained virus response (SVR) is obtained, and this reduces incidence of HCC by over 80%, even when cirrhosis is established. Continuous interferon therapy does not diminish HCC risk when SVR is not obtained. After resection of HCC, antiviral treatment reduces late recurrence related to development of new cancers rather than residual disease, and this improves patient survival. The approach to treatment of HCV genotype 1 is changing. "Triple therapy" with pegylated interferon, ribavirin and a direct antiviral, such as telaprevir or boceprevir, improves efficacy during first treatment and retreatment of non-SVR cases. Since hepatocarcinogenesis with HCV is intimately related to continuing hepatic necroinflammatory activity and cirrhosis, it is likely this will further reduce HCC rates by eradicating liver inflammation and preventing cirrhosis.

Introduction: importance and epidemiology of HCV-related HCC

Hepatocellular carcinoma (HCC) is the third most common cause of cancer death worldwide. At least 80% of cases are caused by chronic liver disease resulting from hepatitis B virus (HBV) and/or hepatitis C virus (HCV) infection.[1–3] HCC may be attributed to HCV infection alone or in association with the co-morbidity of combined infections, immunodeficiency, life-time excessive alcohol intake, obesity, type 2 diabetes (T2D), and cigarette smoking. While the incidence appears to be slightly declining in HBV hyper-endemic regions,[1] in countries like Australia and the United States of America [USA] the incidence has risen substantially during the last 2 to 3 decades, partly explained by parallel changes in the prevalence of chronic HCV infection.[4,5] Japan is unique among Asia-Pacific countries in that HCV the most important etiological agent.[3] The epidemic started in the early 1980s related to medical exposures to blood contamination in the 1940s,[6] particularly among men born between 1931 and 1935. There has been a recent decline in its overall incidence, as well as changes in age- and gender-specific incidence.[3,7–9] Modelling the

HCV epidemic in France,[10] Australia[4] and the USA[5] project the incidence of HCV-related HCC attributable to injection drug use (IDU), which became socially popular in the 1960s and 1970s and continues unabated, will not peak until 2020–2025.

In 60–80% of HCV-infected patients, infection persists indefinitely.[11–13] This is associated with variable liver inflammation and hepatocellular injury, together termed chronic hepatitis C (CHC). A small proportion of patients with CHC develop severer forms of fibrosis which may progress to cirrhosis; estimates are 4–20% will have cirrhosis after 20 years.[12,14,15] At least 170 million people worldwide are chronically infected with HCV.[13] Even though only a minority develop cirrhosis and HCC, a considerable number remain at risk in later life.[4,5,10] Thus, HCC is a late complication of HCV infection for many decades. The immune response to HCV, and other host genetic and environmental factors such as age and gender, alcohol consumption, obesity and its metabolic complications of steatosis, insulin resist-ance and T2D all contribute to the necro-inflammatory activity and fibrotic severity of CHC; they also increase the risk of HCC, as discussed in later sections.

In this chapter, I will first summarize HCV virology and effects of HCV proteins on the immune response, liver inflammation, transcriptional regulation, cell signaling and other biological effects relevant to hepatocarcinogenesis (cell cycle regulation, proliferation, differentiation, immortalization, cell death). The evidence that chronic inflammation and cirrhosis are the key factors in HCV-related development of liver cancer will then be considered, as will the evidence that interferon(IFN)-based antiviral therapy suppresses CHC and subsequent risk of HCC, but only when the hepatic inflammatory response is suppressed, ideally with sustained viral response (SVR).

HCV: viral characteristics and effects of viral proteins on mammalian systems

Overview of HCV virology

HCV has been designated as a *Hepacivirus* within the *Flaviviridae* family.[16] It is a spherical enveloped and extensively lipidated particle, about 50 nm

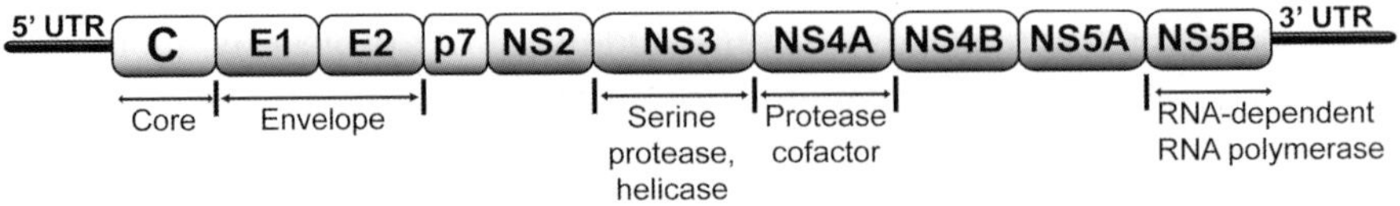

Figure 1. Organisation of the hepatitis C virus genome, including the long open reading frame which encodes structural genes, non-structural (NS) genes and the 5′ and 3′ non-coding (untranslated, UTR) regions.

in diameter. The nucleocapsid contains a small single positive-strand RNA genome of ~9.6 kb with an open reading frame (ORF) flanked by 5′- and 3′-untranslated regions (UTR) (Figure 1). The ORF encodes a polyprotein of ~3000 amino acids, cleaved by cellular and viral proteases into structural (core, p7, envelope proteins E1 and E2) and non-structural (NS) proteins (NS2, 3, 4A, 5A, 5B) (Figure 1). NS3 is a serine protease and helicase for which NS4A is a cofactor, and NS5B is the RNA-dependent RNA polymerase. Excellent reviews of HCV virology have been published,[16–18] including the potential relevance of viral proteins to hepatocarcinogenesis.[19–23]

Based on structural similarity, HCV isolates are classified into 6 main genotypes and several subtypes.[24,25] Within isolates from an infected individual, there may be additional sequence variability, especially in the 5′-UTR and NS5B regions, a phenomenon termed quasispecies. Genotype 1 is the most prevalent strain; genotype 2 is also widely distributed. HCV genotypes 3, 4, 5 and 6 are geographically restricted, being relatively common in South-East Asia (genotypes 3 and 6), Australia/New Zealand (genotype 3) and Egypt/North Africa (genotype 4).[24,25] With the possible exception of genotype 1b, HCV genotype confers relatively minor variation in the pathobiology of liver disease, such as differing profiles of disordered lipid metabolism and hepatic steatosis.[26,27] There are major differences between genotypes in responsiveness to IFN-based antiviral therapy, as reviewed elsewhere.[28]

Methods of study

While HCV infects only humans and chimpanzees, a small animal model has been created in chimeric urokinase-type plasminogen activator (uPa)-severe combined immunodeficient (SCID) mice engrafted with human hepatocytes.[29–31] Such "humanized" murine liver sustains HCV replication. Until recently, studies of viral proteins was confined to expression in cell lines or transgenic mice. These early studies produced a plethora of biological effects on intracellular signalling pathways, metabolism, oxidative stress, proliferation and viability (summarized in Table 1). For understanding the pathogenesis of CHC and HCC, however, several factors challenge the validity of this approach.

First, levels of viral proteins in expression systems are orders of magnitude higher than those in HCV-infected human hepatocytes, replicon systems or whole animals (humans and chimpanzees). Regulated expression systems partly overcome this concern.

Second, cell lines are transformed or immortalized in ways that negate or distort physiological regulation of proliferation, differentiation, and cell death, irrespective of pathways activated or inhibited by viral proteins.

Third, whole virus particles may not exert the same effects as individual proteins because of post-translational changes, physical restriction of access to cellular targets, or because other viral constituents and the immune response to HCV counter such biological effects. Experimental data demonstrating this concern are mentioned later. The same arguments apply to transgenic mouse models which express individual HCV proteins at high levels. As outlined in *Section 3*, some (but not all) such models develop HCC without conspicuous hepatitis or fibrosis, a scenario very different from HCC developing in HCV-infected humans, always associated with longstanding inflammation and usually cirrhosis.

A major advance came with the development of subgenomic and genomic replicons,[32,33] most in the Huh-7 human HCC cell line (reviewed in Ref. 18). These replicon systems allow the study of viral replication and virus-cell interactions, and comprise a convenient test system for testing potential therapeutic compounds.

Production of infectious HCV particles *in vitro* has been achieved by several groups during the last 6 years.[34–41] The full length JFH-1 genome replicates efficiently in Huh-7 cells, with secretion of viral particles that can be subpassaged or infect chimpanzees.[35] The JFH-1 strain was isolated from a patient with fulminant hepatitis C, a very rare syndrome; it

Table 1. Biological effects of HCV proteins in gene expression, replicon and whole virus infection systems.

Protein	Effects	Comments
Entire ORF	Increases ROS production	
HCV polyprotein	Decreases TGF-β transactivation	
Core and whole virus	Suppress innate immunity (TLR, IFN production etc)	See Table 2
	Differential effects on T cells — lymphocyte dysregulation	
	Impairs insulin receptor signaling (causes insulin resistance)	Mechanisms complex — Section 2.7
	Generates both ROS and RNS from mitochondria and ER	Exacerbated by alcohol, steatosis, calcium fluxes
	Induces oxidative stress — up-regulation of anti-oxidant pathways	
	Sensitizes to mitochondrial MPT, apoptosis	
Full length and truncated core	Activates ERK, JNK, AP-1, p38; increases cell proliferation	See Table 3
	Ras activation to prolong MAPK (ERK) activation	
	Increased secretion of growth stimulatory factor	See Table 4
	Suppresses TNF-α-mediated activation of NF-κB	
	Modulates cell death pathways (anti-apoptotic effects)	
	Transcription: among 2000 transcripts in primary human hepatocytes, IL-6, leptin receptor, gp130 and STAT3 increased	
	Interaction with Jak-1 prevents STAT3 activation	
	Signal transduction: cross-talk between androgen receptors and STAT3	
	Suppresses p21 promotor	
	Interacts with Smad3 to block	
	TGF-β-mediated inhibition of proliferation	

(*Continued*)

Table 1. (*Continued*)

Protein	Effects	Comments
E1-E2	ER stress	
NS3/NS4A, 4B	Stimulate fatty acid synthesis by activating SREBP-1	*Section 3*
		Table 4
	Modulate cell death pathways	Table 2
	Inhibition IRF-3 and induction of type 1 IFN	
NS5A	Modulates cell death pathways	Table 4
	Interferes with IFN action	
	ROS generation	
	Signal transduction	
	Transcription	

shows deviation from typical 2a strains.[42] This may be why it does not require adaptive mutations for replication in culture. Another approach has been to employ cDNA constructs of infectious HCV genotype 1b flanked by ribozymes.[18] However, while HCV cell culture systems that generate viral particles are a major advance, limitations include the inability of HCC cell lines to produce lipoproteins required for the secretion, circulation and possibly uptake of whole HCV virions.[17,18]

A more physiological system for HCV replication *in vitro* was developed using non-transformed cultured human fetal hepatocytes.[40,41] It supports HCV replication after addition of infectious serum with diverse genotypes, as well as transfection of *in vitro* transcribed genotype 1a HCV RNA without adaptive mutations. Transfected or infected cultures release infectious HCV in a cyclical pattern for at least 2 months. As in other systems,[17,18] re-infection could be blocked by interferon(IFN)-α and IFN-γ.[40,41]

HCV replication

HCV replication occurs within hepatocytes, although viral transcripts have also been isolated from lymphocytes. As reviewed elsewhere,[17,18] the cellular and molecular pathways include viral attachment, entry into hepatocytes, RNA replication and particle assembly, followed by viral release. Cell entry appears to be a multistep process. It involves tetraspanin CD81, human scavenger receptor SR-B1 (high density lipo-protein receptor) and tight junction molecules claudin-1 and occludin.[43–45] SR-B1 and CD81 are attachment proteins, while claudin 1 and occludins are essential co-receptors for cell entry by clathrin-mediated endocytosis. Glycosaminoglycans and/or low density lipoprotein (LDL) receptors may serve as additional attachment factors. HCV translation and replication start in the cytosol. NS proteins and viral RNA then form replication complexes that appear as a perinuclear membranous web. Following RNA proliferation, viral assembly occurs within the endoplasmic reticulum (ER), with budding into cytoplasmic vesicles. This assembly process and subsequent release occur via the secretory pathway and involve host cell lipid metabolism.[17,45] Thus, cholesterol and fatty acid biosynthesis are critically linked to HCV replication and virus formation,[45] while the association of virus particles with lipids and very low density lipoprotein (VLDL) is required for viral secretion from hepatocytes.[18] Infectious HCV circulates in the form of heterogeneous triglyceride-rich particles.[16–18]

Innate immune responses to HCV

The immune response to HCV is complex.[46–48] It must explain the high rate of viral persistence, the failure of humoral immune responses to neutralise subsequent infections, dysregulation of the hepatic type 1 IFN response and therapeutic efficacy of IFN-α, as well as the worsening effect of immunesuppression on inflammatory and fibrotic liver disease and hepatocarcinogenesis. The innate and adaptive immune responses to HCV have been well reviewed,[46–48] and are summarized in Table 2. Toll-like receptors (TLR), pattern recognition molecules expressed on hepatocytes and immune regulatory cells, activate innate immunity to HCV. Production of type 1 IFNs is an important effector arm. HCV proteins, particularly core and NS3/4A, interact with TLRs on various celltypes.[49] However, using TLR2- and TLR4-transfected cell lines, Hoffmann and colleagues demonstrated that recombinant HCV core protein activated TLR2, while enveloped viral particles did not.[50] They suggested that impaired interaction between the infectious particles and TLR may allow HCV to escape from innate antiviral responses.

Table 2. Effects of HCV on immune response.

Type of immunity	Effects	Comments
INNATE	Blocks TLR signaling (including TLR 2,3,4)	Effects most reproducible for core protein over-expression, less (or absent) for whole virus
	Inhibit expression of IFNs, IFN response factor-1 and ISGs	Partly by blocking TLRs, but possibly at other levels of regulation (Jak-STAT1, iNOS, other signaling pathways)
	Effects on chemokine promoters/ transcriptional regulation Resultant inhibition of cytokine expression	Via MyD88
	Suppresses IFN-α release from plasmacytoid dendritic cells	
	Stimulation of NK cells to release TGF-β and IL-10	Attenuates adaptive immune response
ADAPTIVE	Attenuation of vigorous CD4+ response after acute infection	Precedes chronic HCV infection
	Circulating CD8+ cells exhibit "stunned" phenotype — impaired proliferation, elaboration of IFN-γ, cytotoxicity Lymphocyte dysregulation — core decreases IFN-γ production by CD8+ cells — increases immunoglobulin production by B cells	Unclear if due to direct effect of viral proteins, or block in maturation/migration of HCV-specific CD8+ cells
	Core causes anergic state of stably transfected T cells (decreases IL-2 production)	
	Continuous activation but impaired function of HCV-specific T cells	Possible effect of viral stimulation of PD-1

(*Continued*)

Table 2. (*Continued*)

Type of immunity	Effects	Comments
	Possible effects on regulatory T cells (Tregs)	Not yet well defined
	IL-10 increased — suppresses proliferation of HCV-specific CD4+ and CD8+ cells — inhibits IFN-α production — promotes apoptosis pDCs	Dampens hepatic inflammatory response at cost of impeding antiviral effects: facilitates viral persistence

HCV viral proteins inhibit expression of IFNs by blocking TLR3 signaling, as well as exerting effects on multiple chemokine promoters and transcriptional regulators (via MyD88).[51] In this way, viral proteases could inhibit cytokine expression in infected cells, so countering an effective host cell antiviral response.[51] The entire HCV replicon suppresses IFN response factor (IRF)-1 in cell cultures,[18] while core protein perturbs transcriptional regulation of such IFN-stimulated genes (ISG) as IL-12 and IL-15,[52] thereby dampening an effective innate immune response.[52,53]

Hepatocytes secrete IFN-β, a type 1 IFN which induces an antiviral state that extends to neighbouring uninfected cells.[46] Resultant activation of ISGs has multiple effects that counter HCV infection: suppressing translation, degrading viral RNA, providing feedback amplification of the IFN response through the induction of TLR3, etc. Work with viral proteins indicates that HCV could attenuate the IFN response at several levels (reviewed in Refs. 46–48), thereby subverting innate immune responsiveness and allowing viral persistence; these pathways have not yet been demonstrated in HCV-infected human livers. They include Jak-STAT, iNOS and other intracellular signaling pathways.[54] For example, Lin *et al.*[55] concluded that STAT1 plays an indispensable role in innate HCV antiviral resistance. Immortalized human hepatocytes exhibit a functional antiviral response when infected by HCV *in vitro* via STAT1 induction of the IFN signaling pathway.[56]

HCV can also suppress IFN-α release by plasmacytoid dendritic cells (pDCs) without infecting those cells.[57,58] Natural killer (NK) cells play an important role in liver pathology, and could be connected to the innate immune response by direct cytotoxic effects or cytokine release.[46] *In vitro*, NK cells from HCV-infected individuals over-express cytokines such as transforming growth factor-β (TGF-β) and IL-10 that attenuate the adaptive immune response.[46,59]

Adaptive immune responses to HCV

Depending on age, 15–50% of humans infected with HCV undergo viral clearance.[12,13] This is genetically determined, as shown by the strong association with a polymorphism close to IL-28B, which encodes IFN-lambda3.[60] Spontaneous HCV clearance is associated with a robust HCV-specific CD4+ T cell response [reviewed in Refs. 46–48], with circulating IL-2 and IFN-γ. Conversely, attenuation of this initial vigorous CD4+ T cell response occurs in recurrent viremia after earlier apparent viral control.[61,62] In contrast to the CD4+ response, cytotoxic CD8+ T cells circulate, irrespective of virological outcome. They exhibit a "stunned phenotype" with impaired proliferation, production of IFN-γ and cytotoxicity.[63,64] Whether this inadequate function of CD8+ T cells is mediated by viral factors or is a step in the maturation or migration of HCV-specific CD8+ T cells remains unclear.[48]

Lymphocyte dysregulation is a key feature of chronic HCV infection that could influence the persistence of a chronic inflammatory response.[46–48] HCV core protein differentially affects lymphocyte subpopulations, for example by decreasing IFN-γ production in CD8+ T cells but increasing immunoglobulin production by B cells.[65–67] It also induces an anergic state in stably transfected T cells by decreasing IL-2 production.[64] In chronic HCV infection, there is continuous activation but impaired function of HCV-specific T cells.[63,68] One pathway may be chronic viral antigen stimulation of PD-1.[69,70] Regulatory T cells (Tregs) may also be important.[46–48]

IL-10 production is clearly increased with chronic HCV infection.[46–48] IL-10-producing T cells accumulate at sites of low hepatocyte apoptosis and laminin (matrix) expression, whereas IFN-γ-producing T cells localise to high rates of apoptosis and abundant laminin.[46–48] IL-10 suppresses proliferation of HCV-specific CD4+ and CD8+ T cells *in vitro*,[66] inhibits IFN-α production, promotes apoptosis of pDCs,[71] and down-regulates effector T cell responses to dampen the hepatic inflammatory response, at the cost of impeding antiviral effects.[46–48] These viral effects on immune regulation tend to reduce host tissue inflammation in the liver but facilitate viral persistence.

HCV has a high replication rate and its polymerase lacks a proof-reading strategy. Evolution of escape mutants is an important way in which HCV infection persists, as evident by the diversity of quasispecies during longstanding infection.[16,19,23] Selection is genetically determined by prevailing HLA haplotypes. Further details, and the implications for development of a hepatitis C vaccine, have recently been reviewed.[46]

The immune response and progression of chronic hepatitis C

It is important to understand how HCV infection exerts pro-inflammatory effects in the liver and alters hepatocyte viability. In acute hepatitis C, the onset of hepatitis is temporally related to T cell infiltration, inferring a causal role of immune-mediated cytotoxicity. However, it is less clear that liver damage in CHC is entirely immune mediated.[47,48] For example, CHC progresses more rapidly in patients with immunodeficiency. In the post-liver transplantation context, this is directly related to viral load,[72,73] indicating possible direct effects of viral factors on disease progression.

In CHC, liver histology shows moderate lymphocyte infiltration of parenchyma and portal tracts, the latter often noteworthy for lymphoid follicles and minor bile duct injury.[74] HCV-specific T cells are more abundant in the liver than the blood.[47] High expression of CD95, TNF-α receptor 1 (TNF-R1) and TNF-related apoptosis-inducing ligand (TRAIL) contribute to a high turnover of HCV-specific T cells (reviewed in Refs. 46–48). The secretion of pro-inflammatory cytokines (IL-1, IFN-γ, TNF-α, IL-12) and profibrotic cytokines (TGF-β) activates matrix-depositing stellate cells and periductular fibroblasts to initiate a fibrotic wound healing response associated with apoptosis of some (but not all) HCV-infected hepatocytes.[74]

Effects of viral proteins on metabolic pathways and oxidative stress

HCV proteins, including core, NS3/NS4A and NS5A, have pleotropic effects on gene expression in cell lines (summarized in Table 1) and transgenic mice (*Section 3*) (summarized in Ref. 19). Several intracellular signaling pathways may be involved in disordered lipid metabolism.[75] For example, NS4B activates hepatic fatty acid synthesis via the lipogenic transcription factor, sterol regulatory element binding protein-1 (SREBP-1).[76] HCV protein also impairs insulin receptor signalling by a variety of mechanisms.[77–82] In HCV core protein transgenic mice (discussed later), insulin resistance can be demonstrated *in vivo* and mice develop type 2 diabetes when fed a high fat diet.[77] However, these changes were also associated with high serum levels of TNF-α, a cytokine which perturbs insulin receptor signaling by activating JNK; anti-TNF-α antibody infusion reversed insulin resistance. These data favour cytokine-mediated insulin resistance rather than direct effects of viral proteins on insulin receptor signaling, which accords with patient observations that HCV-related insulin resistance may be due to peripheral defects rather than changes in the liver.[83]

Earlier studies that produced conflicting data about the biological effects of HCV core protein may have been confounded by the large amounts and type (truncated, full length) of protein synthesized. The extensive body of data generated by such studies has recently been reviewed.[20–23] To overcome the problem of over-expression, Li and colleagues regulated core expression in Huh7 cells using a tetracycline-regulated promoter.[75] While core protein had no effect on proliferative capability, it induced a range of anti-oxidant pathways, consistent with the concept that core expression leads to intracellular oxidative stress.[84–86] In turn, oxidative stress can activate several pro-inflammatory, pro-proliferative and cell death pathways, such as extracellular receptor kinase (ERK) or mitogen-activated protein kinase (MAPK), JNK-1/activator protein-1 (AP-1), p38, Fas, and nuclear factor-kappaB (NF-κB).[87,88] *In vitro*, core and NS5A both generate reactive oxygen species (ROS) and reactive nitrogen species (RNS) from mitochondria and ER,[84–86] which sensitizes mitochondria to ionic calcium,[86] ROS-induced membrane permeability transition (MPT) and the mitochondrial cell death pathway. The effects are exacerbated by concomitant ethanol exposure[89] (see later section). Full-length ORF (H77, genotype 1a) expression in the non-transformed human hepatocyte cell line, HH4, also increased intracellular ROS with appropriate anti-oxidant responses.[41] In addition, ORF expression up-regulated genes involved in the innate immune response/inflammation, and down-regulated cell growth genes, with growth inhibition and sensitization to Fas and TRAIL-mediated lysis.[41]

Effects of HCV proteins on hepatocellular proliferation and differentiation

As HCV RNA does not enter the nucleus, HCV cannot directly influence the initiating steps in hepatocarcinogenesis: mutagenesis, DNA repair and genomic instability.[20,23,90,91] However, later steps involve the survival and proliferation of altered clones of dysplastic hepatocytes, which eventually take on the invasive characteristics of neoplastic cells. By altering cellular pathways that produce an imbalance between hepatocyte proliferation, differentiation, immortalization and cell death (by apoptosis), HCV proteins could allow progression of altered hepatocytes to HCC[19–23,92] (depicted in Figure 2). One late step may involve hepatocytes assuming the garb of more primitive (and autonomous) mesenchymal cells, a process termed epithelial-mesenchymal transition (EMT).[93]

Earlier work documenting associations between HCV proteins and cell cycle regulatory pathways produced inconsistent findings.[19–23,92] Implicated pathways include stimulation of transcriptional activity of selected proto-oncogenes (c-myc, Rous sarcoma virus long terminal repeat (LTR), simian virus 40 [SV40]), and activation of pro-proliferative intracellular signaling pathways, such as MAPK via v-H-ras.[94–96] Using a tetracycline on/off regulation system to regulate expression of full-length and truncated core protein, Erhardt *et al.*[97] showed both activated ERK, JNK and p38 kinases with increased cell proliferation in HepG2 cells. Others found effects of core on ERK activation operating upstream at the level of MEK1 or earlier.[96,98] HCV core protein could also modulate liver cell proliferation via activation of Ras/Raf signaling,[96] as well as by exerting anti-apoptotic functions.[99] If core constitutively activates Raf-1, thereby prolonging MAPK activity in response to mitogenic stimuli, this could favour neoplastic transformation of HCV-infected cells.[96]

NF-κB is a pivotal signaling pathway activated both by redox stress and receptors of the TNF superfamily (Fas, TNF-R1, TRAIL death receptors). Because NF-κB regulates pro-inflammatory, anti-apoptotic, and pro-proliferative genes, its activation is of interest to liver inflammation and

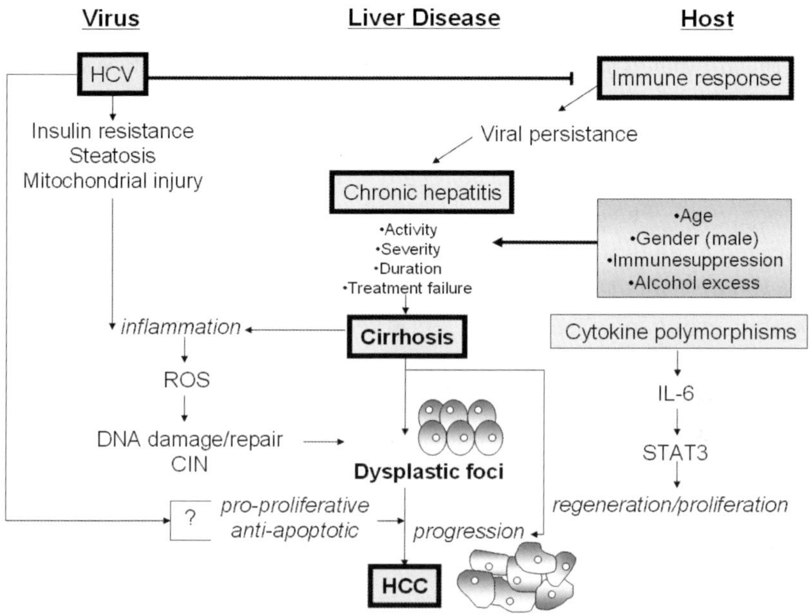

Figure 2. Interactions between virus (HCV) and host determine the severity of liver disease, particularly progression to cirrhosis, and the development of hepatocellular carcinoma. The latter is conceptualised as a multistep process in which DNA is damaged, most likely as a consequence of the inflammatory liver disease and resultant oxidative stress. The major growth pressure for altered hepatocytes to evolve to cancer cells is likely related to the proliferative pressure from cirrhosis, but direct effects of viral proteins on both proliferation and cell death (apoptosis) are possible, while an additional role of host genetic predisposition, such as by high production of the pro-proliferative cytokine IL-6 is starting to emerge (see text).

hepatocarcinogenesis. Work from Karin and others, using diethylnitrosamine (DEN) injection in gene-deleted mice, has indicated that NF-κB activated by IKKβ may protect against hepatocarcinogenesis, acting via negative cross-talk with STAT3.[100–102] In cell lines, over-expression of HCV core protein suppresses TNF-α-mediated activation of NF-κB while activating AP-1 via JNK.[103] Fukutomi and colleagues used HCV core protein expression in Huh-7 cells to demonstrate effects on cell proliferation, DNA synthesis and cell cycle progression.[104] Among numerous genes dysregulated by core expression, wnt-1 and its downstream target WISP-2 were shown to mediate these cell cycle/proliferative effects.[104] A full length HCV replicon stimulated secretion of growth stimulatory factor but a subgenomic replicon devoid of core sequences did not.

To overcome the challenge of interpreting cell cycle data in cancer cells, Ray and colleagues transfected HCV core into primary human hepatocytes.[105] These cells display a morphology resembling poorly differentiated epithelial cells, but continue to secrete albumin after more than 50 passages over 2 years; they show active telomerase. Among nearly 2000 transcripts increased, IL-6, leptin receptor and their gp130 signaling intermediate and STAT3 are candidate pathways for regulation of c-myc and cyclin D1.[106] An effect of HCV on STAT3 as a pro-proliferative pathway for hepatocytes is particularly interesting given recent findings in experimental systems for the roles of IL-6 and STAT3.[100–102] Conversely, other work has shown that interaction between HCV core protein and Jak-1 prevents activation of STAT3; this appears to suppress differentiation of hepatocytes.[107]

HCV proteins may also modulate signaling pathways from other growth and death receptors, such as cross-talk between core and androgen receptors, again via STAT3 activation.[108] This type of interaction could be mechanistically relevant to the male predominance of HCC. Finally, in several cell lines, HCV core protein expression suppressed the p21 promoter; the region responsive to core appears to be located downstream of the p53 binding site.[109] However, in experimental systems core does not interact with p21 or other cell cycle regulators directly. Suppression of cell cycle inhibitors, such as p21, is another potential mechanism whereby HCV proteins could favour hepatocellular proliferation (Figure 2).

TGF-β mediates G1 phase arrest by activating the p21 promoter; core (but not NS3) abrogated these effects.[110] Cheng *et al.*[110] found that expressing intact HCV polyprotein in cell lines decreased TGF-β transactivation. Further, core and NS3 physically interact with Smad3 to block TGF-β-mediated transcriptional activity [reviewed in Ref. 21]. It has been suggested that structural variants of core protein which arise during long-term HCV infection interact with Smad3. This inhibits the TGF-β pathway that opposes cell proliferation and favours hepatocyte differentiation.[111] These findings have recently been extended to selective effects on TGF-β-mediated EMT.[112] Others have found that CHC is associated with *increased production* of TGF-β2, while regulated HCV core expression and the full length JFH-1 genome expressed in HCC cells produced similar effects.[113] The many potential effects of HCV proteins on cell proliferation are summarized in Table 3.

Effects of HCV proteins on cell death pathways

In cell systems, HCV proteins, particularly core but also NS3 and NS5A, modulate cell death pathways (summarized in Table 4). Tumor suppressor p53 has been much studied (sometimes with conflicting results[21,92]), as well as its key target gene, the cell cycle inhibitor, p21. Ray and colleagues found HCV core expression abrogated TNF-α-mediated apoptosis,[114] and suggested the mechanism could be sustained expression of cellular FADD-like interleukin-1β-converting enzyme-like inhibitory protein (c-FLIP).[115] In HCV-immortalized human hepatocytes, *inhibition of core protein expression induced apoptosis*, with enhanced expression of p53 and correspondingly increased pro-apoptotic Bax and decreased anti-apoptotic Bcl-XL.[116] Other pathways have also been implicated.[116,117] As opposed to inhibitory effects on TNF-R1 and p53, Chou *et al.*[118] found that core sensitizes Huh7 cells to TRAIL- but not Fas-mediated apoptosis, and this was dependent on mitochondrial apoptosis signalling via caspase 9. NS5A expression in cell lines sequestered p53 in cytoplasm,[119] down-regulated p21,[120] activated STAT3 via Jak-1,[121] and inhibited TNF-α-mediated (but not Fas-mediated) apoptosis.[122,123]

HCC in transgenic mice expressing HCV proteins

A Tokyo group first described two lines of C57B6 mice in which high-level HCV core (genotype 1b) expression was ensured by placing the gene downstream of an HBV transcriptional regulator.[124] Core protein was expressed in hepatic nuclei of these mice. Both lines developed steatosis early in life.[125] In humans, steatosis has been attributed directly to genotype 3, not genotype 1 HCV,[26,27] while C57B6 mice are also unusually susceptible to steatosis.[102] At no stage did HCV core transgenic mice show liver inflammation, and ALT was not elevated.[125] At 16 months of

Table 3. Effects of HCV proteins on cell proliferation, differentiation and immortalization.

Mediator	Effect	Comment
Core, NS3/4, NS5A	Stimulation of proto-oncogenes (c-myc, Ras)	Some evidence for constitutive Ras activation; Activates Raf-1
	Activation of pro-proliferative mitogen-activated protein kinases (ERK, JNK/AP-1, p38)	Increased proliferation of HepG2 cells. Conflicting findings, particularly on level of MAPK activation — ?upstream of MEK
Core	Suppresses TNF-α-mediated NF-κB activation	Oxidative stress activates NF-κB: net effect unclear
	Activates AP-1 by activating JNK	Pro-proliferative transcription factor
	Among numerous up-regulated genes, wnt-1 and downstream WISP-2 mediated cell cycle/proliferative effects	
	In immortalised primary human hepatocytes, up-regulates IL-6, gp 130 and STAT-3	Candidate pathways for up-regulation of c-myc and cyclin D1
	Direct interaction between core and Jak-1 prevents STAT3 activation to suppress hepatocyte differentiation	STAT3 has complex effects on cell survival and proliferation (discussed in Refs. 100–102)
	Suppressed p21 promoter (cell cycle inhibitor under p53 regulation) — site is downstream of p53 binding site	Does not interact directly with p21 or other cell cycle regulators
	Cross-talk between core and androgen receptors via STAT3 activation	Possible relevance to male predominance of HCC
Full length replicon	Stimulates DNA synthesis, cell cycle progression	Effect lost with deletion of core sequences
	Stimulates secretion of growth stimulatory factor	
	Decreases TGF-β transactivation	Loss of anti-proliferative effect
	Increases production of TGF-β2	Also found in CHC

(*Continued*)

Table 3. (*Continued*)

Mediator	Effect	Comment
Core and NS3	Physically interact with Smad3	Inhibits TGF-β pathway that opposes proliferation and favours differentiation of hepatocytes

Note: Effects of viral proteins on anti-apoptotic function and suppression of cell cycle inhibitors, such as p21, also favour enhanced cell cycle activity and cell proliferation.

Table 4. Effects of HCV proteins on cell death pathways.

Mediator	Effect	Comment
Core	p53	Effects on cell cycle via p21, and on apoptosis
	Blocks TNF-α-mediated apoptosis	Possibly by sustained expression of c-FLIP (see text)
	Inhibition of core expression in immortalized human hepatocytes induced apoptosis	Enhanced expression of p53 and downstream Bax, decreased anti-apoptotic Bcl-XL
	Sensitizes Huh7 cells to TRAIL (not Fas) mediated apoptosis	Depends on caspase 9 activation (mitochondrial pathway)
NS5A	Sequesters p53 in cytoplasm	
	Inhibited TNF-α but not Fas-mediated apoptosis	
	Activated STAT3 via Jak-1	

For more detailed information, see excellent reviews by Liang,[19] Berasin[20] and Kasprzak.[21]

age, 15–30% of male mice (no females) developed liver tumors, first as adenomas, later as HCC in a "nodule-in-nodule" manner.[124] Other transgenic mice expressing NS protein, the entire HCV polyprotein or core protein have been described,[126,127] as reviewed elsewhere.[19] Older males expressing HCV polyprotein developed significant numbers of liver tumors (adenomas and HCCs),[126] but this phenotype appeared "milder" 5 years later, unless animals were co-administered iron to worsen oxidative stress.[127] Many other lines of HCV transgenic mice do not develop hepatic tumors or any other liver pathology [reviewed in Ref. 19]

While the observation that HCC develops in a proportion (30–45%) of older, male HCV core or polyprotein transgenic mice might infer a direct pathogenic relationship between HCV and liver cancer, further experiments have shown that such animals exhibit oxidative stress associated with steatosis,[128] associated with degenerative changes in mitochondria and mutation of mitochondrial DNA.[124] The synergistic effect of iron overload also appeared related to mitochondrial injury and age-related steatosis.[127] Further, HCV core transgenic mice with deleted peroxisome proliferation-activator receptor-alpha (PPAR-α) (a transcription factor involved with regulation of fatty acid oxidation genes) were protected against development of HCC.[129] In mice, sustained PPAR-α activation is associated with liver tumors, but PPAR-α agonist fibrates do not cause HCC in humans, so this may be a species effect. It seems possible that steatosis and related oxidative stress rather than HCV protein expression is what leads to hepatocarcinogenesis in some transgenic mouse models; similar increases in HCC are found with dietary steatosis in C57B6 mice.[102]

Liver inflammation is not conspicuous in most HCV core transgenic models.[19,124,126,130] However, Tsutsumi and colleagues[131] demonstrated increased hepatic expression of TNF-α and IL-1β with related activity of JNK and AP-1; NF-κB was not activated. While the relevance of selective AP-1 but not NF-κB activation in HCV core protein transgenic mice to HCV-related hepatocarcinogenesis is unclear, some recently work in carcinogen models has led to the suggestion that STAT3 and JNK activation in the presence of impaired (or abrogated) NF-κB activation favours hepatocarcinogenesis.[100,101]

To avoid the potential issue of HCV core expression during development,[19] Chang *et al.*[132] developed a conditional expression HCV core transgenic mouse regulated by the tetracycline transactivator. Such core transgenic mice were lean but 20–30% of hepatocytes showed steatosis. Livers showed up-regulation of transcripts for SREBP, 3-hydroxy-3-methylglutaryl-Coenzyme A synthase and other genes involved with lipid transport and metabolism, as well as those involved in mitochondrial function (cytochrome c oxidase subunit II). Among 3 groups of HCV core protein transgenic mice,[132] those with intermediate core expression (not high or low expression) showed steatosis, complement-dependent inflammation and liver fibrosis, but no liver tumors.

Consistent with *in vitro* work (see later section), HCV core-E1-E2 transgenic mice were relatively refractory to Fas-induced apoptosis.[126] After injection with DEN, these mice developed larger HCCs than controls; this was attributable to differences in hepatocyte apoptosis rather than proliferation. In another study of HCV polyprotein transgenic mice animals failed to develop HCC and there was no liver inflammation.[130] However, crossing HCV transgenic mice with Mdr2-gene deleted mice (which develop inflammation-associated HCC) led to varying outcomes depending on the genetic background. N2 generation DEN-treated $Mdr2^{-/-}$.HCV-transgenic female mice (75% FVB/N genome, 25% C57B6) developed significantly larger tumors than DEN-treated $Mdr2^{-/-}$ mice, in parallel with enhanced inflammatory gene expression. However, N7 generation (99% FVB/N, 1%C57B6) mice showed no differences in tumor development between $Mdr2^{-/-}$.HCV-Tg and $Mdr2^{-/-}$ mice. These findings were interpreted as indicating that, depending on host genetic background, the HCV transgene accelerated inflammation-associated hepatocarcinogenesis.

As opposed to the diverse biological/signaling activities when expressed in cell lines (discussed earlier), HCV NS5A transgenic mice are phenotypically normal to 24 months.[133]

Alcohol interaction with HCV protein expression

Alcohol is a synergistic factor for CHC disease severity and HCC risk. Mechanisms whereby excessive alcohol exposure could influence hepatocarcinogenesis are therefore of interest. Both HCV core and NS5A proteins localize to mitochondria and ER *in vitro* and generate ROS and reactive nitrogen species in expression systems[84–86] and transgenic mice.[134] This sensitizes mitochondria to alcohol-induced MPT.[89,134] Alcohol markedly increased lipoperoxide levels in HCV core transgenic mice,[134] a proposed mechanism by which chronic excessive alcohol consumption increases liver injury and HCC risk in CHC.[135] Hepatocyte-specific NS5A expression also induces TLR4, and this could mediate the interaction between alcohol-induced endotoxemia to cause synergistic liver injury and HCC. The stem/progenitor cell marker, Nanog, was up-regulated by TLR4, and mediated hepatocarcinogenesis in endotoxin-treated mice.[136]

Structural variability of HCV and hepatocarcinogenesis

Genotype 1b

The concept that viral determinants drive hepatocarcinogenesis would be strengthened by a link between HCV structural variation and HCC risk. A relationship between genotype 1b and HCC was proposed 20 years ago, but early observations were confounded by co-associations with age and duration of infection, and there were negative studies.[137] In a more recent prospective study of CHC-cirrhosis cases,[138] genotype 1b (hazard ratio [HR] 3.0), male gender (HR 2) and age >60 years (HR 6) were independent predictors of HCC. The course of hepatitis C after liver transplantation may be more aggressive with HCV genotype 1b,[139] which could indicate more severe necroinflammatory disease with this genotype. A meta-analysis of 57 case-control and cohort studies reported HCC incidence in relation to HCV genotype,[140] with particular focus on 21 studies in which age-adjusted risk was estimated. There was considerable study heterogeneity. Age-adjusted relative risk (RR) of HCC increased for genotype 1b (1.63 to 1.78, depending which studies were excluded); it was 2.46 among thse without cirrhosis at study entry. Available data still do not allow exclusion of all confounding variables (alcohol intake, cigarette smoking, occult HBV), and the contention that HCV genotype 1b plays a role in hepatocarcinogenesis by causing more active necroinflammatory liver disease and more rapid progression to cirrhosis is plausible but unproven.

Core mutations

Core protein sequence variation could influence processes pertinent to hepatocarcinogenesis, as indicated by effects on TGF-β-mediated differentiation and anti-proliferative effects, and NF-κB activation (*Section 2.8*). Akuta and colleagues[141] found relationships between amino acid substitutions in core protein, response to Peg-IFN/ribavirin therapy, and risk of HCC during >10 year follow-up among genotype 1b cases associated with non-SVR. Advanced fibrosis stage and non-wildtype core amino acid composition were independent risk factors for HCC.[141] In a more recent Japanese study (genotype 1, 10 year follow-up, 27% SVR),[142] core residues at 70 and 91 were determined pre-treatment. Core mutations were among 6 independent factors correlating with HCC risk (age, male, non-SVR, fibrotic severity, ALT elevation). Others have reported that amino acid substitutions in core protein are not associated with HCC.[43] If core mutations influence HCC risk, their importance seems minimal relative to host and disease variables.

Other viral proteins

Nishise and colleagues determined NS3 protein amino-terminus for patients infected with genotype 1b.[44] After adjusting for age and fibrosis stage, those with group B secondary structure had five-fold increased rate of HCC after adjusting for age and fibrosis stage. No mechanism has been proposed.

Host factors influencing HCC as an outcome of chronic hepatitis C

Constitutional and environmental factors

Age: Age is a powerful independent risk factor for HCC.[37,145–148] In CHC, older age can be related to longer duration of infection, older age at onset, and increased risk of cirrhosis. While age is not known to influence the hepatic inflammatory response, a recent Japanese study found that HCV-related HCC in old women was often associated with less liver inflammation and less severity of liver disease than younger patients.[9]

Gender: Incidence of HCV infection, chronicity and rates of cirrhosis all increase about 2-fold in men.[4–7,11–13] As a complication of CHC (except in very old Japanese women[8,9]), male predominance of HCC reflects that of non-inflammatory forms of cirrhosis (hemochromatosis, alcoholic cirrhosis, etc). Thus, gender influences hepatocarcinogenesis; experimental studies over 40 years have shown direct links to sex steroid levels [reviewed in Ref. 101]. Recently it has been proposed that the relative protection of female mice against DEN-induced HCC is due to estrogen-mediated suppression of IL-6.[101] The influence of gender on cytokine expression is mentioned later.

Family history and genetic factors: The Brescia HCC study found that family history of liver cancer increased risk of HCC (OR 2.4).[146] There was synergism between family history of liver cancer, HCV infection and heavy alcohol intake. It is evident from many studies that risk of HCV-related HCC in Japanese people resident in Japan is higher than most other countries [reviewed in Refs. 7 and 147]. Whether host genetic factors, such as cytokine polymorphisms could be involved or a high rate of occult HBV infection (discussed later) is an important area for future research.

Gene expression profiles have been examined in relation to the outcome of Peg-IFN and ribavirin combination therapy. Two different groups can be discerned, those with up-regulated and those with down-regulated ISGs.[149] Non-response (NR) to treatment was high in the ISG up-regulated group. This was also associated with a polymorphism of IL-28B known to influence recovery from acute hepatitis C and the response of CHC to combination antiviral therapy.[60,149–151] Thus, host genetic factors are critical in determining the hepatic inflammatory response to HCV, as well as response to antiviral treatment, both highly relevant to HCV-related hepatocarcinogenesis.

Alcohol: Several but not all studies show an increased risk of HCC among CHC patients who have drunk to excess over a sustained period.[152–154] Most studies indicate less than 5 standard drinks per day (50 g ethanol/day) does not increase cirrhosis risk,[155–159] but lifetime exposure is more important.[152,158] The association with alcohol may be via metabolic effects that increase oxidative stress,[135] as mentioned earlier; facilitation of viral replication and enhanced necroinflammatory activity have also been suggested. The weight of evidence is that HCC risk is largely attributable to a higher rate of fibrotic progression to cirrhosis. Conversely, discontinuation of excessive alcohol intake may actually further increase HCC risk.[153,160,161] Thus, previous excessive alcohol intake remains a risk factor for HCC after SVR to antiviral therapy.[162]

Obesity: Numerous studies have shown that obesity and steatosis (often associated) is a powerful risk factor for fibrosis progression in CHC.[163–165] There is debate about whether steatosis *per se* or insulin resistance is the key factor enhancing fibrotic progression; more recent evidence suggests the latter. Obesity is an independent risk factor for HCC, irrespective of primary etiology.[160,166,167] A large Japanese study has recently confirmed a strong relationship between body mass index

(BMI) and HCC risk in CHC,[167] while steatosis has also been associated with higher rates of HCC.[168]

Diabetes: Chronic HCV infection is a powerful independent risk factor for type 2 diabetes.[169,170] Proposed mechanisms include effects of HCV proteins on pathways of insulin receptor signaling, on mitochondrial and lipid metabolism, and effects on peripheral tissues (muscle, adipose) secondary to chronic systemic inflammation. Insulin resistance, a key pathophysiological determinant of type 2 diabetes, worsens fibrotic severity of CHC,[170,171] and this would be expected to increase risk of HCC. Several (but not all) studies have confirmed that diabetes is an independent risk factor for HCV-related HCC,[173,174] and similar association is found for other causes of cirrhosis.[174–178] Diabetes also increases risk of HCC recurrence after surgical resection.[179] Since diabetes and HCC are both late complications of advanced cirrhosis, the mechanistic significance of this link remains unclear.

HBV co-infection: Active HBV infection (HBsAg sero-positive with detectable HBV DNA) in the presence of CHC increases both activity and severity of chronic hepatitis,[180,181] and acts synergistically to increase HCC risk.[182,183] For occult HBV infection (HBsAg negative, anti-HBc positive, HBV DNA detectable in liver and occasionally in serum) the situation is less clear [reviewed in Ref. 22]. Some CHC cohort studies have found anti-HBc positivity is an independent risk factor for HCC,[159] and for HCC recurrence after resection.[184] One study found that anti-HBc positivity was an independent risk factor for HCC, but detectable serum HBV DNA among those with occult HBV infection did not increase the risk.[185] Occult HBV appears to be very common in case series from Japan where the rate of HCV-associated HCC seems to be about double that in Europe, North America and Australia.[7,138,146,154,159,186,187]

Cigarette smoking: At least two studies have also found a significant, albeit weak association between cigarette smoking and HCC risk in patients with CHC.[188,189]

Immunosuppression

After solid organ transplantation (lung, kidney, heart, liver — other than for HCC) for patients with chronic HCV infection (particularly genotype 1b), the course of CHC is often accelerated with high rates of liver failure and HCC.[190,191] Among peri-operative determinants of hepatitis C severity after liver transplantation, unusually high viral load appears most important.[73] In turn, this is related to the extent and type of immunosuppression used in the early post-transplant period. For example, glucocorticoids worsen hepatitis C recurrence in association with high levels of viremia (>10^7 IU/mL). In cell culture, corticosteroids up-regulate occludin and SCRB1 to facilitate hepatocellular re-uptake of HCV, thereby increasing propagation of HCV 5–10-fold.[192]

HIV coinfection also accelerates fibrotic progression of CHC to cirrhosis and increases risk of HCC,[191] often at a young age.[194,195] While there is some evidence that lower CD4+ count increases the rate of fibrotic progression,[195] nearly half the HIV-infected patients who die from liver disease have CD4+ count >200 cell/mL.[194] There appears to be more active "hepatitis" in these cases, again strengthening the link between liver inflammation and HCC.

Hepatitis disease "activity", hepatocellular proliferation and cirrhosis are risk factors for HCC with chronic HCV infection

Cirrhosis

Cohort studies repeatedly show that cirrhosis is usually present at diagnosis of HCV-related HCC.[147,153,196–198] Conversely, there are few cases in which surrounding liver at the time of HCC resection or autopsy fails to exhibit cirrhosis (F4) or advanced (bridging) fibrosis (F3).[147,199] In those with cirrhosis, the highest risk for HCC is among those with the most advanced disease, as reflected by Child-Pugh-Turcotte score, serum albumin, severity of portal hypertension etc. Similarly, increased liver stiffness as determined by transient elastography, which correlates closely with fibrotic severity of CHC,[200] is a powerful prospective determinant of HCC onset; HR was 16 [CI 3.7–75] when liver stiffness measurement exceeded 16.7 kPa,[201] which is strongly predictive of cirrhosis. With factors that increase the risk of HCV-related HCC, such as immunosuppression, HIV or HBV co-infection, obesity and diabetes,

CHC is usually more active and more severe, typically with established cirrhosis. Likewise, cirrhosis and poor liver function are the key risk factor for development of HCC after SVR.[148,162,202,203]

HCV-related cirrhosis is a slowly progressive disease, that may be accelerated by other causes of liver disease. In many series, HCC is the first complication to develop and is the dominant cause of mortality.[187,204] The annual incidence of HCC among HCV-infected persons with cirrhosis has been estimated as 3.6% from a long-term, prospective European study.[204] It may be higher in Japan, where some estimates exceed 6% per annum.[7,147,187,205,206]

Activity

The inflammatory "activity" of chronic hepatitis is indicated by histological changes in the liver, including patterns of lobular and portal tract inflammation and hepatocyte injury/cell death (apoptosis). In the absence of biopsy, serum alanine transaminase (ALT) levels are a surrogate marker. In addition to the factors described in Section 6, the collective evidence from cohort studies indicates that disease activity plays an important role in determining fibrotic progression of CHC.[185,207–209] At one end of the spectrum, cases with normal ALT have ~50% slower rates[210,211] and relatively low risk of cirrhosis. Hepatitis activity (ALT level) has been a risk factor for HCC development in many Japanese studies,[141,143,186,209,212] including after SVR to interferon,[148,162,202,203] and recurrence after surgical resection.[184] During repeated course of IFN therapy, failure to suppress ALT to below 1.5 times the upper limit of normal [$\times$ N] was associated with ~10-fold higher risk of HCC.[212]

Hepatocellular proliferation

Hepatocytes are physiologically resting cells, only entering the cell cycle when primed by cytokines, such as those released during liver inflammation. In chronic hepatitis and cirrhosis, hepatocytes are constantly being injured and replaced; as such, they exhibit increased expression of cell cycle genes. Such "replicative pressure" contributes to the multistep pathway of hepatocarcinogenesis,[213] either by allowing clones of altered dysplastic hepatocytes to expand, or by facilitating replication of "hepatic precursor" cells as a reserve compartment for liver regeneration.[213–215] In early work, we compared hepatic expression of the cell cycle marker, Ki67 in HCV-related cirrhotic livers between cases which 2 years or later developed HCC and those that did not.[216] Cases leading to HCC exhibited greater proliferative activity, a finding confirmed by others using different markers, such as silver-stained nucleolar organiser region,[217] and hepatic proliferating cell nuclear antigen expression; the latter increased HCC risk 6-fold among patients with CHC-cirrhosis.[218]

Pro-inflammatory pathways and gene expression profiles in HCV-related HCC

The concept that chronic inflammation is pivotal to hepatocarcinogenesis is supported by clinical correlations and experimental studies. The evidence is strongest for chronic hepatitis B, where adoptive transfer experiments show the need for HBV-specific cytotoxic T lymphocytes.[22,31,219,220]

Cytokines and HCC

Several cytokines and their intracellular signaling pathways have been studied in relation to HCV-related HCC. A polymorphism in IL-1β (but not of TNF-α) has been noted in Japanese patients with HCV-HCC.[221] The 31T/T phenotype increased the OR 2.63. High serum IL-6 levels have been associated with HCC risk for CHB,[222] but data for CHC are inconsistent. Some findings indicate this association is confined to women.[223] Others found associations between serum IL-6 (but not all studies) and IL-18 in patients with HBV- or HCV-related HCC compared to uncomplicated cirrhosis.[222–225] Another study found serum IL-18 levels correlated with HCC invasiveness and survival.[225] Among 219 patients coming to transplantation (predominantly for CHC), there was significant association between the IL-6 high-producer phenotype and HCC; OR was 3.74 in females and 14.8 in males.[226] These findings support the concept that more inflammatory chronic liver disease increases the risk of hepatocarcinogenesis.[20,23,224]

TGF-β, via its type 1 receptor (TGF-R1), signals through Smad3. There are two phosphoisoforms, C-terminal (pSmad3C) and linker-phosphorylated Smad3 (pSmad3L); the latter is catalyzed by JNK-1, also activated by TGF-β. pSmad3C up-regulates p21 to suppress hepatocellular proliferation, but JNK/pSmad3L promotes extracellular matrix deposition. In CHC biopsies, hepatocellular pSmad3L immunostaining increased with necroinflammatory grade and fibrotic stage,[227] while antiproliferative pSmad3C diminished. More than half of patients with strong pSmad3L positivity developed HCC within 12 years, versus ~10% showing low pSmad3L positivity.

Hepatocarcinogenic interactions between IL-6 and TGF-β have also been suggested.[228] Hepatic progenitor/stem cells express STAT3, Oct4 and Nanog, together with the differentiation proteins, TGF-R2 and embryonic liver foldrin (ELF). HCCs contained cells that expressed progenitor cell markers but lacked TGF-R2 and ELF expression, while elf knockout mice developed spontaneous HCC with abundant expression of IL-6 and its signaling intermediate, STAT3. The authors suggested that HCC could arise from an IL-6-driven transformed stem cell with inactivated TGF-β signaling.

In a search for host genetic factors involved with HCC development among HCV-infected individuals, a University of Tokyo study found 31 SNPs in 29 genes significantly associated with HCC;[229] three (SCYB14, GFRA1 and CRHR2) were confirmed in a secondary screen. SCYB14 is also known as CXCL14 and belongs to the cytokine gene family, encoding secreted proteins involved in immune-regulatory and inflammatory processes.

COX-2

Cyclo-oxygenase-2 (COX-2) activity has also been shown to correlate with HCC risk in CHC. Twenty-nine patients with stage 1 HCC underwent curative resections and were followed for median 5 years (range 2–13 years); COX-2 expression score in surrounding liver correlated with serum ALT. Higher COX-2 expression in cirrhotic liver was a risk factor for HCC recurrence/development of new tumors.[230]

Gene expression profiles

Host genetic factors are critical in determining the hepatic inflammatory response to chronic HCV infection,[46–48] as well as the response to antiviral treatment. Several studies have examined the transcriptosome of HCC derived from HCV-infected human livers and compared the results with HBV-related HCC.[231–234] While genes involved with inflammation predominated in hepatitis B, expression of anti-inflammatory response genes is more conspicuous in CHC.[231] Rather similar data showing down-regulation of immune system genes has been noted in early components of nodule-in-nodule HCC, mostly cases of CHC.[232] Heat shock protein-70 (HSP70), a stress-response protein, was the predominant up-regulated gene. Delpuech *et al.*[233] noted over-expression of TGF-β-induced genes. Mas *et al.* compared differentially expressed genes (DEG) between HCV-cirrhosis, HCV-HCC and surrounding cirrhotic liver.[235] Characteristic gene signatures were over-expression of genes mediating cell proliferation, cell death and inflammation for cirrhosis *versus* normal liver, cell death, cell cycle, DNA replication and immune response in early HCC, with DNA repair genes also expressed in advanced HCC. A set of genes was identified that could predict whether or not cirrhotic tissue was associated with HCC.[235]

Effects of HCV anti-viral therapy on risk of HCC

Antiviral response determines risk of HCC

Although there has been only one RCT,[205] the weight of accumulated evidence from retrospective and prospective cohort studies indicates that effective antiviral therapy of CHC reduces HCC risk substantially. The first HCV treatment was IFN monotherapy. This was only modestly effective but was much used in Japan. In the late 1990s, IFN/ribavirin combination became the standard of care, substantially improving SVR rates, and during the last 5 years, pegylated(Peg)-IFN-alpha/ribavirin has been regarded as optimal therapy.[28,236–239] A small number of (mostly older) studies found effects of IFN *versus* no treatment,[205] irrespective of treatment response, but this has not been demonstrated in the Peg-IFN era. Conversely, least 12 studies have reported on rates of HCC according to treatment outcome and pre-treatment histological severity (reviewed in Refs. 3,47,240,241). These data are summarized in Table 5. The vast majority of these studies, including thousands of treated cases from Japan,[47,240–246] have observed that rates of HCC are substantially reduced only among those with a response to antiviral therapy, most impressively with SVR.[3,47,154,197,206,241–253] There is also evidence that SVR prolongs life expectancy.[254,255]

In the Japanese studies, HCC rates are lowest in those with both viral and biochemical response, and intermediate when there is biochemical response without SVR (Table 5). Biochemical response was defined as normalization of serum ALT, providing further evidence of a relationship between necro-inflammatory activity and hepatocarcinogenesis. The beneficial effect of antiviral therapy against development of HCC in patients with CHC may be even greater with use of Peg-IFN/ribavirin (combination treatment) using currently recommended doses of both agents and response-driven treatment duration (reviewed in Refs. 28,256–258); recent data support this contention.[239,263]

Some workers have claimed that IFN administration to patients with CHC exerts anti-proliferative effects.[262] In the author's view, this may be simply a response to the diminished hepatocellular injury that follows anti-viral effects of IFN. On the other hand, a reduction of c-kit-positive hepatic progenitor cells was noted in 16 cases of CHC in which there was no response to IFN-based antiviral treatment.[264] *In vitro*, IFN-α had dose-dependent anti-proliferative effects on similar progenitor cells of rodent origin, and this effect was confirmed by administration of Peg-IFN to mice placed on a choline-deficient diet. There were concomitant changes in apoptosis and differentiation markers.[264]

The global impression from studies reporting beneficial effects of antiviral therapy of CHC on development of HCC is that SVR confers at least 80% protection (Table 5) [reviewed in Refs. 3,237–240;254–258]. Non-SVR can be divided into complete non-response or null response (NR), when no substantial reduction in viral load is observed during 12 weeks of treatment, and various types of partial response;[28,237,238] the latter include post-treatment relapse, viral breakthrough during treatment, and more than 2 log reduction in serum HCV RNA titre at week 12 but with still detectable HCV RNA. Earlier data indicate a reduced risk of HCC in the response/relapse category compared with NR and untreated

Table 5. Effect of antiviral treatment on development of HCC in chronic hepatitis C patients.

Author (Year)[Ref.]	No. treated or followed	Median follow-up (yrs)	Agent(s) used	SVR	*Developed Response/ relapse	HCC Nonresponders	Untreated	Liver histology
Benvegnu (1998)[250]	88	6	IFN		!5.6%		27%	Cirrhosis
Imai (1998)[242]	419	4	IFN	0.7%	5.8%	14%	12%	20% cirrhosis
Kasahara (1998)[256]	1022	7	IFN	1.6%	3%	7.9%	NS	NS: ?~10% cirrhosis
Okanoue (1999)[254]	1148	2.7	IFN	1%	3%	7%	NS	F3 636; cirrhosis 40
Takimoto (2002)[257]	652	4.5	IFN	0.3%	0.75%	2.3%	NS	NS
Kashigawi (2003)[258]	351	5.7	IFN	1.5%	NS	8.2%	NS	NS
Coverdale (2004)[154]	384	9.4	IFN	2%	4%	11%	10%	~25% with F3 or cirrhosis
Shiratori (2005)[187]	345	6.8	IFN	17%	!!31%	!!31%	47%	All cirrhosis
Hung (2006)[252]	132	3	IFN	6.8%	NS	26%	NS	All cirrhosis

(*Continued*)

Table 5. *(Continued)*

Author (Year)Ref.	No. treated or followed	Median follow-up (yrs)	Agent(s) used	SVR	*Developed HCC Response/ relapse	Nonresponders	Untreated	Liver histology
Yu (2006)[259]	1,619	5	IFN(1057), IFN/ Ribavirin (760)	1.7%	NS	11%	9.6%	NS
Cardoso (2010)[239]	307	3.5	PegIFN/ ribavirin	1.24/100 person-years	!!5.85/100 person-years	!!5.85/100 person-years	NR	F3 127; cirrhosis 180
Morgan (2010)[196]	#526	7	PegIFN/ ribavirin	1.4%	6.5%	9.1%	NR	~30% cirrhosis

*Data (%) are the proportion of those in stated treatment outcome group.
!In this study, the only comparison was treatment vs no treatment
!!Note, in these studies, response was only characterized as SVR or non-SVR
#All previous non-SVR to IFN or IFN/ribavirin
IFN, interferon. NS, not stated. NR, not relevant (not included in this study)

cases (Table 5), but these data are mostly limited to retrospective cohort observations. Japanese cases designated as biochemical but not virological responders might fall into a similar category.[162,184,185,208,209,230,254]

Risk factors for HCC after sustained viral response

Instances of HCC developing after SVR are confined to a few hundred cases [reviewed in Ref. 147] (Table 5), which compares favorably with the rate of 3–6% per annum in untreated CHC-cirrhosis or non-responders to antiviral therapy.[187,256–258] These cases involve men aged 65 years or older, are reported more commonly from Japan, and patients are more likely to have had cirrhosis and poor liver function at the time of treatment.[148,162,202,203] Continued ALT elevation, a life-time history of alcohol abuse, occult HBV infection, diabetes or obesity are other risk factors.[148,162,202,203] An implication for clinical practice is that SVR to antiviral therapy should not be regarded as 100% protective against development of HCC. Continued surveillance for early onset of HCC is indicated, particularly among older men with other risk factors.[147]

Long-term IFN treatment fails to prevent HCC

Despite the experimental and putative anti-hepatocarcinogenic effects of Peg-IFN, continued administration of this agent to patients without SVR fails to reduce HCC risk. Three large multicentre studies confirm that for those with non-SVR to earlier antiviral therapy, long-term Peg-IFN has no beneficial effects and should no be used in this high risk group for HCC.[265,266] Instead, results with triple therapy are more encouraging for obtaining an anti-viral response, as discussed later.

Treatment of HCV infection prevents HCC recurrence after surgery

There have been attempts to prevent recurrence of HCC after hepatic resection, and particularly to avert the development of new cancers after more than 1 year of follow-up. The most studied approach has been use of interferon and other antiviral agents;[267–275] reviewed in Refs. 240,274,275.

For CHC, there have been several RCTs (Table 6) and one meta-analysis[275] of IFN therapy after resection of HCC. Such treatment confers considerable efficacy against late recurrence of HCC (Table 6) after either ablation or surgical resection of a "curable" HCC (OR 0.26). Eradication of HCV (SVR) appears to be important for this beneficial effect of preventing development of new HCCs,[275] and there is now strong evidence that this prolongs survival (OR 0.31).[275]

The only other agents with reported efficacy against HCC recurrence after surgical resection are acyclic retinoids and vitamin K analogs.[276–279] Their mechanism of action is not related to suppression of necroinflammatory activity. After 1 year of use, the protective efficacy is prolonged for several years.[275] Development of these agents appears to be have been discontinued, possibly because of a high rate of adverse effects.

Future perspectives and outstanding challenges

Preventing HCV infection is an important step towards prevention of HCC. Transmission in healthcare settings is now entirely preventable and therefore is unacceptable,[285] but the biggest challenge is vaccine development because the primary mode of HCV spread is now IDU. On the other hand, effective antiviral therapy of CHC substantially reduces HCC risk, even at the stage of cirrhosis.[286] The results of phase 3 studies of new direct antiviral agents, such as the NS3/4 protease inhibitors, telaprevir and boceprevir, in combination with Peg-IFN and ribavirin (triple therapy) indicate improved efficacy for SVR against HCV genotype 1 infections.[287,288] This efficacy extends to re-treatment of cases with non-SVR; ~50% obtained SVR after 24 weeks of triple therapy, versus only 15% for Peg-IFN/ribavirin retreatment.[289] Even patients with previous NR to antiviral therapy had ~25% SVR after re-treatment with Peg-IFN/ribavirin/telaprevir, and similar results have recently been published with Peg-IFN/ribavirin/boceprevir. Since this group of HCV genotype 1 patients often have cirrhosis and are at particularly high risk of HCC, it will be important to document whether effective antiviral treatment at this late stage reduces liver cancer risk. At another end of the spectrum, the efficacy of triple therapy for SVR in treatment-naïve genotype 1 CHC is in the range of 60–70%,[287,288] inferring improved potential for protection against hepatocarcinogenesis.

Table 6. Efficacy of interferon treatment in preventing late recurrence of HCC after ablation or surgical resection.

Author (year)[Ref.]	Total, or number treated vs untreated	Treatment course	Median follow-up (yrs)	Outcomes
Ikeda (2000)[267]	10 vs 10	IFNβ 6 MIU 2/wk for 36 mo	2.8	Reduced recurrence
Miyaguchi (2002)[272]	22 vs 24	IFNα 3 MIU 3/wk 16 wk	1	Reduced recurrence and improved survival
Kubo (2002)[273]	15 vs 15	IFNα 6 MIU/d 2 wk, then 2–3/wk 88 wk	2	Reduced late recurrence and improved survival
Mazzaferro (2006)[268]	80	IFNα (3 MIU, 3/wk) 48 wk	4	Reduced late recurrence
Nishiguchi (2005)[269]	15 vs 15	IFNα 6 MIU/d 2 wk, then 2–3/wk 88 wk	2	Reduced recurrence and improved survival
Lin (2004)[270]	13	IFNα 3 MIU, various frequency, to 18 mo	2	Reduced 1 and 4 yr recurrence
Shirotori (2003)[271]	49 vs 25	IFNα 6 MIU 3/wk 48 wk	7	(Ablation therapy) Improved long-term survival; no effect on first recurrence
Suou (2001)[280]	18 vs 22	IFNα, total dose 480 MIU	4	SVR 33%; reduced recurrence
Hung (2005)[281]	20 vs 40	IFN/ribavirin 6–12 mo	3	SVR 50%; reduced recurrence
Sagaguchi (2005)[282]	24 vs 33	IFNα, total dose 504 MIU	4	SVR 4%; reduced recurrence
Jeong (2007)[283]	42 vs 42	IFNα, total dose 480 MIU	7	SVR 69%; reduced recurrence
Kudo (2007)[284]	43 vs 84	IFNα and Peg-IFN, total dose 1320 MIU	5	SVR 5%; reduced recurrence

See Meta-analysis by Singal *et al.*[295] for more detailed analysis of survival and overall efficacy.

For overall prevention of HCV-related HCC, a priority is to identify cases of both acute and chronic hepatitis C in the community and consider intervention with curative antiviral therapy before development of chronic HCV infection (in acute cases),[290,291] or chronic HCV infection before advanced cirrosis evolves. Curbing co-morbidity from heavy drinking, overweight/insulin resistance and cigarette smoking should also slow disease progression and HCC risk for HCV-infected persons. Another desirable development would be to design pharmacological approaches to interrupt hepatocarcinogenesis in damaged and inflamed livers infected with HCV. However, logical approaches to the design of such chemoprevention requires an improved understanding of the multistep development of primary liver cancer. In particular, we need to learn how chronic liver inflammation occurs in HCV infection, how viral proteins coupled to the inflammatory response promote proliferation and de-differentiation of altered hepatocytes, and how this leads to disordered elimination of damaged cells and/or expansion of hepatic precursor cells.

Acknowledgements

The author is grateful to Betty Rooney, Derrick vanRooyen and Narci Teoh for assistance with preparation of the manuscript.

References

1. Yuen MF, Hou JL, Chutaputti A. (2009) Asia Pacific Working Party on Prevention of Hepatocellular Carcinoma. Hepatocellular carcinoma in the Asia Pacific region. *J Gastroenterol Hepatol* **24**:346–53.
2. Lim SG, Mohammed R, Yuen MF *et al.* (2009) Prevention of hepatocellular carcinoma in hepatitis B virus infection. *J Gastroenterol Hepatol* **24**:1352–7.
3. Ueno Y, Sollano JD, Farrell GC. (2009) Prevention of hepatocellular carcinoma complicating chronic hepatitis C. *J Gastroenterol Hepatol* **24**:531–6.
4. Law MG, Dore GJ, Bath N *et al.* (2003) Modelling hepatitis C virus incidence, prevalence and long-term sequelae in Australia, 2001. *Int J Epidemiol* **32**:725–6.

5. Davis GL, Alter MJ, El-Serag H *et al.* (2010) Aging of hepatitis C virus (HCV)-infected persons in the United States: A multiple cohort model of HCV prevalence and disease progression. *Gastroenterology* **138**:513–21.
6. Saito I, Miyamura T, Ohbayashi A *et al.* (1990) Hepatitis C virus infection is associated with the development of hepatocellular carcinoma. *Proc Natl Acad Sci USA* **87**:6547–9.
7. Tanaka Y, Hanaka K, Mizokami M *et al.* (2002) A comparison of the molecular clock of hepatitis C virus in the United States and Japan predicts that hepatocellular carcinoma incidence in the United States will increase over the next two decades. *Proc Natl Acad Sci USA* **99**:15584–9.
8. Tanaka H, Imai Y, Hiramatsu K *et al.* (2008) Declining incidence of hepatocellular carcinoma in Osaka, Japan, from 1990 to 2003. *Ann Intern Med* **148**:820–6.
9. Takata A, Kuromatsur R, Ando E *et al.* (2010) HCC develops even in the early stage of chronic liver disease in elderly patients with HCV infection. *Int J Mol Med* **26**:249–56.
10. Deuffic-Burban S, Deltenre P, Louvet A *et al.* (2008) Impact of viral eradication on mortality related to hepatitis C: A modelling approach in France. *J Hepatol* **49**:175–83.
11. Tong MJ, El-Farra NS, Reikes AR *et al.* (1995) Clinical outcomes after transfusion-associated hepatitis C. *N Engl J Med* **332**:1463–6.
12. Thomas DL, Seeff LB. (2005) Natural history of hepatitis C. *Clin Liver Dis* **9**:383–98.
13. Alter MJ. (2007) Epidemiology of hepatitis C virus infection. *World J Gastroenterol* **13**:2436–41.
14. Dore GJ, Freeman AJ, Law M *et al.* (2002) Is severe liver disease a common outcome for people with chronic hepatitis C? *J Gastroenterol Hepatol* **17**:423–30.
15. Sweeting MJ, De Angelis D, Neal KR *et al.* (2006) Estimated progression rates in three United Kingdom hepatitis C cohorts differed according to method of recruitment. *J Clin Epidemiol* **59**:144–52.
16. Purcell R. (1997) The hepatitis C virus: Overview. *Hepatology* **26**:11S–14S.
17. Burlone ME, Budkowska A. (2009) Hepatitis C virus cell entry: Role of lipoproteins and cellular receptors. *J Gen Virol* **90**:1055–70.
18. Saito S, Heller T, Yoneda M *et al.* (2007) Lifestyle-related diseases of the digestive system: A new in vitro model of hepatitis C virion production:

Application of basic research on hepatitis C virus to clinical medicine. *J Pharm Sci* **105**:138–44.

19. Liang TJ, Heller T. (2004) Pathogenesis of hepatitis C-associated hepatocellular carcinoma. *Gastroenterology* **127**:S62–S71.
20. Berasin C, Castillo J, Perugorria MJ *et al.* (2009) Inflammation and liver cancer: New molecular links. *Ann NY Acad Sci* **1155**:206–21.
21. Kasprzak A, Adamek A. (2008) Role of hepatitis C virus proteins (C, NS3, NS5A) in hepatitis oncogenesis. *Hepatol Res* **38**:1–26.
22. Fung J, Lai CL, Yuen MF. (2009) Hepatitis B and C virus-related carcinogenesis. *Eur Soc Clin Micro Infect Dis* **15**:964–70.
23. Castello G, Scala S, Palmieri G *et al.* (2010) HCV-related hepatocellular carcinoma: From chronic inflammation to cancer. *Clin Immunol* **134**:237–50.
24. Zein NN. (2000) Clinical significance of hepatitis C virus genotypes. *Clin Microbiol Rev* **13**:223–35.
25. Simmonds P, Bukh J, Combet C *et al.* (2005) Consensus proposals for a unified system of nomenclature of hepatitis C virus genotypes. *Hepatology* **42**:962–73.
26. Hui JM, Kench J, Farrell GC *et al.* (2002) Genotype-specific mechanisms for hepatic steatosis in chronic hepatitis C infection. *J Gastroenterol Hepatol* **17**:873–81.
27. Negro F, Sanyal AJ. (2009) Hepatitis C virus, steatosis and lipid abnormalities: Clinical and pathogenic data. *Liver Int* **29**(Suppl 2):13–25.
28. Teoh NC, Farrell GC, Chan HLY. (2010) Individualisation of antiviral therapy for chronic hepatitis C. *J Gastroenterol Hepatol* **25**:1206–16.
29. Mercer DF, Schiller DE, Elliott JF *et al.* (2001) Hepatitis C virus replication in mice with chimeric human livers. *Nat Med* **7**:927–33.
30. Chayama K, Hayes CN, Hiraga N *et al.* (2010) Animal model for study of human hepatitis viruses. *J Gastroenterol Hepatol* **26**:13–8.
31. Bissig KD, Wieland SF, Tran P *et al.* (2010) Toward small animal models for the study of human hepatitis viruses. *J Clin Invest* **120**:924–30.
32. Krieger N, Lohmann V, Bartenschlager R. (2001) Enhancement of hepatitis C virus RNA replication by cell culture-adaptive mutations. *J Virol* **75**:1437–49.
33. Blight KJ, McKeating JA, Marcotrigiano J *et al.* (2003) Efficient replication of hepatitis C virus genotype 1a RNAs in cell culture. *J Virol* **77**:3181–90.

34. Heller T, Saito S, Auerbach J *et al.* (2005) An *in vitro* model of hepatitis C virion production. *Proc Natl Acad Sci USA* **102**:2579–83.
35. Wakita T, Pietschmann T, Kato T *et al.* (2005) Production of infectious hepatitis C virus in tissue culture from a cloned viral genome. *Nat Med* **11**:791–6.
36. Lindenbach BD, Meuleman P, Ploss A *et al.* (2006) Cell culture-grown hepatitis C virus is infectious *in vivo* and can be recultured *in vitro*. *Proc Natl Acad Sci USA* **103**:3805–9.
37. Lindenbach BD, Evans MJ, Syder AJ *et al.* (2005) Complete replication of hepatitis C virus in cell culture. *Science* **309**:623–6.
38. Yi M, Villanueva RA, Thomas DL *et al.* (2006) Production of infectious genotype 1a hepatitis C virus (Hutchinson strain) in cultured human hepatoma cells. *Proc Natl Acad Sci USA* **103**:2310–5.
39. Kato T, Matsumura T, Heller T *et al.* (2007) Production of infectious hepatitis C virus of various genotypes in cell cultures. *J Virol* **81**:4405–11.
40. Lázaro CA, Chang M, Tan W *et al.* (2007) Hepatitis C virus replication in transfected and serum-infected cultured human fetal hepatocytes. *Am J Pathol* **170**:478–89.
41. Tang W, Lázaro CA, Campbell JS *et al.* (2007) Responses of non-transformed human hepatocytes to conditional expression of full-length hepatitis C virus open reading frame. *Am J Pathol* **171**:1831–46.
42. Kato T, Furusaka A, Miyamoto M *et al.* (2001) Sequence analysis of hepatitis C virus isolated from a fulminant hepatitis patient. *J Med Virol* **64**:334–9.
43. Harris HJ, Davis C, Mullins JGL *et al.* (2010) Claudin asscociation with CD81 defines hepatitis C virus entry. *J Biol Chem* **10**:1–15.
44. Evans MJ, von Hahn T, Tscherne DM *et al.* (2007) Claudin-1 is a hepatitis C virus co-receptor required for a late step in entry. *Nature* **446**:801–5.
45. Kapadia SB, Barth H, Baumert T *et al.* (2007) Initiation of hepatitis C virus infection is dependent on cholesterol and cooperativity between CD81 and scavenger receptor B type 1. *J Virol* **81**:374–83.
46. Rehermann B. (2009) Hepatitis C virus versus innate and adaptive immune responses: A tale of coevolution and coexistence. *J Clin Invest* **119**:1745–54.
47. Bowen DG, Walker CM. (2005) Adaptive immune responses in acute and chronic hepatitis virus infection. *Nature* **436**:946–52.

48. Hiroishi K, Ito T, Imawari M. (2008) Immune responses in hepatitis C virus infection and mechanisms of hepatitis C virus persistence. *J Gastroenterol Hepatol* **23**:1473–82.
49. Dolganiuc A, Oak S, Kodys K *et al.* (2004) Hepatitis C core and non-structural proteins trigger toll-like receptor 2-mediated pathways and inflammatory activation. *Gastroenterology* **127**:1513–24.
50. Hoffmann M, Zeisel MB, Jilg N *et al.* (2009) Toll-like receptor 2 senses hepatitis C virus core protein but not infectious viral particles. *J Innate Immun* **1**:446–54.
51. Sillanpää M, Kaukinen P, Melén K *et al.* (2008) Hepatitis C virus proteins interfere with the activation of chemokine gene promoters and downregulate chemokine gene expression. *J Gen Virol* **89**:432–43.
52. Ciccaglione AR, Stellacci E, Marcantonio C *et al.* (2007) Repression of interferon regulatory factor 1 by hepatitis C core protein results in inhibition of antiviral and immunomodulatory genes. *J Virol* **81**:202–14.
53. Lin W, Kim SS, Yeung E *et al.* (2006) Hepatitis C virus core protein blocks interferon signalling by interaction with the STAT1 SH2 domain. *J Virol* **80**:9226–35.
54. Miller K, McArdle S, Gale MJ Jr *et al.* (2004) Effects of the hepatitis C virus core protein on innate cellular defense pathways. *J Interferon Cytokine Res* **24**:391–402.
55. Lin W, Choe WH, Hiasa Y *et al.* (2005) Hepatitis C virus expression suppresses interferon signalling by degrading STAT1. *Gastroenterology* **128**:1034–41.
56. Kanda T, Steele R, Ray R *et al.* (2007) Hepatitis C virus infection induces the beta interferon signaling pathway in immortalized human hepatocytes. *J Virol* **81**:12375–81.
57. Dolganiuc A, Kodys K, Kopasz A *et al.* (2003) Hepatitis C virus core and non-structural protein 3 proteins induce pro-and anti-inflammatory cytokines and inhibit dendritic cell differentiation. *J Immunol* **70**:5615–24.
58. Dolganiuc A, Chang S, Kodys K *et al.* (2006) Hepatitis C virus (HCV) core protein-induced, monocyte-mediated mechanisms of reduced IFN-alpha and plasmacytoid dendritic cell loss in chronic hepatitis C. *J Immunol* **177**:6758–68.
59. Jinushi M, Takehara T, Tatsumi T *et al.* (2004) Negative regulation of NK cell activities by inhibitory receptor CD94/NKG2A leads to altered NK

cell-induced modulation of dendritic cell functions in chronic hepatitis C virus infection. *J Immunol* **173**:6072–81.
60. Thomas DL, Thio CL, Martin MP *et al.* (2009) Genetic variation in IL28B and spontaneous clearance of hepatitis C virus. *Nature* **461**: 798–801.
61. Gerlach JT, Diepolder HM, Jung MC *et al.* (1999) Recurrence of hepatitis C virus after loss of virus-specific CD4+ T-cell response in acute hepatitis. *Gastroenterology* **117**:933–41.
62. Nascimbeni M, Mizukoshi E, Bosmann M *et al.* (2003) Kinetics of CD4+ and CD8+ memory T-cell responses during hepatitis C virus rechallenge of previously recovered chimpanzees. *J Virol* **77**:4781–93.
63. Wedemeyer H, He XS, Nascimbeni M *et al.* (2002) Impaired effector function of hepatitis C virus-specific CD8+ T cells in chronic hepatitis C virus infection. *J Immunol* **169**:3447–58.
64. Sundström S, Ota S, Dimberg LY *et al.* (2005) Hepatitis C virus core protein induces an anergic state characterized by decreased interleukin-2 production and perturbation of mitogen-activated protein kinase responses. *J Virol* **79**:2230–9.
65. Yao ZQ, Eisen-Vandervelde A, Waggoner SN *et al.* (2004) Direct binding of hepatitis C virus core to gC1qR on CD4+ and CD8+ T cells leads to impaired activation of Lck and Akt. *J Virol* **78**:6409–19.
66. Accapezzato D, Francavilla V, Paroli M *et al.* (2004) Hepatic expansion of a virus-specific regulatory CD8(+) T cell population in chronic hepatitis C virus infection. *J Clin Invest* **113**:963–72.
67. Kanda T, Steele R, Ray R *et al.* (2009) Inhibition of intrahepatic gamma interferon production by hepatitis C virus non-structural protein 5A in transgenic mice. *J Virol* **83**:8463–9.
68. Cox AL, Mosbruger T, Mao Q *et al.* (2005) Cellular immune selection with hepatitis C virus persistence in humans. *J Exp Med* **201**:1741–52.
69. Urbani S, Amadei B, Tola D *et al.* (2006) PD-1 expression in acute hepatitis C virus (HCV) infection is associated with HCV-specific CD8 exhaustion. *J Virol* **80**:11398–403.
70. Nakamoto N, Kaplan DE, Coleclough J *et al.* (2008) Functional restoration of HCV-specific CD8 T cells by PD-1 blockade is defined by PD-1 expression and compartmentalization. *Gastroenterology* **134**:1927–37.

71. Auffermann-Gretzinger S, Keeffe EB, Levy S. (2001) Impaired dendritic cell maturation in patients with chronic, but not resolved, hepatitis C virus infection. *Blood* **97**:3171–6.
72. Roche B, Samuel D. (2007) Risk factors for hepatitis C recurrence after liver transplantation. *J Viral Hepat* **14**:89–96.
73. Shackel NA, Jamias J, Rahman W *et al.* (2009) Early high peak hepatitis C viral load levels independently predict hepatitis C-related liver failure post-liver transplantation. *Liver Tanspl* **15**:709–18.
74. Clouston AD, Powell EE, Walsh MJ *et al.* (2005) Fibrosis correlates with a ductular reaction in hepatitis C: Roles of impaired replication, progenitor cells and steatosis. *Hepatology* **41**:809–18.
75. Li K, Prow T, Lemon SM *et al.* (2002) Cellular response to conditional expression of hepatitis C virus core protein in Juj7 cultured human hepatoma cells. *Hepatology* **35**:1237–46.
76. Park CY, Jun HJ, Wakita T *et al.* (2009) Hepatitis C virus non-structural 4B protein modulates sterol regulatory element-binding protein signalling via the Akt pathway. *J Biol Chem* **284**:9237–46.
77. Shintani Y, Fjuie H, Miyoshi H *et al.* (2004) Hepatitis C virus infection and diabetes: Direct involvement with the virus in the development of insulin resistance. *Gastroenterology* **126**:840–8.
78. Pazienza V, Clément S, Pugnale P *et al.* (2007) The hepatitis C virus core protein of genotypes 3a and 1b downregulates insulin receptor substrate 1 through genotype-specific mechanisms. *Hepatology* **45**:1164–71.
79. Pazienza V, Clément S, Pugnale P *et al.* (2009) Gene expression profile of Huh-7 cells expressing hepatitis C virus genotype 1b or 3a core proteins. *Liver Int* **29**:661–9.
80. Banerjee A, Saito K, Ait-Goughoulte M *et al.* (2008) Hepatitis C virus core protein upregulates serine phosphorylation of insulin receptor substrate-1 and impairs the downstream akt/protein kinase B signalling pathway for insulin resistance. *J Virol* **82**:2606–12.
81. Banerjee A, Meyeer K, Mazumdar B *et al.* (2010). Hepatitis C virus differentially modulates activation of forkhead transcription factors and insulin-induced metabolic gene expression. *J Virology* **84**:5936–46.
82. Yao ZQ, Prayther D, Trabue C *et al.* (2008). Differential regulation of SOCS-1 signalling in B and T lymphocytes by hepatitis C virus core protein. *Immunology* **125**:197–207.

83. Milner KL, van der Poorten D, Trenell M *et al.* (2010) Chronic hepatitis C is associated with peripheral rather than hepatic insulin resistance. *Gastroenterology* **138**:932–41.
84. Wang T, Weinman SA. (2006) Causes and consequences of mitochondrial reactive oxygen species generation in hepatitis C. *J Gastroenterol Hepatol* **21**:S34–S7.
85. Li Y, Boehning DF, Qian T *et al.* (2007) Hepatitis C virus core protein increases mitochondrial ROS production by stimulation of Ca2+ uniporter activity. *FASEB J* **21**:2474–85.
86. Dionisio N, Garcia-Mediavilla MV, Sanchez-Campos S *et al.* (2009) Hepatitis C virus NS5A and core proteins induce oxidative-mediated calcium signalling alterations in hepatocytes. *J Hepatol* **50**:872–82.
87. Singh R, Czaja MJ. (2007) Regulation of hepatocyte apoptosis by oxidative stress. *J Gastroenterol Hepatol* **22**(Suppl 1):S45–S8.
88. Garcia-Ruiz C, Fernandez-Checa JC. (2007) Redox regulation of hepatocyte apoptosis. *J Gastroenterol Hepatol* **22**(Suppl 1):S38–S42.
89. Tsutsumi T, Suzuke T, Moriya K *et al.* (2003) Hepatitis C virus core protein activates ERK and p38 MAPK in cooperation with ethanol in transgenic mice. *Hepatology* **38**:820–8.
90. Hoeijmakers JK. (2009) DNA damage, aging and cancer. *N Engl J Med* **361**:1475–85.
91. Nishimura T, Nishida N, Komeda T *et al.* (2006) Genotype stability and clonal evolution of hepatocellular carcinoma assessed by autopsy-based genome-wide microsatellite analysis. *Cancer Genet Cytogenet* **161**:164–9.
92. Ray RB, Ray R. (2001) Hepatitis C virus core protein: Intriguing properties and functional relevance. *FEMS Microbiol Lett* **202**:149–56.
93. Teoh NC. (2010) Pre-"EMT"ing key processes in liver carcinogenesis: Growing evidence for how malignant hepatocytes invade and conquer. *Hepatology* **51**:384–8.
94. Tsuchihara K, Hijikata M, Fukuda K *et al.* (1999) Hepatitis C virus core protein regulates cell growth and signal transduction pathway transmitting growth stimuli. *Virology* **258**:100–7.
95. Spaziani A, Alisi A, Sanna D *et al.* (2006) Role of p38 MAPK and RNA-dependent protein kinase (PKR) in hepatitis C virus core-dependent nuclear delocalization of cyclin B1. *J Biol Chem* **281**:10983–9.

96. Giambartolomei S, Covone F, Levrero M *et al.* (2001) Sustained activation of the Raf/MEK/Erk pathway in response to EGF in stable cell lines expressing the hepatitis C virus (HCV) core protein. *Oncogene* **20**:2606–10.
97. Erhardt A, Hassan A, Heintges T *et al.* (2002) Hepatitis C virus core protein induces cell proliferation and activates ERK, JNK and p38 MAP kinases together with the MAP kinase phosphatase MKP-1 in a HepG2 Tet-Off cell line. *Virology* **292**:272–84.
98. Hayashi J, Aoki H, Moriyama M *et al.* (2000) Hepatitis C virus core protein activates the MAPK/ERK cascade synergistically with tumor promoter TPA, but not with epidermal growth factor or transforming growth factor alpha. *Hepatology* **32**:958–61.
99. Shimotohno K, Watashi K, Tsuchihara K *et al.* (2002) Hepatitis C virus and its roles in cell proliferation. *J Gastroenterol* **37**:S50–S4.
100. He G, Yu GY, Temkin V *et al.* (2010) Hepatocyte IKKbeta/NF-kappaB inhibits tumor promotion and progression by preventing oxidative stress-driven STAT3 activation. *Cancer Cell* **17**:286–97.
101. Naugler WE, Sakurai T, Kim S *et al.* (2007) Gender disparity in liver cancer due to sex differences in MyD88-dependent IL-6 production. *Science* **317**:121–4.
102. Park EJ, Lee JH, Yu GY *et al.* (2010) Dietary and genetic obesity promote liver inflammation and tumorigenesis by enhancing IL-6 and TNF expression. *Cell* **140**:197–208.
103. Shrivastava A, Manna SK, Ray R *et al.* (1998) Ectopic expression of hepatitis C virus core protein differentially regulates nuclear transcription factors. *J Virol* **72**:9722–8.
104. Fukutomi T, Zhou Y, Kawai S *et al.* (2005) Hepatitis C virus core protein stimulates hepatocyte growth: Correlation with upregulation of wnt-1 expression. *Hepatology* **41**:1096–105.
105. Ray RB, Meyer K, Ray R. (2000) Hepatitis C virus core protein promotes immortalization of primary human hepatocytes. *Virology* **271**:197–204.
106. Basu A, Meyer K, Lai KK *et al.* (2006) Microarray analyses and molecular profiling of Stat 3 signaling pathway induced by hepatitis C virus core protein in human hepatocytes. *Virology* **349**:347–58.
107. Hosui A, Takehara T, Ohkawa K *et al.* (2006) Suppressive effect on hepatocyte differentiation of hepatitis C virus core protein. *Biochem Biophys Res Commun* **346**:1125–30.

108. Kanda T, Steele R, Ray R *et al.* (2008) Hepatitis C virus core protein augments androgen receptor mediated signalling. *J Virol* **82**:11066–72.
109. Ray RB, Steele R, Meyer K *et al.* (1998) Hepatitis C virus core protein represses p21WAF1/Cip1/Sid1 promoter activity. *Gene* **208**:231–6.
110. Cheng PL, Chang MH, Chao CH *et al.* (2004) Hepatitis C viral proteins interact with Smad3 and differentially regulate TGF-beta/Smad3-mediated transcriptional activation. *Oncogene* **23**:7821–38.
111. Pavio N, Battaglia S, Boucreux D *et al.* (2005) Hepatitis C virus core variants isolated from liver tumor but not from adjacent non-tumor tissue interact with Smad3 and inhibit the TGF-beta pathway. *Oncogene* **24**:6119–32.
112. Battaglia S, Benzoubir N, Nobilet S *et al.* (2009) Liver cancer-derived hepatitis C virus core proteins shift TGF-beta responses from tumor suppression to epithelial-mesenchymal transition. *PLoS One* **4**:e4355.
113. Hassan M, Selimovic D, Ghozlan H *et al.* (2009) Hepatitis C virus core protein triggers hepatic angiogenesis mechanism including multiple pathways. *Hepatology* **49**:1469–82.
114. Ray RB, Meyer K, Steele R *et al.* (1998) Inhibition of tumor necrosis factor (TNF)-alpha-mediated apoptosis by hepatitis C virus core protein. *J Biol Chem* **273**:2256–9.
115. Saito K, Meyer K, Warner R *et al.* (2006) Hepatitis C virus core protein inhibits tumor necrosis factor alpha-mediated apoptosis by a protective effect involving cellular FLICE inhibitory protein. *J Virol* **80**:4372–9.
116. Meyer K, Basu A, Saito K *et al.* (2005) Inhibition of hepatitis C virus core protein expression in immortalized human hepatocytes induces cytochrome c-independent increase in Apaf-1 and caspase-9 activation for cell death. *Virology* **336**:198–207.
117. Banerjee A, Saito K, Meyer K *et al.* (2009) Hepatitis C core protein and cellular protein HAX-1 promote 5-flurouracil-mediated hepatocyte growth inhibition. *J Virol* **83**:9663–71.
118. Chou AH, Tsai HF, Wu YY *et al.* (2005) Hepatitis C virus core protein modulates TRAIL-mediated apoptosis by enhancing Bid cleavage and activation of mitochondria apoptosis signalling pathway. *J Immunol* **174**:2160–6.
119. Majumder M, Ghosh AK, Steele R *et al.* (2001) Hepatitis C virus NS5A physically associates with p53 and regulates p21/waf1 gene expression in a p53-dependent manner. *J Virol* **75**:1401–7.

120. Ghosh AK, Steele R, Meyer K *et al.* (1999) Hepatitis C virus NS5A protein modulates cell cycle regulated genes and promotes cell growth. *J Gen Virol* **80**:1179–83.
121. Sarcar B, Ghosh AK, Steele R *et al.* (2004) Hepatitis C virus NS5A mediated STAT3 activation requires co-operation of Jak1 kinase. *Virology* **322**:51–60.
122. Ghosh AK, Majumder M, Steele R *et al.* (2000) Hepatitis C virus NS5A protein protects against TNF-alpha mediated apoptotic cell death. *Virus Res* **67**:173–8.
123. Majumder M, Ghosh AK, Steele R *et al.* (2002) Hepatitis C virus NS5A protein impairs TNF-mediated hepatic apoptosis, but not by an anti-FAS antibody, in transgenic mice. *Virology* **294**:94–105.
124. Moriya K, Fujie H, Shintani Y *et al.* (1998) The core protein of hepatitis C virus induces hepatocellular carcinoma in transgenic mice. *Nat Med* **4**:1065–7.
125. Koike K. (2007) Hepatitis C virus contributes to hepatocarcinogenesis by modulating metabolic and intracellular signalling pathway. *J Gastroenterol Hepatol* **22**:S108–S11.
126. Lerat H, Honda M, Beard MR *et al.* (2002) Steatosis and liver cancer in transgenic mice expressing the structural and non-structural proteins of hepatitis C virus. *Gastroenterology* **122**:352–65.
127. Furutani T, Hino K, Okuda M *et al.* (2006) Hepatic iron overload induced hepatocellular carcinoma in transgenic mice expressing the hepatitis C virus polyprotein. *Gastroenterology* **130**:2087–98.
128. Moriya K, Nakagawa K, Santa T *et al.* (2001) Oxidative stress in the absence of inflammation in a mouse model for hepatitis C virus-associated hepatocarcinogenesis. *Cancer Res* **61**:4365–70.
129. Tanaka N, Moriya K, Kiyosawa K *et al.* (2008) PPARα activation is essential for HCV core protein-induced hepatic steatosis and hepatocellular carcinoma in mice. *J Clin Invest* **118**:683–93.
130. Klopstock N, Katzenellenbogen M, Pappo O *et al.* (2009) HCV tumor promoting effect is dependent on host genetic background. *PLoS One* **4**:e5025.
131. Tsutsumi T, Suzuka T, Moriya K *et al.* (2002) Alteration of intrahepatic cytokine expression and AP-1 activation in transgenic mice expressing hepatitis C virus core protein. *Virology* **304**:415–24.

132. Chang ML, Yeh CT, Lin DY *et al.* (2009) Hepatic inflammation mediated by hepatitis C virus core protein is ameliorated by blocking complement activation. *BMC Med Genomics* **2**:51.
133. Majumder M, Steele R, Ghosh AK *et al.* (2003) Expression of hepatitis C virus non-structural 5A protein in the liver of transgenic mice. *FEBS Lett* **555**:528–32.
134. Koike K, Tsutsumi T, Miyoshi H *et al.* (2008) Molecular basis for the synergy between alcohol and hepatitis virus in hepatocarcinogenesis. *J Gastroenterol Hepatol* **23**:S87–S91.
135. Rigamonti C, Mottaran E, Reale E *et al.* (2003) Moderate alcohol consumption increases oxidative stress in patients with chronic hepatitis C. *Hepatology* **38**:42–9.
136. Machida K, Tsukamoto H, Mkrtchyan H *et al.* (2009) Toll-like receptor 4 mediates synergism between alcohol and HCV in hepatic oncogenesis involving stem cell marker Nanog. *Proc Natl Acad Sci U.S.A.* **106**:1548–53.
137. Brechot C. (1997) Hepatitis C virus 1b, cirrhosis and hepatocellular carcinoma. *Hepatology* **25**:772–4.
138. Bruno S, Crosignani A, Maisonneuve P *et al.* (2007) Hepatitis C virus genotype 1b as a major risk factor associated with hepatocellular carcinoma in patients with cirrhosis: A seventeen-year prospective cohort study. *Hepatology* **46**:1350–6.
139. Sheiner PA. (2000) Hepatitis C after liver transplantation. *Seminars in Liver Disease* **20**:201–9.
140. Raimondi S, Bruno S, Mondelli MU *et al.* (2009) Hepatitis C virus genotype 1b as a risk factor for hepatocellular carcinoma development: A meta-analysis. *Hepatology* **50**:1142–54.
141. Akuta N, Suzuki F, Kawamura Y *et al.* (2007) Amino acid substitutions in the hepatitis C virus core region are the important predictor of hepatocarcinogenesis. *Hepatology* **46**:1357–64.
142. Nakamoto S, Imazeki F, Jukai K *et al.* (2010) Association between mutations in the core region of hepatitis virus genotype 1 and hepatocellular carcinoma development. *J Hepatol* **52**:72–8.
143. Fukuhara T, Takeishi K, Toshima T *et al.* (2010) Impact of amino acid substitutions in the core region of HCV on multistep hepatocarcinogenesis. *Hepatol Res* **40**:171–8.

144. Nishise Y, Saito T, Sugarhara K *et al.* (2007) Risk of hepatocellular carcinoma and secondary structure of hepatitis C virus (HCV) NS3 protein amino-terminus, in patients infected with HCV subtype 1b. *J Infect Dis* **196**:1006–9.
145. Tanaka H, Tsukuma H, Yamano H *et al.* (1998) Hepatitis C virus 1b(II) infection and development of chronic hepatitis, liver cirrhosis and hepatocellular carcinoma: A case-control study in Japan. *J Epidemiol* **8**:244–9.
146. Donato F, Gelatti U, Chiesa R *et al.* (1999) A case-control study on family history of liver cancer as a risk factor for hepatocellular carcinoma in North Italy. Brescia HCC Study. *Cancer Causes Control* **10**:417–21.
147. Farrell GC. (1999) Hepatocellular carcinoma after sustained response to interferon in non-cirrhotic hepatitis C: Flaws in the cure, or a clue to the flaws? *J Gastroenterol Hepatol* **14**:833–7.
148. Ikeda K, Saitoh S, Arase Y *et al.* (1999) Effect of interferon therapy on hepatocellular carcinogenesis in patients with chronic hepatitis type C: A long-term observation study of 1,643 patients using statistical bias correction with proportional hazard analysis. *Hepatology* **29**:1124–30.
149. Honda M, Sakai A, Yamashita T *et al.* (2010) Hepatic ISG expression is associated with genetic variation in interleukin 28B and the outcome of IFN therapy for chronic hepatitis C. *Gastroenterology* **139**:499–509.
150. Tillmann HL, Thompson AJ, Patel K *et al.* (2010) A polymorphism near IL28B is associated with spontaneous clearance of acute hepatitis C virus and jaundice. *Gastroenterology* **139**:1586–92.
151. Tanaka Y, Nishida N, Sugiyama M *et al.* (2009) Genome-wide association of IL28B with response to pegylated interferon-alpha and ribavirin therapy for chronic hepatitis C. *Nat Genet* **41**: 1105–9.
152. Khan KN, Yatsuhashi H. (2000) Effect of alcohol consumption on the progression of hepatitis C virus infection and risk of hepatocellular carcinoma in Japanese patients. *Alcohol Alcohol* **35**: 286–95.
153. Donato F, Tagger A, Gelatti U *et al.* (2002) Alcohol and hepatocellular carcinoma: The effect of lifetime intake and hepatitis virus infections in men and women. *Am J Epidemiol* **155**:323–31.
154. Coverdale S, Khan M, Byth K *et al.* (2004) The effects of interferon treatment response on liver complications of chronic hepatitis C: 9-year follow-up study. *Am J Gastroenterol* **99**:636–44.

155. Khan MH, Thomas L, Byth K *et al.* (1998) How much does alcohol contribute to the variability of hepatic fibrosis in chronic hepatitis C? *J Gastroenterol Hepatol* **13**:419–426.
156. Ostapowicz G, Watson KJR, Locarnini SA *et al.* (1998) Role of alcohol in the progression of liver disease caused by hepatitis C virus infection. *Hepatology* **27**:1730–5.
157. Monto A, Patel K, Bostrom A *et al.* (2004) Risks of a range of alcohol intake on hepatitis C-related fibrosis. *Hepatology* **39**:826–34.
158. Hutchinson SJ, Bird SM, Goldberg DJ. (2005) Influence of alcohol on the progression of hepatitis C virus infection: A meta-analysis. *Clin Gastroneterol Hepatol* **11**:1150–9.
159. Dutta U, Byth K, Kench J *et al.* (1999) Risk factors for development of hepatocellular carcinoma among Australians with hepatitis C: a case-control study. *Aust NZ J Med* **29**:300–7.
160. Fan J-G, Farrell GC. (2009) The Asia-Pacific working party for prevention of hepatocellular carcinoma. Prevention of hepatocellular carcinoma in nonviral-related liver diseases. *J Gastroenterol Hepatol* **24**:712–9.
161. Vecchia CL. (2007) Alcohol and liver cancer. *Eur J Cancer Prev* **16**:495–7.
162. Iwasaki Y, Takaguchi K, Ikeda H *et al.* (2004) Risk factors for hepatocellular carcinoma in hepatitis C patients with sustained virologic response to interferon therapy. *Liver Int* **24**:603–10.
163. Hourigan LF, MacDonald GA, Purdie D *et al.* (1999) Fibrosis in chronic hepatitis C correlates significantly with body mass index and steatosis. *Hepatology* **29**:1215–9.
164. Patton HM, Patel K, Behling C *et al.* (2004) The impact of steatosis on disease progression and early and sustained treatment response in chronic hepatitis C patients. *J Hepatol* **40**:484–90.
165. Powell EE, Jonsson JR, Clouston AD. (2005) Steatosis: Co-factor in other liver diseases. *Hepatology* **42**:5–13.
166. Saunders D, Seidel D, Allison M *et al.* (2010) Systematic review: The association between obesity and hepatocellular carcinoma — epidemiological evidence. *Aliment Pharmacol Ther* **31**:1051–63.
167. Ohki T, Tateishi R, Sato T *et al.* (2008) Obesity is an independent risk factor for hepatocellular carcinoma development in chronic hepatitis C patients. *Clin Gastroenterol Hepatol* **6**:459–64.

168. Tanaka A, Uegaki S, Kurihara H *et al.* (2007) Hepatic steatosis as a possible risk factor for the development of hepatocellular carcinoma after eradication of hepatitis C virus with antiviral therapy in patients with chronic hepatitis C. *World J Gastroenterol* **21**:5180–7.
169. Mehta SH, Strathdee SA, Thomas DL. (2001) Association between hepatitis C virus infection and diabetes mellitus. *Epidemiologic Rev* **23**:302–13.
170. Mehta SH, Brancati FL, Strathdee SA *et al.* (2003) Hepatitis C virus infection and incident type 2 diabetes. *Hepatology* **38**:50–6.
171. Hui JM, Sud A, Farrell GC *et al.* (2003) Insulin resistance is associated with chronic hepatitis C virus infection and fibrosis progression. *Gastroenterology* **125**:1695–704.
172. Negro F, Clément S. (2009) Impact of obesity, steatosis and insulin resistance on progression and response to therapy of hepatitis C. *J Viral Hepat* **16**:681–8.
173. Veldt BJ, Chen W, Heathcote EJ *et al.* (2008) Increased risk of hepatocellular carcinoma among patients with hepatitis C cirrhosis and diabetes mellitus. *Hepatology* **47**:1856–62.
174. Lai MS, Hsieh MS, Chiu YH *et al.* (2006) Type 2 diabetes and hepatocellular carcinoma: A cohort study in high prevalence area of hepatitis virus infection. *Hepatology* **43**:1295–302.
175. Davila JA, Morgan RO, Shaib Y *et al.* (2005) Diabetes increases the risk of hepatocellular carcinoma in the United States: A population based case control study. *Gut* **54**:533–9.
176. El-Serag HB, Tran T, Everhart JE. (2004) Diabetes increases the risk of chronic liver disease and hepatocellular carcinoma. *Gastroenterology* **126**:460–8.
177. Starley BQ, Calcagno CJ, Harrison SA. (2010) Nonalcoholic fatty liver disease and hepatocellular carcinoma: A weighty connection. *Hepatology* **51**:1820–32.
178. Torisu Y, Ikeda K, Kobayashi M *et al.* (2007) Diabetes mellitus increases the risk of hepatocarcinogenesis in patients with alcohol cirrhosis: A preliminary report. *Hepatol Res* **37**:517–23.
179. Teoh NC, Fan JG. (2008) Diabetes mellitus and prognosis after curative therapy for hepatocellular carcinoma: Alas, still grave for those who are hyperglycemic. *J Gastroenterol* Hepatol **23**:1633–4.
180. Weltman MD, Brotodihardjo A, Crewe EB *et al.* (1995) Coinfection with hepatitis B & C or B, C & D viruses results in severe chronic liver disease and responds poorly to interferon-α treatment. *J Viral Hepatitis* **2**:39–45.

181. Gaeta GB, Precone DF, Cozzi-Lepri A *et al.* (2006) Multiple viral infections. *J Hepatology* **44**:S108–113.
182. Tagger A, Donato F, Ribero ML *et al.* (1999) Case-control study on hepatitis C virus (HCV) as a risk factor for hepatocellular carcinoma: the role of HCV genotypes and the synergism with hepatitis B virus and alcohol. Brescia HCC study. *Int J Cancer* **81**:695–9.
183. Donato F, Boffetta P, Puoti M. (1998) A meta-analysis of epidemiological studies on the combined effect of hepatitis B and C virus infections in causing hepatocellular carcinoma. *Int J Cancer* **75**:347–54.
184. Iwadou S, Nouso K, Kuwaki K *et al.* (2010) Time-dependent analysis of predisposing factors for the recurrence of hepatocellular carcinoma. *Liver Int* **30**:1027–32.
185. Adachi S, Shibuya A, Miura Y *et al.* (2008) Impact of occult hepatitis B virus infection and prior hepatitis B virus infection on development of hepatocellular carcinoma in patients with liver cirrhosis due to hepatitis C virus. *Scand J Gastroenterol* **43**:849–56.
186. Tanaka H, Tsukuma H, Yamano H *et al.* (2004) Prospective study on the risk of hepatocellular carcinoma among hepatitis C virus-positive blood donors focusing on demographic factors, alanine aminotransferase level at donation and interaction with hepatitis B virus. *Int J Cancer* **112**:1075–80.
187. Shiratori Y, Ito Y, Yokosuka O *et al.* (2005) Antiviral therapy for cirrhotic hepatitis C: Association with reduced hepatocellular carcinoma development and improved survival. *Ann Intern Med* **142**:105–14.
188. Fujita Y, Shibata A, Ogimoto I *et al.* (2006) The effect of interaction between hepatitis C virus and cigarette smoking on the risk of hepatocellular carcinoma. *Brit J Cancer* **94**:737–9.
189. Pessione F, Ramond MJ, Peters L *et al.* (2003) Five-year survival predictive factors in patients with excessive alcohol intake and cirrhosis. Effect of alcoholic hepatitis, smoking and abstinence. *Liver Int* **23**:45–53.
191. Chiang YJ, Wang HH, Lui KL *et al.* (2008) Hepatocellular carcinoma following renal transplantation: experience in northern Taiwan. *Tansplant Proc* **40**:2397–9.
192. Hoffmann CJ, Subramanian AK, Cameron AM *et al.* (2008) Incidence and risk factors for hepatocellular carcinoma following solid organ transplantation. *Transplantation* **86**:784–90.

192. Ciesek S, Steinmann E, Iken M *et al.* (2010) Glucocorticosteroids increase cell entry by hepatitis C virus. *Gastroenterology* **138**:1875–84.
193. Di Benedetto F, De Ruvo N, Berretta M *et al.* (2008) Hepatocellular carcinoma in HIV patients treated by liver transplantation. *Eur J Surg Oncol* **34**:422–7.
194. Salmon-Ceron D, Lewden C, Morlat P *et al.* (2005) Liver disease as a major cause of death among HIV infected patients: role of hepatitis C and B viruses and alcohol. *J Hepatol* **43**:911–2.
195. Reiberger T, Ferlitsch A, Seighart W *et al.* (2009) HIV-HCV co-infected patients with low CD4+ cell nadirs are at risk for faster fibrosis progression and portal hypertension. *J Viral Hepat* **17**:400–9.
196. Morgan TR, Ghany MG, Kim HY *et al.* (2010) Outcome of sustained virological responders with histologically advanced chronic hepatitis C. *Hepatology* **52**:833–44.
197. Heathcote EJ. (2004) Prevention of hepatitis C virus-related hepatocellular carcinoma. *Gastroenterology* **127**(Suppl 1):S294–S302.
198. Colombo M. (1999) Natural history and pathogenesis of hepatitis C virus related hepatocellular carcinoma. *J Hepatol* **31**:25–30.
199. Yeh MM, Daniel HD, Torbenson M. (2010) Hepatitis C-associated hepatocellular carcinomas in non-cirrhotic livers. *Mod Pathol* **23**:276–83.
200. Wong VW-S, Chan HL-Y. (2010) Transient elastography. *J Gastroenterol Hepatol* **25** [in press].
201. Masuzaki R, Tateishi R, Yoshida H *et al.* (2009) Prospective risk assessment for hepatocellular carcinoma development in patients with chronic hepatitis C by transient elastrography. *Hepatology* **49**:1954–61.
202. Tsuda N, Yuki N, Mochizuki K *et al.* (2004) Long-term clinical and virological outcomes of chronic hepatitis C after successful interferon therapy. *J Med Virol* **74**:406–13.
203. Ikeda M, Fujiyama S, Tanaka M *et al.* (2005) Risk factors for development of hepatocellular carcinoma in patients with chronic hepatitis C after sustained response to interferon. *J Gastroenterol* **40**:148–56.
204. Sangiovanni A, Prati GM, Fasani P *et al.* (2006) The natural history of compensated cirrhosis due to hepatitis C virus: A 17-year cohort study of 214 patients. *Hepatology* **43**:1303–10.
205. Nishiguchi S, Kuroki T, Nakatani S *et al.* (1995) Randomised trial of effects of interferon-alpha on incidence of hepatocellular carcinoma in chronic active hepatitis C. *Lancet* **346**:1051–5.

206. Yoshida H, Shiratori Y, Moriyama M *et al.* (1999) Interferon therapy reduces the risk for hepatocellular carcinoma: National surveillance program of cirrhotic and noncirrhotic patients with chronic hepatitis C in Japan. *Ann Intern Med* **131**:174–81.
207. Yano M, Kumada H, Kage M *et al.* (1996) The long-term pathological evolution of chronic hepatitis C. *Hepatology* **23**:1334–40.
208. Tarao K, Rino Y, Ohkawa S *et al.* (2002) Close associated between high serum alanine aminotransferase levels and multicentric hepatocarcinogenesis in patients with hepatitis C virus-associated cirrhosis. *Cancer* **94**:1787–95.
209. Miyakawa T, Tarao K, Ohshige K *et al.* (2009) High serum alanine aminotransferase levels for the first three successive years can predict very high incidence of hepatocellular carcinoma in patients with Child Stage A HCV-associated liver cirrhosis. *Scand J Gastroenterol* **44**:1340–8.
210. Poynard T, Bedossa P, Opolon P. (1997) Natural history of liver fibrosis progression in patients with chronic hepatitis C. The OBSVIRC, METAVIR, CLINIVIR and DOSVIRC groups. *Lancet* **349**:825–32.
211. Poynard T, Ratziu V, Charlotte F *et al.* (2001) Rates and risk factors of liver fibrosis progression in patients with chronic hepatitis C. *J Hepatol* **34**:730–9.
212. Moriyama M, Matsumura H, Aoki H *et al.* (2005) Decreased risk of hepatocellular carcinoma in patients with chronic hepatitis C whose serum alanine aminotransferase levels became less than twice the upper limit of normal following interferon therapy. *Liver Int* **25**:85–90.
213. Teoh N. (2009) Proliferative drive and liver carcinogenesis: Too much of a good thing? *J Gastroenterol Hepatol* **24**:1817–25.
214. Gordon JW, Harold G, Mathers LY. (1994) Transgenic mouse models of hepatocellular carcinoma. *Hepatology* **19**:538–9.
215. Dan YY, Yeoh GC. (2008) Liver stem cells: A scientific and clinical perspective. *J Gastroenterol Hepatol* **23**:687–98.
216. Dutta U, Kench J, Byth K *et al.* (1998) Hepatocellular proliferation and development of hepatocellular carcinoma: A case-control study in chronic hepatitis C. *Hum Pathol* **29**:1279–84.
217. Borzio M, Trerè D, Borzio F *et al.* (1998) Hepatocyte proliferation rate is a powerful parameter for predicting hepatocellular carcinoma development in liver cirrhosis. *Mol Pathol* **51**:96–101.

218. Donato MF, Arosio E, Del Ninno E *et al.* (2001) Colombo M. High rates of hepatocellular carcinoma in cirrhotic patients with high liver cell proliferative activity. *Hepatology* **34**:523–8.
219. Chisari FV, Isogawa M, Wieland SF (2010) Pathogenesis of hepatitis B virus infection. *Pathol Biol (Paris)* **58**:258–66.
220. Villa E, Fattovich G. No inflammation? No cancer! Clear HBV early and live happily. *J Hepatol* **52**:768–70.
221. Wang Y, Kato N, Hoshida H *et al.* (2010) Interleukin-1beta gene polymorphisms associated with hepatocellular carcinoma in hepatitis C virus infection. *Hepatology* **37**:65–71.
222. Wong VW, Yu J, Cheng AS *et al.* (2009) High serum interleukin-6 level predicts future hepatocellular carcinoma development in patients with chronic hepatitis B. *Int J Cancer* **124**:2766–70.
223. Nakagawa H, Maeda S, Yoshida H *et al.* (2009) Serum IL-6 levels and the risk for hepatocarcinogenesis in chronic hepatitis C patients: An analysis based on gender differences. *Int J Cancer* **125**:2264–9.
224. Porta C, De Amici M, Quaglini S *et al.* (2008) Circulating interleukin-6 as a tumor marker for hepatocellular carcinoma. *Ann Oncol* **19**:353–8.
225. Tangkijvanich P, Thong-Ngam D, Mahachai V *et al.* (2007) Role of serum interleukin-18 as a prognostic factor in patients with hepatocellular carcinoma. *World J Gastroenterol* **13**:4345–9.
226. Falleti E, Fabris C, Toniutto P *et al.* (2009) Interleukin-6 polymorphisms and gender: Relationship with the occurrence of hepatocellular carcinoma in patients with end-stage liver disease. *Oncology* **77**:304–13.
227. Matsuzaki K, Murata M, Yoshida K *et al.* (2007) Chronic inflammation associated with hepatitis C virus infection perturbs hepatic transforming growth factor β signalling, promoting cirrhosis and hepatocellular carcinoma. *Hepatology* **46**:48–57.
228. Tang Y, Kitisin K, Jogunoori W *et al.* (2008) Progenitor/stem cells give rise to liver cancer due to aberrant TGF-β and IL-6 signaling. *Proc Natl Acad Sci U.S.A.* **105**:2445–50.
229. Kato N, Ji G, Wang Y *et al.* (2005) Large-scale search of single nucleotide polymorphisms for hepatocellular carcinoma susceptibility genes in patients with hepatitis C. *Hepatology* **42**:846–53.
230. Morinaga S, Tarao K, Yamamoto Y *et al.* (2007) Overexpressed cyclo-oxygenase-2 in the background liver is associated with the clinical course

of hepatitis C virus-related cirrhosis patients after curative surgery for hepatocellular carcinoma. *J Gastroenterol Hepatol* **22**:1249–55.

231. Honda M, Kanedo S, Kawai H *et al.* (2001) Differential gene expression between chronic hepatitis B and C hepatic lesion. *Gastroenterology* **120**:955–66.
232. Chuma M, Sakamoto M, Yamazaki K *et al.* (2003) Expression profiling in multistage hepatocarcinogenesis: Identification of HSP70 as a molecular marker of early hepatocellular carcinoma. *Hepatology* **37**:198–207.
233. Delpuech O, Trabut JB, Carnot F *et al.* (2002) Identification, using cDNA a macroarray analysis, of distinct expression profiles associated with pathological and virological features of hepatocellular carcinoma. *Oncogene* **21**:2926–37.
234. Lee CF, Ling ZQ, Zhao T *et al.* (2008) Distinct expression patterns in hepatitis B virus- and hepatitis C virus-infected hepatocellular carcinoma. *World J Gastroenterol* **14**:6072–7.
235. Mas VR, Maluf DG, Archer KJ *et al.* (2009) Genes involved in viral carcinogenesis and tumor initiation in hepatitis C virus-induced hepatocellular carcinoma. *Mol Med* **15**:85–94.
236. Poynard T, McHutchison J, Manns M *et al.* (2002) Impact of pegylated interferon alfa-2b and ribavirin on liver fibrosis in patients with chronic hepatitis C. *Gastroenterology* **122**:1303–13.
237. McCaughan GW, Omata M. (2007) The Asia Pacific Association for the Study of the Liver (APASL) Hepatitis C Working Party. APASL Consensus Statements on the diagnosis, management and treatment of hepatitis C virus infection. *J Gastroenterol Hepatol* **22**:615–33.
238. Ghany MG, Strader DB, Thomas DL *et al.* (2009) Diagnosis, management and treatment of chronic hepatitis C: An update. *Hepatology* **49**:1335–74.
239. Cardoso A-C, Moucari R, Figueiredo-Mendes C *et al.* (2010) Impact of peginterferon and ribavirin therapy on hepatocellular carcinoma: Incidence and survival in hepatitis C patients with advanced fibrosis. *J Hepatol* **52**:652–7.
240. Farrell GC, Fan JG. (2009) Prevention of hepatocellular carcinoma. In: Al Knawy B, Reddy KR, Bolondi L. Hepatocellular carcinoma: A practical approach. *Informa Healthcare* 36–63.
241. Bruno S, Stroffolini T, Colombo M *et al.* (2007) Sustained virological response to interferon-alpha is associated with improved outcome in HCV-related cirrhosis: A retrospective study. *Hepatology* **45**:579–87.

242. Kuwana K, Ichida T, Kamimura T *et al.* (1997) Risk factors and the effect of interferon therapy in the development of hepatocellular carcinoma: A multivariate analysis of 343 patients. *J Gastroenterol Hepatol* **12**:149–55.
243. Imai Y, Kawata S, Tamura S *et al.* (1998) Relation of interferon therapy and hepatocellular carcinoma in patients with chronic hepatitis C. Osaka hepatocellular carcinoma prevention study group. *Ann Intern Med* **129**:94–9.
244. Shindo M, Ken A, Okuno T (1999) Varying incidence of cirrhosis and hepatocellular carcinoma in patients with chronic hepatitis C responding differently to interferon therapy. *Cancer* **85**:1943–50.
245. Tanaka K, Sata M, Uchimura Y *et al.* (1998) Long-term evaluation of interferon therapy in hepatitis C-associated cirrhosis. Does IFN prevent development of hepatocellular carcinoma? *Oncol Rep* **5**:205–8.
246. Okanoue T, Itoh Y, Minami M *et al.* (1999) Interferon therapy lowers the rate of progression to hepatocellular carcinoma in chronic hepatitis C but not significantly in advanced stage: A retrospective analysis of 1148 patients. Viral hepatitis therapy study group. *J Hepatol* **30**:653–9.
247. Bonino F, Oliveri F, Colombatto P *et al.* (1997) Impact of interferon-alpha therapy on the development of hepatocellular carcinoma in patients with liver cirrhosis: Results of an international survey. *J Viral Hepat* **4**(Suppl 2):79–82.
248. Fattovich G, Giustina G, Degos F *et al.* (1997) Effectiveness of interferon alfa on incidence of hepatocellular carcinoma and decompensation in cirrhosis type C. European Concerted Action on Viral Hepatitis (EUROHEP). *J Hepatol* **27**:201–5.
249. Valla DC, Chevallier M, Marcellin P *et al.* (1999) Treatment of hepatitis C virus-related cirrhosis: A randomized, controlled trial of interferon alfa-2b versus no treatment. *Hepatology* **29**:1870–5.
250. Benvegnù L, Chemello L, Noventa F *et al.* (1998) Retrospective analysis of the effect of interferon therapy on the clinical outcome of patients with viral cirrhosis. *Cancer* **83**:901–9.
251. Cammà C, Giunta M, Andreone P *et al.* (2001) Interferon and prevention of heptocellular carcinoma in viral cirrhosis: An evidence-based approach. *J Hepatology* **34**:593–602.
252. Hung CH, Lee CM, Lu SN *et al.* (2006) Long-term effect of interferon alpha-2b plus ribavirin therapy on incidence of hepatocellular carcinoma in patients with hepatitis C virus-related cirrhosis. *J Viral Hepat* **13**:409–14.

253. Gramenzi A, Andreone P, Fiorino S *et al.* (2001) Impact of interferon therapy on the natural history of hepatitis C virus related cirrhosis. *Gut* **48**:843–8.
254. Okanoue T, Itoh Y, Kirishima T *et al.* (2002) Transient biochemical response in interferon therapy decreases development of hepatocellular carcinoma for five years and improves long-term survival of chronic hepatitis C patients. *Hepatol Res* **23**:62–77.
255. Yoshida H, Arakawa Y, Sata M *et al.* (2002) Interferon prolonged life expectancy among chronic hepatitis C patients. *Gastroenterology* **123**:483–91.
256. Kasahara A, Hayashi N, Mochizuki K *et al.* (1998) Risk factors for hepatocellular carcinoma and its incidence after interferon treatment in patients with chronic hepatitis C. *Hepatology* **27**:1394–402.
257. Takimoto M, Ohkoshi S, Ichida T *et al.* (2002) Interferon inhibits progression of liver fibrosis and reduces the risk of hepatocarcinogenesis in patients with chronic hepatitis C: A retrospective multicenter analysis of 652 patients. *Dig Dis Sci* **47**:170–6.
258. Kashiwagi K, Furusyo N, Kubo N *et al.* (2003) A prospective comparison of the effect of interferon-alpha and interferon-beta treatment in patients with chronic hepatitis C on the incidence of hepatocellular carcinoma development. *J Infect Chemother* **9**:333–40.
259. Yu ML, Lin SM, Chuang WL *et al.* (2006) A sustained virological response to interferon or interferon/ribavirin reduces hepatocellular carcinoma and improves survival in chronic hepatitis C: A nationwide, multicentre study in Taiwan. *Antivir Ther* **11**:985–94.
260. George SL, Bacon BR, Brunt EM *et al.* (2009) Clinical, virologic, histologic, and biochemical outcomes after successful HCV therapy: A 5-year follow-up of 150 patients. *Hepatology* 729–38.
261. Veldt BJ, Heathcote EJ, Wedemeyer H *et al.* (2008) Sustained virologic response and clinical outcomes in patients with chronic hepatitis C and advanced fibrosis. *Ann Intern Med* **147**:677–84.
262. Donato MF, Degott C, Arosio E *et al.* (2005) Interferon-alpha suppresses liver cell proliferation in patients with chronic hepatitis C virus infection. *J Viral Hepat* **12**:499–506.
263. Lok AS, Seeff LB, Morgan TR *et al.* (2009) Incidence of hepatocellular carcinoma and associated risk factors in hepatitis C-related advanced liver disease. *Gastroenterology* **136**:138–48.

264. Lim R, Knight B, Patel K *et al.* (2006) Antiproliferative effects of interferon alpha on hepatic progenitor cells *in vitro* and *in vivo*. *Hepatology* **43**:1074–83.
265. Fartoux L, Degos F, Trepo C *et al.* (2007) Effect of prolonged interferon therapy on the outcome of heaptitis C virus-related cirrhosis: A randomized trial. *Clin Gastroenterol Hepatol* **5**:502–7.
266. Di Bisceglie AM, Shiffman ML, Everson GT *et al.* (2008) Prolonged therapy of advanced chronic hepatitis C with low-dose peginterferon. *N Engl J Med* **359**:2429–41.
267. Ikeda K, Arase Y, Saitoh S *et al.* (2000) Interferon beta prevents recurrence of hepatocellular carcinoma after complete resection or ablation of the primary tumor. A prospective randomized study of hepatitis C virus-related liver cancer. *Hepatology* **32**:228–32.
268. Mazzaferro V, Romito R, Schiavo M *et al.* (2006) Prevention of hepatocellular carcinoma recurrence with alpha-interferon after liver resection in HCV cirrhosis. *Hepatology* **44**:1543–54.
269. Nishiguchi S, Tamori A, Kubo S. (2005) Effect of long-term postoperative interferon therapy on intrahepatic recurrence and survival rate after resection of hepatitis C virus-related hepatocellular carcinoma. *Intervirology* **48**:71–5.
270. Lin SM, Lin CJ, Hsu CW *et al.* (2004) Prospective randomized controlled study of interferon-alpha in preventing hepatocellular carcinoma recurrence after medical ablation therapy for primary tumors. *Cancer* **100**:376–82.
271. Shiratori Y, Shiina S, Teratini T *et al.* (2003) Interferon therapy after tumor ablation improves prognosis in patients with hepatocellular carcinoma associated with hepatitis C virus. *Ann Intern Med* **138**:299–306.
272. Miyaguchi S, Watanabe T, Takahashi H *et al.* (2002) Interferon therapy for hepatocellular carcinoma patients with low HCV RNA levels. *Hepatogastroenterology* **49**:724–9.
273. Kubo S, Nishiguchi S, Hirohashi K *et al.* (2002) Randomized clinical trial of long-term outcome after resection of hepatitis C virus-related hepatocellular carcinoma by post-operative interferon. *Br J Surg* **89**:418–22.
274. Clavien PA. (2007) Interferon: The magic bullet to prevent hepatocellular carcinoma recurrence after resection? *Ann Surg* **245**:843–5.
275. Singal AK, Freeman DH Jr, Anand BS. (2010) Meta-analysis: Interferon improves outcomes following ablation or resection of hepatocellular carcinoma. *Aliment Parmacol Ther* **32**:851–8.

276. Muto Y, Moriwaki H, Saito A. (1996) Prevention of second primary tumors by an acyclic retinoid in patients with hepatocellular carcinoma. *N Engl J Med* **340**:1046–7.
277. Takai K, Okuno M, Yasuda I *et al.* (2005) Prevention of second primary tumors by an acyclic retinoid in patients with hepatocellular carcinoma. Updated analysis of the long-term follow-up data. *Intervirology* **48**:39–45.
278. Kakizaki S, Sohara N, Sato K *et al.* (2007) Preventive effects of vitamin K on recurrent disease in patients with hepatocellular carcinoma arising from hepatitis C virus infection. *J Gastroenterol Hepatol* **22**:518–22.
279. Mizuta T, Ozaki I, Eguchi Y *et al.* (2006) The effect of menatetrenone, a vitamin K2 analog, on disease recurrence and survival in patients with hepatocellular carcinoma after curative treatment: A pilot study. *Cancer* **106**:867–72.
280. Suou T, Mitsuda A, Koda M *et al.* (2001) Interferon alpha inhibits intrahepatic recurrence in hepatocellular carcinoma with chronic hepatitis C: A pilot study. *Hepatol Res* **20**:301–11.
281. Hung CH, Lee CM, Wang JH *et al.* (2005) Antiviral therapy after nonsurgical tumor ablation in patients with hepatocellular carcinoma associated with hepatitis C virus. *J Gastroenterol Hepatol* **20**:1553–9.
282. Sakaguchi Y, Kudo M, Fukunuga T *et al.* (2005) Low-dose, long-term, intermittent interferon-alpha-2b therapy after radical treatment by radiofrequency ablation delays clinical recurrence in patients with hepatitis C virus-related hepatocellular carcinoma. *Intervirology* **48**:64–70.
283. Jeong SC, Aikata H, Katamura Y *et al.* (2007) Effects of a 24-week course of interferon-alpha therapy after curative treatment of hepatitis C virus-associated hepatocellular carcinoma. *World J Gastroenterol* **13**:5343–50.
284. Kudo M, Sakaguchi Y, Chung H *et al.* (2007) Long-term interferon maintenance therapy improves survival in patients with HCV-related hepatocellular carcinoma after curative radiofrequency ablation. A matched case-control study. *Oncology* **72**(Suppl 1):132–8.
285. Alter MJ. (2008) Healthcare should not be a vehicle for transmission of hepatitis C virus. *J Hepatol* **48**:2–4.
286. Forns X, Bruix J. (2010) Treating hepatitis C in patients with cirrhosis: The effort is worth it. *Hepatology* **52**:624–6.
287. McHutchinson JG, Everson GT, Gordon SC *et al.* (2009) Telaprevir with peginterferon and ribavirin for chronic HCV genotype 1 infection. *N Engl J Med* **360**:1827–38. Erratum in: *N Engl J Med* **361**:1516.

288. Kwo PY, Lawitz EJ, McCone J *et al.* (2010) Efficacy of boceprevir, an NS3 protease inhibitor, in combination with peginterferon alfa-2b and ribavirin in treatment-naive patients with genotype 1 heaptitis C infection (SPRINT-1): An open-label, randomised, multicentre phase 2 trial. *Lancet* **376**:705–16.
289. McHutchinson JG, Manns MP, Muir AJ *et al.* (2010) Telaprevir for previously treated chronic HCV infection. *N Engl J Med* **362**:1292–303.
290. Wiegand J. (2008) Newly acquired hepatitis C — many hurdles from diagnosis until treatment initiation. *J Gastroenterol Hepatol* **23**:1782–4.
291. Dore GJ, Hellard M, Matthews GV *et al.* (2010) Effective treatment of injecting drug users with recently acquired hepatitis C virus infection. *Gastroenterology* **138**:123–35.

Chapter 9

Advances in the Interventional Therapies for Hepatocellular Carcinoma

Carmen Chi Min Cho*, Joyce Wai Yi Hui
and Simon Chun Ho Yu

Department of Imaging and Interventional Radiology, Prince of Wales Hospital, Shatin, Hong Kong, China

Hepatocellular carcinoma (HCC) is one of the most common malignancies worldwide. Surgical treatment, including hepatic resection and liver transplantation, is the most effective therapy and is considered potentially curative. However, less than 20% of HCC can be treated surgically because of multicentric tumors, early vascular invasion, extra hepatic metastasis, shortage of donor organs, poor hepatic reserve or other co-morbidities precluding major surgery. In such instances, a variety of interventional treatments can be offered in order to improve the prognosis of the patient.

Introduction

It is generally accepted that for patients with few and small tumors, local ablation therapies are ideal, provided that there is adequate hepatic reserve. There is a wide variety of minimally invasive ablative therapies available, although radiofrequency ablation (RFA) is currently recognized as the preferred treatment option. Some techniques are relatively novel while other more established therapies are undergoing continual technical advances. In this chapter, focus will be on these newer technologies

* Corresponding author. Email: ccm193@ha.org.hk

although more study is required before these become standard treatments or supersede RFA.[1]

In cases where the tumor characteristics preclude the patient from surgery or local ablative treatments, i.e. larger and multifocal tumors, patients may choose between transhepatic arterial chemoembolization (TACE) or selective internal radiation therapy (SIRT). Although randomized controlled trials comparing these two modalities are lacking, TACE is the most widely used.[1] In the next section, the rationale and efficacy of these two treatments will be described and in particular, more recent advances regarding chemoembolization will be discussed.

Transhepatic arterial chemoembolization

It has been clinically proven by randomized controlled trials and meta-analyses that TACE is an effective treatment for unresectable HCC as it delays tumor progression and improves survival when compared with supportive treatment or systemic chemotherapy.[2–5] It has also been shown that hepatectomy with adjuvant TACE is beneficial in improving survival outcomes.[6]

The purpose of TACE is twofold: firstly to de-arterialize the tumor and secondly to selectively deliver chemotherapeutic agents into the tumor. Many different regimens of TACE are in use but despite these variations, the common denominator of this procedure is the intra-arterial infusion of a chemotherapeutic agent in an emulsion with iodized oil and particle embolization. Controversies exist as to which particles or chemotherapeutic agents to use and whether chemotherapeutic agents provide any beneficial effect at all. Whether there is a superior TACE protocol remains open to debate despite many clinical trials investigating this topic.

Although TACE is widely regarded as the treatment of choice for tumors unsuitable for resection or local therapy, ongoing efforts are being made in attempt to improve its efficacy. One such technique is using drug eluting microbeads (DEB) in lieu of a drug-oil emulsion. The process of emulsification between a chemotherapeutic agent and iodized oil is very unstable and the two components begin to separate as soon as they are injected into the hepatic arterial circulation. The ultimate goal of using drug eluting microbeads is to obtain the highest sustained concentration of drugs within the tumor, with the lowest concentration in the peripheral blood. This should optimize the antitumoral effect while improving the tolerance and lower the rate of side effects. Currently, there is a range of drug eluting microbeads available with varying particle sizes and compositions. The soft and deformable spheres usually consist of a macromer derived from polyvinyl alcohol (PVA) which can be delivered through conventional or microcatheters and can be loaded with chemotherapeutic agents, commonly doxorubicin (Figure 1). The findings of present studies indicate that using drug loaded particles is a highly effective treatment with a low rate of side effects.[7–10] An advantageous pharmacokinetic profile has been observed in patients undergoing TACE using drug eluting microbeads, with the peak plasma concentration of chemotherapeutic agent being significantly lower than conventional TACE[7,9] (Figure 2). These preliminary results are promising and warrant the development of randomized controlled studies to establish its role against conventional TACE.

Apart from using drug eluting microbeads, another formulation which appears to improve biodistribution properties, is the addition of ethanol to iodized oil (Lipiodol ethanol mixture). A recent *in vivo* study has shown that the use of this mixture is associated with a greater embolic effect as indicated by a higher degree of Lipiodol retention, without an increase in

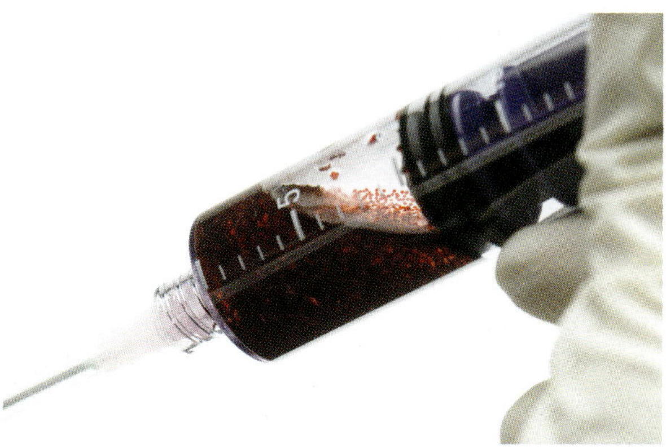

Figure 1. Drug eluting beads loaded with doxorubicin composed of PVA polymer.

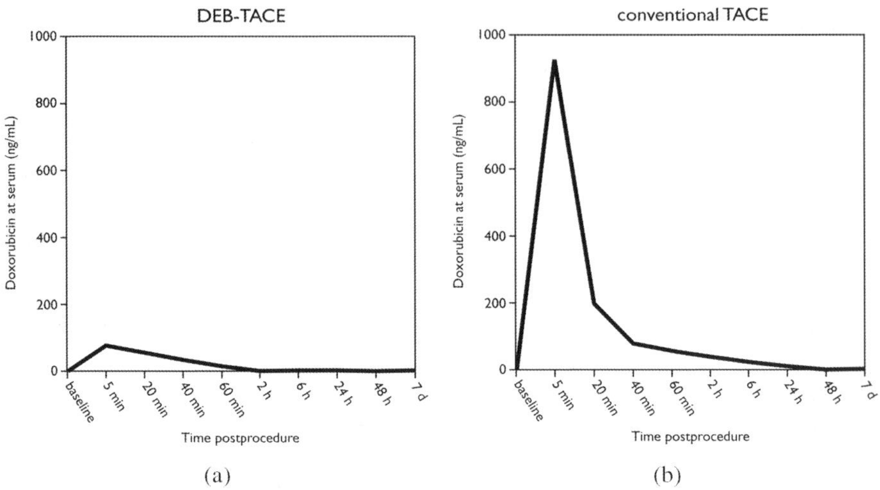

Figure 2. Measurements of doxorubicin levels in the peripheral blood at different time points in DEB-TACE patients (a) and in conventional TACE (b).

lung shunting or decomposition rate, compared with other ethanol-free regimens.[11]

Other more novel but promising therapies are also undergoing clinical trials including the locoregional delivery of antiangiogenic factors[12,13] and immunotherapeutic agents such as OK-432 and TNP-470 in conjunction with TACE.[13] However, randomized controlled trials in patients are lacking and conclusive evidence of the efficacy of these techniques is not yet available.

Selective internal radiotherapy

SIRT or radioembolization is a minimally invasive transcatheter therapy through which radioactive microspheres are infused into the hepatic arteries that supply the tumor, the technique being similar to that of TACE. Two main radioembolic devices (^{90}Y, ^{188}Rh) are currently available, with ^{90}Y being the most commonly used. Once infused, these microspheres selectively implant within the tumor arterioles. Embedded within the arterioles, the impregnated microspheres emit high energy and low penetrating radiation to the tumor selectively. Unlike external beam therapy, radioembolization can deliver high cumulative radiation doses to targeted hepatic segments without the clinical manifestation of radiation-induced liver disease (RILD). The major contraindication for the use of ^{90}Y microspheres, which is particular to this treatment, is the presence of hepatopulmonary shunting which would result in excessive radiation being delivered to the lungs. Therefore pretreatment ^{99m}Tc macro-aggregated albumin (MAA) scan is required in all patients being considered for this treatment.

Although the use of SIRT dates back to the early 1960s, only recently has its therapeutic safety and efficacy been recognized and promising results have emerged from recent clinical trials. A consensus panel report from the Radioembolization Brachytherapy Oncology Consortium concluded that there is sufficient evidence to support the safe and effective use of this loco-regional therapy in HCC patients.[14] Nevertheless, randomized controlled trials comparing ^{90}Y therapy to other treatments are lacking and further study is required in order to establish its role against other established treatments, in particular TACE.

Local ablation therapies

Radiofrequency ablation

RFA involves creating thermal injury to target tissue through electromagnetic energy deposition. An alternating electric field is generated within the patient. Because of the relatively high electrical resistance of tissue compared with the metal electrodes, there is agitation of the ions present in the target tissue that surrounds the electrode. This then results in frictional heat and coagulation necrosis.

It is well accepted that RFA is more effective in treating liver tumors when compared with the seminal ablation technique of percutaneous ethanol injection (PEI). In fact, five randomized trials comparing RFA versus PEI for the treatment of early-stage HCC consistently showed that RFA leads to better local control.[15–18] Additionally, two meta-analyses confirmed that treatment with RFA offers a distinct survival benefit as compared with PEI, establishing it as the standard percutaneous technique. Even so, RFA does have its limitations. Histological data from explanted liver specimens in patients who underwent RFA showed that large tumor size and presence of large abutting vessels significantly reduce the efficacy of RFA. Abutting vessels cause rapid heat loss due to perfusion-mediated tissue cooling otherwise known as the heat sink effect. Treatment of lesions near the liver surface, in proximity to the gastrointestinal tract or adjacent to the porta hepatis, also create risk of major complications. Because of these drawbacks, novel ablative techniques have been developed in an attempt to overcome some of the limitations of RFA.

Laser ablation

The term laser ablation (LA) refers to tissue destruction by conversion of absorbed light, usually infrared, into heat. Infrared energy penetrates tissue for a distance of 12–15 mm, although heat is conducted beyond this range, allowing a larger zone of tissue to be ablated. Penetration has been shown to be increased in malignant tissue compared with normal parenchyma.[19] Cell death from coagulative necrosis occurs at temperatures above 60°C, while temperatures above 100°C cause vaporization from evaporation of tissue water. Overheating above 300°C will lead to carbonization, which in turn decreases optical penetration of the infrared rays.

The most widely utilized device for LA techniques is the Nd-YAG (neodynium: yttrium-aluminium-garnet) laser with a wavelength of 1064 nm. More recently, more compact and less expensive diode lasers with shorter wavelengths of 800–900 nm have been used, although the lower tissue penetration produces a smaller volume of destruction. Flexible quartz fibres with diameters from 300–600 μm deliver light into target tissues. Conventional bare tip diameter create a near spherical lesion of about 15-mm diameter but have been largely replaced by interstitial fibres which have flat or cylindrical diffusing tips, providing a much larger ablative areas of up to 50 mm in diameter.[20,21] The use of beam-splitting devices allows the use of up to four fibres at once with corresponding increase in ablative volume, although this requires multiple fibres to be placed and only works at lower powers. Increased laser power produces better light transmission and larger ablative zones. However, it also carries a higher risk of overheating and carbonization of tissue. The use of water-cooled laser application sheaths allows a higher power output while preventing carbonization and the use of multiple water-cooled higher power fibres allows ablative zones of up to 80 mm in diameter.[22]

Like other ablative techniques, different imaging modalities have been used to guide percutaneous LA, including ultrasound and computed tomography, the choice of which is determined by local experience and resource availability. The use of magnetic resonance (MR) guidance is only feasible with LA systems as it is entirely metal free and does not produce any radiofrequency interference. MR-guided LA, often in conjunction with liver-specific contrast material, is advantageous in that it offers real-time thermal mapping that allows the operator to visualize the size, location, and temperature of the ablative zone.[23,24] Thermal imaging can be performed with most MR systems with changes in temperature demonstrated as increased magnetic field. Different MR sequences can be used to measure changes in tissue temperature, all of which are best used in conjunction with subtraction techniques i.e. pretreatment image subtraction from heating image. Additionally, the use of open MR magnets allows real-time imaging of needle placement in a multiplanar fashion unlimited by presence of bone or gas unlike ultrasound. The disadvantage of an open magnet is its lower field and gradient strength thereby reducing image quality and increasing scan time.[25]

The inherent properties of RFA and LA are similar in that they share similar mechanisms of causing cell death and also similar limitations including the heat sink effect. Data regarding long-term survival rates for LA is scarce which reflects the relative novelty of this treatment. Only one randomized control prospective study compared LA with RFA which showed no significant difference in overall survival rates for up to five years, but a statistically higher survival rate for RFA over LA for Child A patients and nodules $\leq$ 25mm.[26] Nevertheless, results for water-cooled higher power MR guided LA have been promising and further data from randomized trials are required to determine long-term survival rates and before LA can be established as standard treatment.

Microwave ablation

Microwave ablation includes all electromagnetic methods of inducing tumor destruction with frequencies greater than or equal to 900 kHz. Microwaves cause rapid molecular rotation in cells and other materials containing water which then generates heat, leading to coagulation necrosis.

Percutaneous microwave coagulation therapy (MCT) is a well-established minimally invasive technique for small HCCs and metastatic liver tumors (Figure 3). It offers a theoretical advantage over RFA in that its treatment effect is less affected by nearby vessels. Nonetheless, previous literature, including one RCT comparing the effectiveness of MCT with that of RFA,[27] revealed that RFA was the favored ablative technique with respect to local recurrence and complication rates.

However, these studies were based on conventional single probe techniques, and new devices have since been developed which appear to overcome the limitation of the small coagulation volume in early experiences. In particular, probes with multiple antennas, either straight or

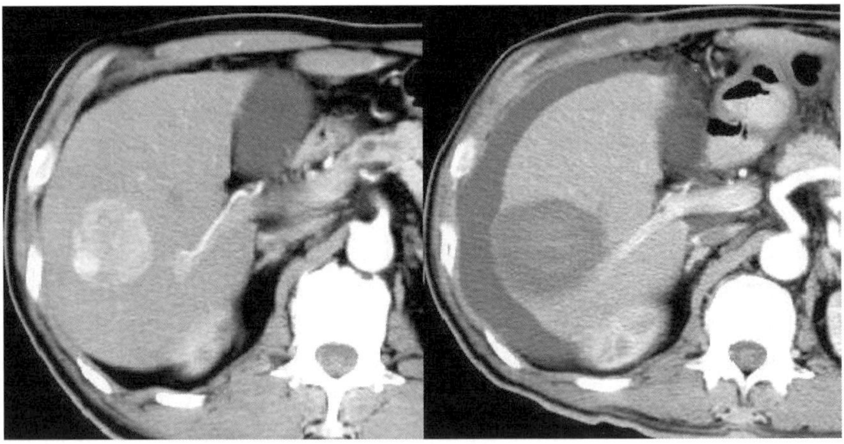

(a) (b)

Figure 3. Contrast CT images of a patient with HCC treated with microwave ablation. Pretreatment scan (a) shows an arterially enhancing tumor in the right hepatic lobe. Two-month post-treatment scan (b) demonstrates a necrotic area in the corresponding site but no viable tumor.

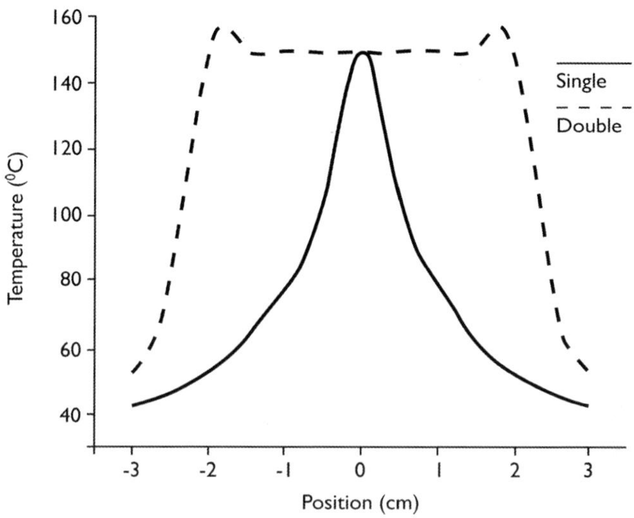

Figure 4. Graph showing relative temperature distribution for single and double microwave sources. The temperature between two antennae is consistently higher across the ablation zone due to thermal synergy.

looped, are becoming more popular and have shown promising results. The thermal synergy provided by three simultaneous antennas allows the zone of ablation to be larger than the sum of its parts, i.e. three single-antenna ablations[28] (Figure 4). In addition, simultaneously powering three antennas decreases the total ablation time by 67%.[29] Another device using a cooled-shaft antenna enables delivery of greater microwave energy, thereby increasing the zone of coagulation without risk of skin burns and increased pain[30] (Figure 5). These new techniques potentially allow the effective treatment of larger liver tumors in a shorter span of time.

With these new advances, continual study and comparison with other ablative techniques is warranted to define the role of MCT in treatment of liver tumors.

Irreversible electroporation

Electroporation is a technique which increases the cell membrane permeability by altering the transmembrane potential and subsequently

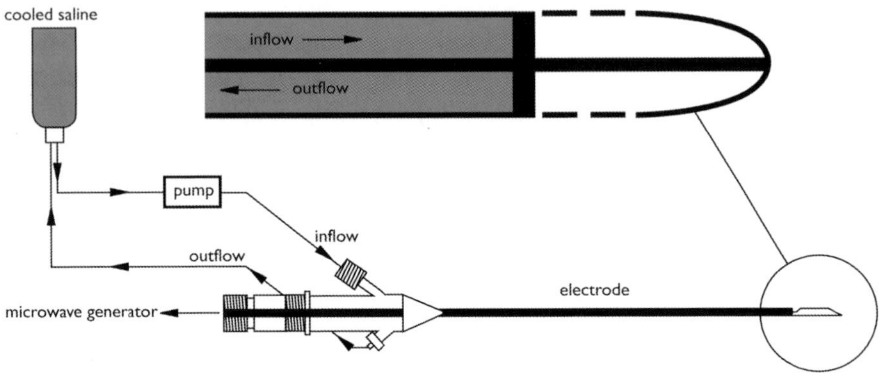

Figure 5. Schematic diagram of cooled shaft antenna which consists of a steady flow pump. The 4°C saline solution circulates within the lumen of the antenna shaft so that it maintains a mean temperature of 10°C ± 2°C.

disrupting cell membrane integrity, allowing the transport of molecules via nano-sized, pores. This process has been used for drug delivery into cells when utilized in a *reversible* fashion. Irreversible electroporation (IE) has been introduced to cause cell death, previously applied to effectively kill microbial organisms.[31] The process has subsequently been studied with encouraging results on healthy tissue cells.[32,33] Unlike established thermal ablation techniques such as RFA and MCT, IE induces tissue death by changing the permeability of the cell membrane. Therefore, it is not affected by the heat sink effect. This implies that IE has the ability to sharply delineate the tumor area from surrounding healthy tissues. Complete tissue death can be achieved even in cases where the ablation zone is adjacent to a large vessel. Furthermore, IE can create tissue death in micro-to milli-second range. For example, ablation of a 3 × 4 cm volume would take 8 minutes compared to conventional techniques which require at least 30 minutes.

Percutaneous irreversible electroporation has been successfully utilized *in vivo* and in select human patients to treat tumors in a broad range of organs, including liver, pancreas kidney, lymph node, and lung. The technique uses ultrasound or CT guidance to position electrodes around the targeted tumor. The number of electrodes used is determined by the

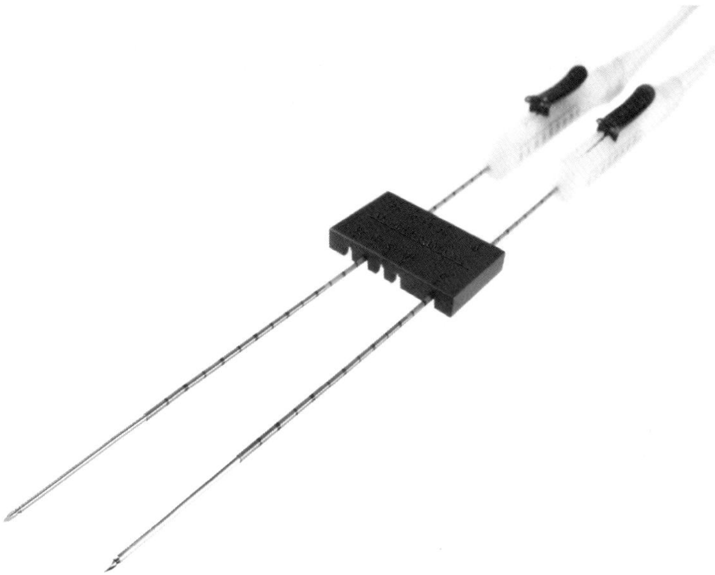

Figure 6. Probes used for irreversible electroporation (Courtesy of ANGIODYNAMICS®, Inc.).

size and shape of the tumor (Figure 6). During the procedure, the ablation zone can be continuously monitored using ultrasound.[34]

In a recent cohort study including 69 separate tumors of the liver, kidney or lung were treated with IE. No mortalities occurred although transient ventricular arrhythmia was encountered in four patients. This may be circumvented with electrocardiographically-synchronized delivery.[35]

IE is still a novel technology with ongoing trials evaluating its clinical safety and efficacy in tumor ablation. The initial results have been encouraging although its role in treatment of HCC has yet to be established.

High intensity focused ultrasound

High intensity focused ultrasound (HIFU) is a non-invasive procedure which can precisely heat and destroy pathogenic tissue. It has been developed for the treatment of uterine fibroids and has been successfully applied for the destruction of solid tumors of the bone, brain, breast, liver, pancreas, rectum, kidney, testes, and prostate. HIFU was first approved for the treatment of HCC in China in 1999.[36]

In HIFU therapy, ultrasound beams are focused on diseased tissue and due to the significant energy deposition at the focus, temperature within the tissue rises from 65° to 85°C, destroying cells by coagulation necrosis. Real-time US guidance allows precise ablation of lesions of any shape without damage to surrounding structures. Its non-invasive characteristics allow HIFU to treat large tumors and multicentric tumors. Even lesions located <1 cm from major blood vessels including the IVC, hepatic and portal veins, can be successfully ablated without any blood vessel injury.[37] This ability provides an advantage over other local ablation techniques which require percutaneous insertion of an instrument and are generally indicated for patients with less than three tumors and a tumor size of less than 3 cm. Close proximity to major vessels may also preclude treatment with these more invasive techniques.

In a recent study, both short-term and long-term therapeutic effectiveness were shown to be significantly greater in patients with advanced HCC receiving HIFU compared to control patients. Although these results are similar to other regional ablative techniques such as RFA, the patients recruited had rather comparatively late-stage HCC.[38]

Complications of HIFU included low grade fever, transient local pain, derangement of liver enzymes, and minor skin burns. No severe complications such as liver failure or bleeding occurred. There are certain disadvantages of HIFU: firstly it is a time-consuming procedure, taking on average of 3–4 hrs for one operation; secondly, it is labor intensive work, necessitating up to five medical staff to complete the procedure.

Although early results show that the survival results for HIFU are comparative to other regional ablative techniques such as RFA, HIFU offers the advantage of being less invasive and the ability to treat large tumors in close proximity to major vessels or other vital structures. It holds a promising potential, especially for treating late-stage disease.

References

1. Clark HP, Carson WF, Kavanagh PV *et al.* (2005) Staging and current treatment of hepatocellular carcinoma. *Radio Graphics* **23**:S3–23.

2. Llovet JM, Real MI, Montana X *et al.* (2002) Arterial embolization or chemoembolization versus symptomatic treatment in patients with unresectable hepatocellular carcinoma: A randomized control trial. *Lancet* **359**:1734–9.
3. Lo CM, Ngan H, Tso WK *et al.* (2001) Randomized controlled trial of transarterial lipiodol chemoembolization for hepatocellular carcinoma: Is there room for new studies? *Clin Gastroenterol* **32**:383–9.
4. Camma C, Schepis F, Orlando A *et al.* (2002) Transarterial chemoembolization for unresectable hepatocelluar carcinoma: Meta-analysis of randomized trial. *Radiology* **224**:47–54.
5. Llovet JM, Bruix J. (2003) Systematic review of randomized trials for unresectable hepatocellular carcinoma: Chemoembolization improves survival. *Hepatology* **37**:429–42.
6. Chong Z, Cuo RP, Li JQ. (2009) A randomized controlled trial of hepatectomy with adjuvant transcatheter chemoemoblization versus hepatectomy alone for stage IIIA hepatocellular carcinoma. *Journal of cancer research and clinical oncology* **135**:1437–45.
7. Guido P, Pietro Q, Claudio M *et al.* (2008) Transhepatic arterial chemoembolization with Oxaliplatin-eluting microspheres for unresectable hepatic tumours. *Anticancer Research* **28**:3835–42.
8. Kettenbach J, Stadler A, V. Katzler I *et al.* (2008) Drug-loaded microspheres for the treatment of liver cancer: Review of current results. *Cardiovasc Intervent Radiol* **31**:468–76.
9. Varela M, Real MI, Burrel M *et al.* (2007) Chemoembolization of hepatocellular carcinoma with drug eluting beads: Efficacy and doxorubicin pharmacokinetics. *Journal of Hepatology* **46**:474–81.
10. Malagari K, Chatzimichael K, Alexopoulou E *et al.* (2008) Transarterial chemoembolization of unresectable hepatocellular carcinoma with drug eluting beads: Results of an open-label study of 62 patients. *Cardiovasc Intervent Radiol* **21**:269–80.
11. Yu SCH, Leung TWT, Lau WY *et al.* (2008) A comparison of three transarterial lipiodol-based formulations for hepatocellular carcinoma: *In vivo* biodistribution study in humans. *Cardiovasc Intervent Radiol* **31**:289–98.
12. Qi XH, Wu ZM, Liu Q *et al.* (2008) Study of heptatic arterial infusion of endostar combined with TACE on advanced hepatocellular carcinoma. *Chinese-German J of Clin Onco* **7**:568–70.

13. Maataoui A, Qian J, Vossoughi D *et al.* (2005) Transarterial chemoembolization alone and in combination with other therapies: A comparative study in an animal HCC model. *Eur Radiol* **15**:127–33.
14. Ibrahim SM, Lewandowski RJ, Sato KT *et al.* (2008) Radioembolization for the treatment of unresectable hepatocellular carcinoma: A clinical review. *World Journal of Gastroenterology* **14**:1664–9.
15. Lencioni R, Allgaier HP, Cioni D *et al.* (2003) Small hepatocellular carcinoma in cirrhosis: Randomized comparison of radiofrequency thermal ablation versus percutaneous ethanol injection. *Radiology* **228**:235–40.
16. Lin SM, Lin CJ, Lin CC *et al.* (2004) Radiofrequency ablation improves prognosis compared with ethanol injection for hepatocellular carcinoma ≤4 cm. *Gastroengerology* **127**:1712–23.
17. Shiina S, Teratani T, Obi S *et al.* (2005) A randomized controlled trial of radiofrequency ablation versus ethanol injection, and percutaneous acetic acid injection to treat hepatocellular carcinoma of 3 cm of less. *Gut* **54**:1151–6.
18. Brunello F, Veltri A, Carucci P *et al.* (2008) Radiofrequency ablation versus ethanol injection for early hepatocellular carcinoma: A randomized controlled trial. *Scand J Gastroenterol* **43**:727–35.
19. Goldberg SN, Grassi CJ, Cardella JF *et al.* (2005) Image-guided tumor ablation: Standardization of terminology and reporting crtieria. *Radiology* **235**:728–39.
20. Huang GT, Wang TH, Sheu JC *et al.* (1991) Low-power laserthermia for the treatment of small hepatocellular carcinoma. *Eur J Cancer* **27**:1622–7.
21. Muralidharan V, Malcontenti-Wilson C, Christophi C. (2002) Interstitial laser hyperthermia for colorectal liver metastases: The effect of thermal sensitization and the use of a cylindrical diffuser tip on tumor necrosis. *J Clin Laser Med Surg* **20**:189–96.
22. Vogl TJ, Straub R, Zangos S *et al.* (2004) MR-guided laser-induced thermotherapy (LITT) of liver tumours: Experimental and clinical data. *Int J Hyperthermia* **20**:713–24.
23. Joarder R, de Jode M, Lamb GA *et al.* (2001) The value of MnDPDP enhancement during MR guided laser interstitial thermoablation of liver tumors. *J Magn Reson Imaging* **13**:37–41.
24. Gedroyc WM. (2005) Magnetic resonance guidance of thermal ablation. *Top Magn Reson Imaging* **16**:339–53.
25. Gough Palmer AL, Gedroyc WM. (2008) Laser ablation of hepatocellular carcinoma-A review. *World J Gastroenterol* **14**:7170–4.

26. Ferrari FS, Megliola A, Scorzelli A *et al.* (2007) Treatment of small HCC through radiorequency ablation and laser ablation. Comparison of techniques and long-term results. *Radiol Med (Torino)* **112**:337–93.
27. Shibata T, Iimuro Y, Yamamoto Y *et al.* (2002) Small hepatocellular carcinoma: Comparison of radio-frequency ablation and percutaneous microwave coagulation therapy. *Radiology* **223**:331–7.
28. Wright AS, Lee FT Jr, Mahvi DM. (2003) Hepatic microwave ablation with multiple antennae results in synergistically larger zones of coagulation necrosis. *Ann Surg Oncol* **40**:275–83.
29. Brace CL, Laeseke PF, Sampson LA *et al.* (2007) Microwave ablation with multiple simultaneously powered small-gauge triaxial antennas: Results from an *in vivo* swine liver model. *Radiology* **244**:151–6.
30. Kuang M, Lu MD, Xie XY *et al.* (2007) Liver cancer: Increased microwave delivery to ablation zone with cooled-shaft antenna-experimental and clinical studies. *Radiology* **242**:914–23.
31. Oshima T, Sato M. (2004) Bacterial sterilization and intracellular protein release by a pulsed electric field. *Adv Biochem Eng Biotechnol* **90**:113–33.
32. Edd JF, Horowitz L, Davalos R *et al.* (2006) *In vivo* results of a new focal tissue ablation technique: Irreversible electroporation. *IEEE Trans Biomed Eng* **53**:1409–15.
33. Rubinsky B, Onik G, Mikus P. (2007) Irreversible electroporation: A new ablation modality-clinical implications. *Technol Cancer Res Treat* **6**:37–48.
34. Lee EW, Loh CT, Kee ST. (2007) Imaging guided percutaneous irreversible electroporation: Ultrasound and immunohistological correlation. *Tech Cancer Res & Treat* **6**:287–93.
35. Thomson KR, Cheung W, Ellis SJ *et al.* (2011) Investigation of the safety of irreversible electroporation in humans. *J Vasc Interv Radiol* **22**(5):612–21.
36. Wu F, Chen WZ, Bai J. (1999) A preliminary study of high intensity focused ultrasound in the treatment of hepatocellular carcinoma. *Chin J Ultrasound* **8**:213–6.
37. Zhang L, Zhu H, Jin CB. (2009) High intensity focused ultrasound (HIFU): Effective and safe therapy for hepatocellular carcinoma adjacent to major hepatic veins. *Eur Radiol* **19**:437–45.
38. Li YY, Sha WH, Zhou YJ *et al.* (2007) Short and long term efficacy of high intensity focused ultrasound therapy for advanced hepatocellular carcinoma. *J Gastroenterol Hepatol* **22**:2148–54.

Section III

Mediators in Chronic Inflammation and Cancers

Chapter 10

Exploration of Cytokine Signaling in Clinical Management of Hepatocellular Carcinoma

Xuelian Zhao and Xin Wei Wang*

Liver Carcinogenesis Section, Laboratory of Human Carcinogenesis, Centre for Cancer Research, National Cancer Institute, Bethesda, MD, USA

Chronic infection and inflammation contribute to about 25% of all cancer cases worldwide. Specifically, hepatocellular carcinoma (HCC), the frequent malignant cancer with the third leading cause of cancer death, is a representative malignancy showing a strong association with chronic inflammatory disease. HCC develops almost exclusively in cirrhotic livers resulting from viral hepatitis, alcoholic or fatty liver disease. Several clinical studies indicate that >85% of HCCs retain markers for HBV and/or HCV. Cytokines, the most common mediators linking inflammation and cancer, show altered expression in cirrhotic disease and HCC, which can be categorized as pro- or anti-carcinogenesis. Thus, understanding the signaling pathway and the exploration of cytokine-based clinical management is representing a promising therapeutic strategy. In this chapter, we provide a general overview of the connection of inflammation and HCC and highlight the process of translating basic science to clinical managements by introducing two cytokines — tumor necrosis factor alpha (TNF-α) and interleukin 6 (IL-6). Though promising, current cytokine-based therapies are at an early stage, for example, TNF-α have both pro- and anti-tumor effects, which lead to contradictory strategies in clinic applications. As our understanding of the

* Corresponding author. Email: wangx@intra.nci.nih.gov

mechanistic connections between inflammation and cancer development accumulate, the cytokine-based clinical management should be more specific and efficient in HCC prognosis, diagnosis and treatment.

Introduction

General introduction of cytokines

Cytokines are diverse group of secreted or membrane-bound proteins that are mainly synthesized by different immune cells, including monocytes, macrophages, dendritic cells, T and B lymphocytes.[1] Besides, many epithelial cells are also capable of producing cytokines. In addition to the roles in inflammation and immunity, cytokines control many different cellular functions including proliferation, differentiation and cell survival/apoptosis. Cytokines can be classified into two groups: pro-inflammatory or anti-inflammatory. Pro-inflammatory cytokines, including IFNγ, IL-1, IL-6 and TNF-α *et al*., are predominantly derived from the innate immune cells and T helper 1 (Th1) cells. Anti-inflammatory cytokines, including IL-10, IL-4, IL-13 and IL-5 *et al*., are synthesized from Th2 immune cells. In this chapter, we focus on TNF-α and IL-6 and discuss their potentials in the clinical management of HCC.

Chronic inflammation and HCC

The connection between chronic inflammation and cancer has been recognized for several decades, such as the close association between chronic ulcerative colitis and colon cancer as well as the association between chronic hepatitis and HCC.[2] Epidemiological studies have established that many tumors occur in association with chronic infectious diseases. Meanwhile, persistent inflammation in the absence of infections also increases the risk and accelerates the development of cancer. HCC is one of the most common solid organ malignancies worldwide and is more frequently diagnosed at an advanced stage, which makes it as a leading cause of cancer-related mortality. Among those inflammatory-related cancers, HCC is one clear example showing strong association with inflammation.

A full study of the inflammatory pathways in HCC would reveal key molecules which may be utilized as therapeutic as well as anti-inflammatory targets.

Cytokines as mediators of chronic inflammation and HCC

The mediators that link inflammation and HCC are widely explored due to their great potential in future clinical investigations. Accumulating evidence indicates that certain transcriptional factors (e.g., NF-κB and STAT3), cytokines, chemokines and growth factors [e.g., TNF-α, IL-6, interferons, transforming growth factor beta (TGF-β) or epidermal growth factor receptor (EGFR)] as well as tumor-associated microenvironment are involved in HCC development. Among those mediators, cytokines have been suggested as key mediators in inflammatory-related HCC development. In this chapter, we will explore four main risk factors that could promote liver inflammation and tumorigenesis and will update the roles of key cytokines that contribute to these processes.

Virus association — chronic hepatitis B or C infections

Hepatitis B (HBV) and C (HCV) viral infections are the predominant etiological factors that are associated with the development of HCC, resulting from the induction of chronic inflammation. Although the exact mechanisms underlying the transition from HBV and HCV-induced chronic hepatitis to HCC remain elusive, aberrant expression of cytotoxic cytokines is thought to be critically involved.[3–5] Our recent study including mainly HBV cirrhotic patients has identified a gene signature correlated with the risk of metastatic HCC. This signature showed a marked increase in Th2 cytokines, implying an anti-inflammatory status in patients with metastatic HCC.[6] Most recently, another study indicated that the proinflammatory and homeostatic cytokines lymphotoxin (LT) α and β, two members of TNF superfamily, and the receptor (LTβR) are upregulated in HBV- or HCV-induced hepatitis and HCC. This study revealed that hepatocytes are the major LT-responsive liver cells, and LTβR inhibition in LTα, β-transgenic mice with hepatitis suppresses HCC formation. Thus, cytokine LT signaling represents a pathway involved in hepatitis-induced HCC.

Chemical carcinogens-aflatoxin

Aflatoxin exposure is another major risk factor for the development of HCC. Aflatoxins are toxins produced by the moulds *Aspergillus flavus* and *A. parasiticus*.[7] Epidemiological studies indicate that areas of endemic HBV are often found to also have high levels of the food borne contaminant aflatoxin.[8] HBV infection and aflatoxin exposure appear to have synergistic effects on the risk of HCC.[9]

Alcohol abuse

In 2004, the World Health Organization (WHO) concluded that alcohol accounts for approximately 1.8 million deaths per year. Long-term alcohol exposure is also one of the major risk factors of liver cirrhosis and HCC. It has been shown that altered cytokines have an important role in triggering the malignant growth. For example, an alcohol-induced induction of TNF-α expression and activation creates a cytokine pattern that promotes carcinogenesis.[10] A recent study indicates that IL-17$^+$ cells are significantly elevated in alcoholic liver disease and HCC.[11] IL-17, along with IL-22, is produced by Th17 cells, which represent a newly identified subset of T helper cells.[12–14] IL-17 is suggested to stimulate hepatocytes to produce C-reactive protein and promote hepatocyte survival.[15] In addition, Th17 cells may also promote HCC growth *via* production another cytokine of IL-22 that stimulates liver tumor cell proliferation.[16] Therefore, blocking or modulation of IL-17 might be a potential therapeutic strategy to treat alcohol-related liver diseases including HCC.

Obesity

Obesity is another HCC risk factor. Obesity is a major health problem worldwide, which increases the risk of developing several chronic diseases such as coronary heart disease, type II diabetes and nonalcoholic fatty liver disease (NAFLD). Epidemiological data indicate that obesity is strongly associated with the incidence and mortality of HCC. Recent studies have also demonstrated that either dietary or genetic obesity is a potent *bona fide* liver tumor promoter in mice. It is interesting to note that tumor-promoting cytokines IL-6 and TNF are required for obesity-promoted HCC development.[17]

Cytokines: from basic science research to translational and clinical research

It is notable that HCC develops almost exclusively in cirrhotic livers, which are resulted from either viral hepatitis or alcohol abuse induced chronic liver inflammation. Evidence suggests a dysregulation of inflammatory signaling in the development of HCC from advanced fibrosis and cirrhosis. Since inflammatory conditions are present before the occurring of the malignant change, understanding the physiological function of cytokines, which play a central role in connecting inflammation to cancer, as well as their precise roles in the pathogenesis, is important in clinical era. Here, we focus on two cytokines, i.e., TNF and IL-6, as examples for translating basic research to potential clinical applications.

Tumor necrosis factor

Receptors and signaling

TNF is a kind of inflammatory cytokines that exert a major role in the immune regulation and inflammatory responses.[18] There are two types in TNF class, i.e., TNF-α and TNF-β. TNF-α is the most common type with a dominant role in inducing cell death, inflammation, and preventing tumorigenesis. TNF-α binds to TNF receptor for its activation. There are two TNF receptors on the cell surface, i.e., TNF receptor type 1 (TNFR1) (also known as CD120a; p55/60) and TNF receptor type 2 (TNFR2) (also known as CD120b; p75/80), which can bind to TNF.[19,20] TNFR1, a type I transmembrane glyprotein identified in 1989, is expressed in most cells and can be fully activated by the membrane-integrated TNF or its soluble form released after proteolytic cleavage. TNFR2, found in 1990, is primarily expressed in hematopoietic lineage and endothelial cells and is proved to be only activated by the membrane-integrated form of TNF. Compared with TNFR1, TNFR2 lacks a death domain (DD).

TNFR1 activates multiple intracellular cascades including the transcriptional factor nuclear factor κB (NF-κB), the mitogen-activated protein kinase (MAPK), JNK, P38 and ERK pathways. TNFR1 mediates the signaling by recruiting proteins such as TNFR1-associated death domain (TRADD), TRAF2 and TRAF5 adaptor protein and protein kinase RIP1.[21] In the NF-κB pathway, TRADD recruits the ubiquitin ligases TNF receptor–associated factors TRAF2, TRAF5 and cellular inhibitors of apoptosis cIAP1 and cIAP2. TRAF2 also recruits the protein kinase IKK. IκBα binds to NF-κB, which is phosphorylated by IKK and degraded, causing the release of NF-κB. Consequently, NF-κB mediates the transcription of many proteins involved in cell death and inflammatory response. TNFR1 is also involved in death signaling because of existed DD located intracellularly. Nevertheless, TRADD can recruit the caspase-8 and cause cell apoptosis.[22] Activation of the TNFR2 members via their ligands also exerts a wide range of cellular responses. TNFR2 always functions together with TNFR1 through recruiting the E3 ligase –IAP1 which can ubiquitinate and degrade c-IAP2 and the adaptor protein TRAF. Indeed, membrane bound-TNF can bind both TNFR1 and TNFR2, and can show more efficiency to induce cell death than the soluble form of TNF.[23]

Biological activity and rationale for clinical development

TNF-α is a critical inflammatory cytokine involved in inflammation, tumor progression, cell death and cell survival. It was firstly identified as a powerful anti-tumor cytokine. However, evidence shows that it also acts as a tumor promoting factor. The contradictory roles of TNF-α on tumor probably reflect the difference between chronic local administration and acute high-dose local administration. High dose administration induced hemorrhagic tumor necrosis while chronically produced TNF-α was a key mediator of tumor-related inflammation.[24] So, TNF-α is a universal effectors involved in host defense and inflammation. *In vitro* study showed that TNF-α was found to be selectively toxic to tumor cells.[25] It was also reported that TNF-α is a key effecter molecule in $CD8^+$ T cells and NK cells-mediated cancer cell killing.[26] These data showed that TNF-α had a strong anti-tumor activity and it could become an important therapeutic target for cancer. However, systemic TNF-α treatment was closely related to serious toxicity, even raising the possibility that it could enhance tumor growth.[27] Considering its tumor promoting activity, inhibition of TNF-α by administrating anti-TNF antibodies or other TNF antagonists might be an effective tool in cancer therapy.

Gastrointestinal & hepatological diseases-related clinical trials

Numerous TNF-related clinical trials were conducted in the last 20 years. Because of its toxicity, it has not been widely used. Several studies by combining TNF with various agents have demonstrated significant anti-tumor activities. In 2006, a novel nanoparticle colloidal gold based delivery system bound with TNF was attempted in patients with advanced-stage solid malignancies including HCC. The principle of the study is that the diameter of the fenestrae of normal blood vessels ranges from 2 to 7 nm, the larger 27 nm colloidal gold nanoparticle, bound with anti-cancer therapeutic TNF, may redistribute its therapeutic payload away from healthy tissues and passively accumulate within solid tumors. The study of TNF-bound colloidal gold (CYT-6091) was initiated to determine its anti-tumor effects and its long-term toxicity. In this trial, 108 patients were stratified according to disease types and then received colloidal gold-bound TNF IV with beginning dose of 50 $\mu g\,m^{-2}$ and increased by 50 $\mu g\,m^{-2}$ 12–78 hours prior to surgery. Patients then undergo standard-care surgery. Tumor and normal tissues are removed for analysis of anti-tumor effects. Patients are followed 3 years for analysis of long-term toxicities and response to the treatment. Early clinical data showed that TNF bounded to the novel nanotechnology of colloidal gold did accumulate preferentially within tumors. In contrast to systemic administration of recombinant TNF, there appear to be no significant toxicities associated with colloidal gold delivery of TNF (NCT00436410).[28] Given the improved efficiency with combination therapy in this trial, the applications of the colloidal gold technology may involve conjugating other active agents before long.

Recently, a phase Ib dose-escalation study of recombinant asparagine-glycine-arginine-human TNF (NGR-hTNF) in combination with doxorubicin was initiated in patients with advanced or metastatic highly vascularised solid tumors to determine the safety and antivascular effect of escalating doses of NGR-hTNF (NCT00878111). NGR-hTNF is a vascular targeting agent exploiting a tumor-homing peptide (NGR) that selectively binds to aminopeptidase N/CD13, which is overexpressed on endothelial cells of newly formed tumor blood vessels. Cohorts of 15 patients were given NGR-hTNF (0.2–0.4–0.8–1.6 μg m^{-2}) and doxorubicin (60–75 mg m^{-2}), both given intravenously every 3 weeks. The preliminary data demonstrate that NGR-hTNF plus doxorubicin was administered safely and showed promising antivascular effect in patients pre-treated with anthracyclines. Based on tolerability, the dose level of 0.8 μg m^{-2} NGR-hTNF plus doxorubicin 75 mg m^{-2} was selected for phase II development.[29–32]

Based on the hypothesis that variant cytokine alleles might contribute to interindividual difference in HBV or HCV inflammatory responses and account for HCC outcome, recently, at least three trials were initiated in HBV or HCV-positive patients. One completed study demonstrated that carrying the TNF308.2 allele correlated with disease severity and hepatic fibrosis, which may contribute to higher HCC risk.[33]

IL-6

Receptors and signaling

Since its discovery and cloning at early 1980s by Dr. Tadamitsu Kishimoto and his colleagues, IL-6 has experienced enormous changes in its nomenclature as well as its biological significances and clinical impacts. IL-6 was initially suggested as a B cell stimulatory factor because it could stimulate immature B cells into immunoglobulin-producing cells. It was soon recognized that IL-6 acted as a myeloma/plasmacytoma growth factor and a hepatocyte stimulating factor, and was found to be involved in various diseases, including chronic inflammation and hemopoietic malignancies. Those findings immediately drew attentions of many immunologists and cancer researchers.[34–36] To date, IL-6 has been demonstrated to play important roles in inflammation regulation,[37] immune response and hematopoiesis,[38] metabolism,[39] and many other essential biological processes.[40]

Upon its activation by a variety of stimuli, such as cytokines, TNF, platelet-derived growth factor, and certain bacterial and viral components, IL-6 is produced by a number of antigen-presenting cells (e.g., dendritic cells and macrophages) as well as non-hematopoietic cells (keratinocytes, fibroblasts, and astrocytes). IL-6 utilizes its specific receptor complex IL-6R (also known as CD126) and a commonly shared signaling glycoprotein 130 (gp130, also known as CD130) as co-receptors possibly in a form of hexmeric complexes, each of which combines two heterotrimers of IL-6, IL-6R and gp130.[41] The formation of cytokine receptor, i.e., a cytokine-specific receptor plus a common signal transducer, seems to be shared by other cytokine systems.[42,43] In contrast to ubiquitously expressed gp130, IL-6R is mainly expressed by hepatocytes and leukocytes,[44,45] reminiscent of IL-6's regulation of acute phase protein response in the liver.[46] The physiological functions and activities of IL-6 will be discussed in the next section. Even without the presence of IL-6R, cells can still be responsive to IL-6 through a "trans-signaling" process mediated by soluble IL-6R (sIL-6R).[47] sIL-6R is generated by either metalloproteinase-mediated cleavage of membrane bound IL-6R or alternative splicing regulation occurring at pre-mRNA level. Through these mechanisms, sIL-6R migrates and binds to IL-6 and gp130 to form a functional complex, and thereby confers IL-6R-lacking cells with IL-6-responsiveness.

The downstream signaling following IL-6/IL-6R/gp130 formation includes but not limited to the JAK-STAT pathway, the MAP Kinase-NF-IL6 pathway, and the Negative Feedback pathway (SOCS).[48] In JAK-STAT pathway, IL-6 activates the Janus family of kinases (JAKs) bound to cytoplasmic domain of gp130, which in turn phosphorylates signal transducer and activator of transcription (STAT)-3 and promotes its nuclear relocalization and transcriptional regulation. Other downstream effectors of activated JAKs include the phosphoinositol 3 kinase (PI3K)-protein kinase B (pkB/Akt) pathway.[49,50] IL-6 also activates Ras-dependent MAP kinases through gp130, which phosphorylates nuclear factor (NF)-IL6 transcription factor at threonine 235. The activated NF-IL6 is bound to the IL-6-responsive elements in the promoters of acute phase genes, and positively regulates their expression. Besides, NF-IL6 seems to activate the gene expression of IL-6 by recognizing and binding to a 14 bp dyad sequence in the promoter region, therefore providing a positive feedback loop.[51] IL-6 induced expression of suppressor of cytokine signals (SOCS), on the other hand, represses IL-6-activated JAK-STAT pathway and thereby is involved in the negative feedback regulation of IL-6.

Besides IL-6 signaling itself, the extensive interaction with other signaling pathways, such as TGF-beta, cyclooxygenase (COX)-2, Wnt/wingless, and NF-κB pathways, contribute to the tumorigenic activity of IL-6 in liver cancer and other cancer types.[52]

Biological activity and rationale for clinical development

IL-6 has a wide variety of biologic effects, which includes acute phase reactants in liver, in inflammation regulation, immune response, metabolism, cell survival, proliferation, differentiation, and angiogenesis. All of these functions strongly suggest the high relevance of IL-6 and its downstream signaling in tumorigenesis. In fact, many tumor types have been shown to have a high expression level of IL-6 with STAT-3 persistently activated,[53,54] and the IL-6 level in circulation is associated with high risk of HCC in patients with chronic hepatitis B infection.[55] Furthermore, evidence is emerging to expose the intrinsic and direct links between IL-6 and cell transformation/tumor initiation. IL-6-mediated activation of STAT-3 has been shown to be crucial for malignant transformation, cell motility, cell growth, and maintenance/self-renewal of cancer stem cell populations in lung, prostate, HCC, and breast cancer.[56,57] IL-6 has also been suggested to play roles in bone metastasis and cancer progression. Those evidences strongly argue for the potential of targeting IL-6 in cancer therapy, which have led to a number of clinical trials as discussed below.

Gastrointestinal & hepatological diseases-related clinical trials

To date, no clinical data exist for anti-IL-6 administration to patients with gastrointestinal or hepatological diseases. However, a phase I/II study of CNTO 328 in patients with solid tumors has currently been approved by FDA (NCT00841191). CNTO 328 (siltuximab), developed by Centocor, is a human-mouse chimeric monoclonal antibody that specifically binds human IL-6 with high affinity. The purpose of this study is to determine the recommended dose of CNTO 328 monotherapy, in patient with malignant solid tumors and to estimate the clinical benefit of CNTO 328 monotherapy in patients with ovarian cancer and with KRAS mutant tumors. Despite the lack of clinical data, numerous pre-clinical models have strongly suggested the anticancer utility of CNTO 328 administration in the context of advanced malignancy. Zaki *et al.* have shown that CNTO 328 could completely inhibit IL-6 induced serum amyloid A (SAA) production in a dose-dependent manner.[58] They also showed that treatment of tumor-induced cachexia nude mice with systemic administration of CNTO 328 inhibited body weight loss, indicating the suppression of cachexia by CNTO 328.[59] Besides its own effect, two studies by Voorhees and colleagues also suggested strong rationale for the clinical development of the CNTO 328/dexamethasone and CNTO 328/bortezomib combination for patients with myeloma.[60,61] Compared to other two previously conducted trials in patients with advanced multiple myeloma (MM) and patients with renal cell carcinoma (RCC), current clinical trial of CNTO 328 is a new one produced with changed process. Considering it's first administration to patients, the planned trial will attempt to demonstrate safety and confirm those findings of anti-cancer activity in patients.

Concluding remarks and future perspectives

The link between inflammation and cancer has been well accepted. Although numerous cytokines as central mediators of the connection, were demonstrated clinically significant against certain malignancies, tumor specific, or even tumor stage specific inflammatory subtypes or cytokines/cytokine profiles, truly represent the biology of tumorigenesis. All these await to be assessed and utilized as a valuable tool in prognosis, diagnosis, and treatment of HCC or other malignancies.

References

1. Budhu A, Wang XW. (2006) The role of cytokines in hepatocellular carcinoma. *J Leukoc Biol* **80**:1197–213.

2. Hussain SP, Hofseth LJ, Harris CC. (2003) Radical causes of cancer. *Nat Rev Cancer* **3**:276–85.
3. Lee SH, Park SG, Lim SO *et al.* (2005) The hepatitis B virus X protein up-regulates lymphotoxin alpha expression in hepatocytes. *Biochim Biophys Acta* **1741**:75–84.
4. Vainer GW, Pikarsky E, Ben-Neriah Y. (2008) Contradictory functions of NF-κB in liver physiology and cancer. *Cancer Lett* **267**:182–8.
5. Haybaeck J, Zeller N, Wolf MJ *et al.* (2009) A lymphotoxin-driven pathway to hepatocellular carcinoma. *Cancer Cell* **16**:295–308.
6. Budhu A, Forgues M, Ye QH *et al.* (2006) Prediction of venous metastases, recurrence and prognosis in hepatocellular carcinoma based on a unique immune response signature of the liver microenvironment. *Cancer Cell* **10**:99–111.
7. Wogan GN. (1992) Aflatoxins as risk factors for hepatocellular carcinoma in humans. *Cancer Res* **52**:2114s–8s.
8. Groopman JD, Johnson D, Kensler TW. (2005) Aflatoxin and hepatitis B virus biomarkers: A paradigm for complex environmental exposures and cancer risk. *Cancer Biomark* **1**:5–14.
9. Ross RK, Yuan JM, Yu MC *et al.* (1992) Urinary aflatoxin biomarkers and risk of hepatocellular carcinoma. *Lancet* **339**:943–6.
10. Tilg H, Diehl AM. (2000) Cytokines in alcoholic and nonalcoholic steatohepatitis. *N Engl J Med* **343**:1467–76.
11. Lemmers A, Moreno C, Gustot T *et al.* (2009) The interleukin-17 pathway is involved in human alcoholic liver disease. *Hepatology* **49**:646–57.
12. Stockinger B, Veldhoen M. (2007) Differentiation and function of Th17 T cells. *Curr Opin Immunol* **19**:281–286.
13. Dong C. (2008) Regulation and pro-inflammatory function of interleukin-17 family cytokines. *Immunol Rev* **226**:80–86.
14. Ouyang W, Kolls JK, Zheng Y. (2008) The biological functions of T helper 17 cell effector cytokines in inflammation. *Immunity* **28**:454–67.
15. Patel DN, King CA, Bailey SR *et al.* (2007) Interleukin-17 stimulates C-reactive protein expression in hepatocytes and smooth muscle cells via p38 MAPK and ERK1/2-dependent NF-κB and C/EBP beta activation. *J Biol Chem* **282**:27229–38.
16. Radaeva S, Sun R, Pan HN *et al.* (2004) Interleukin 22 (IL-22) plays a protective role in T cell-mediated murine hepatitis:IL-22 is a survival factor for hepatocytes via STAT3 activation. *Hepatology* **39**:1332–42.

17. Park EJ, Lee JH, Yu GY *et al.* (2010) Dietary and genetic obesity promote liver inflammation and tumorigenesis by enhancing IL-6 and TNF expression. *Cell* **140**:197–208.
18. Locksley RM, Killeen N, Lenardo MJ. (2001) The TNF and TNF receptor superfamilies: Integrating mammalian biology. *Cell* **104**:487–501.
19. Tanabe K, Matsushima-Nishiwaki R, Yamaguchi S *et al.* (2010) Mechanisms of tumor necrosis factor-alpha-induced interleukin-6 synthesis in glioma cells. *J Neuroinflammation* **7**:16.
20. Martinez-Moczygemba M, Huston DP. (2003) Biology of common beta receptor-signaling cytokines: IL-3, IL-5, and GM-CSF. *J Allergy Clin Immunol* **112**:653–65.
21. Bouwmeester T, Bauch A, Ruffner H *et al.* (2004) A physical and functional map of the human TNF-α/NF-κB signal transduction pathway. *Nat Cell Biol* **6**:97–105.
22. Micheau O, Tschopp J. (2003) Induction of TNF receptor I-mediated apoptosis via two sequential signaling complexes. *Cell* **114**:181–90.
23. Grell M, Wajant H, Zimmermann G *et al.* (1998) The type 1 receptor (CD120a) is the high-affinity receptor for soluble tumor necrosis factor. *Proc Natl Acad Sci USA* **95**:570–5.
24. Balkwill F. (2009) Tumour necrosis factor and cancer. *Nat Rev Cancer* **9**:361–71.
25. Colotta F, Peri G, Villa A *et al.* (1984) Rapid killing of actinomycin D-treated tumor cells by human mononuclear cells. I. Effectors belong to the monocyte-macrophage lineage. *J Immunol* **132**:936–44.
26. Prevost-Blondel A, Roth E, Rosenthal FM *et al.* (2000) Crucial role of TNF-alpha in CD8 T cell-mediated elimination of 3LL-A9 Lewis lung carcinoma cells *in vivo*. *J Immunol* **164**:3645–51.
27. Leibovich SJ, Polverini PJ, Shepard HM *et al.* (1987) Macrophage-induced angiogenesis is mediated by tumour necrosis factor-alpha. *Nature* **329**:630–2.
28. Powell AC, Paciotti GF, Libutti SK. (2010) Colloidal gold: A novel nanoparticle for targeted cancer therapeutics. *Methods Mol Biol* **624**:375–84.
29. Gregorc V, Citterio G, Vitali G *et al.* (2010) Defining the optimal biological dose of NGR-hTNF, a selective vascular targeting agent, in advanced solid tumours. *Eur J Cancer* **46**:198–206.
30. Gregorc V, Santoro A, Bennicelli E *et al.* (2009) Phase Ib study of NGR-hTNF, a selective vascular targeting agent, administered at low doses in

combination with doxorubicin to patients with advanced solid tumours. *Br J Cancer* **101**:219–24.

31. Gregorc V, Zucali PA, Santoro A *et al.* (2010) Phase II study of asparagine-glycine-arginine-human tumor necrosis factor alpha, a selective vascular targeting agent, in previously treated patients with malignant pleural mesothelioma. *J Clin Oncol* **28**:2604–11.
32. van Laarhoven HW, Fiedler W, Desar IM *et al.* (2010) Phase I clinical and magnetic resonance imaging study of the vascular agent NGR-hTNF in patients with advanced cancers (European Organization for Research and Treatment of Cancer Study 16041). *Clin Cancer Res* **16**:1315–23.
33. Jeng JE, Tsai HR, Chuang LY *et al.* (2009) Independent and additive interactive effects among tumor necrosis factor-alpha polymorphisms, substance use habits, and chronic hepatitis B and hepatitis C virus infection on risk for hepatocellular carcinoma. *Medicine (Baltimore)* **88**:349–57.
34. Andus T, Geiger T, Hirano T *et al.* (1987) Recombinant human B cell stimulatory factor 2 (BSF-2/IFN-beta 2) regulates beta-fibrinogen and albumin mRNA levels in Fao-9 cells. *FEBS Lett* **221**:18–22.
35. Gauldie J, Richards C, Harnish D *et al.* (1987) Interferon beta 2/B-cell stimulatory factor type 2 shares identity with monocyte-derived hepatocyte-stimulating factor and regulates the major acute phase protein response in liver cells. *Proc Natl Acad Sci USA* **84**:7251–5.
36. Kawano M, Hirano T, Matsuda T *et al.* (1988) Autocrine generation and requirement of BSF-2/IL-6 for human multiple myelomas. *Nature* **332**:83–5.
37. Gabay C. (2006) Interleukin-6 and chronic inflammation. *Arthritis Res Ther* **8**(Suppl 2):S3.
38. Hirano T, Taga T, Matsuda T *et al.* (1990) Interleukin 6 and its receptor in the immune response and hematopoiesis. *Int J Cell Cloning* **8**(Suppl 1):155–66.
39. Krook A. (2008) IL-6 and metabolism-new evidence and new questions. *Diabetologia* **51**:1097–99.
40. Ara T, Declerck YA. (2010) Interleukin-6 in bone metastasis and cancer progression. *Eur J Cancer* **46**:1223–31.
41. Boulanger MJ, Chow DC, Brevnova EE *et al.* (2003) Hexameric structure and assembly of the interleukin-6/IL-6 alpha-receptor/gp130 complex. *Science* **300**:2101–4.

42. Russell SM, Keegan AD, Harada N *et al.* (1993) Interleukin-2 receptor gamma chain: A functional component of the interleukin-4 receptor. *Science* **262**:1880–3.
43. Obiri NI, Debinski W, Leonard WJ *et al.* (1995) Receptor for interleukin 13. Interaction with interleukin 4 by a mechanism that does not involve the common gamma chain shared by receptors for interleukins 2, 4, 7, 9, and 15. *J Biol Chem* **270**:8797–804.
44. Hibi M, Murakami M, Saito M *et al.* (1990) Molecular cloning and expression of an IL-6 signal transducer, gp130. *Cell* **63**:1149–57.
45. Saito M, Yoshida K, Hibi M *et al.* (1992) Molecular cloning of a murine IL-6 receptor-associated signal transducer, gp130, and its regulated expression *in vivo*. *J Immunol* **148**:4066–71.
46. Kamimura D, Ishihara K, Hirano T. (2003) IL-6 signal transduction and its physiological roles: The signal orchestration model. *Rev Physiol Biochem Pharmacol* **149**:1–38.
47. Scheller J, Rose-John S. (2006) Interleukin-6 and its receptor: From bench to bedside. *Med Microbiol Immunol* **195**:173–83.
48. Kishimoto T. (2005) Interleukin-6: From basic science to medicine — 40 years in immunology. *Annu Rev Immunol* **23**:1–21.
49. Zhang J, Li Y, Shen B. (2003) PI3-K/Akt pathway contributes to IL-6-dependent growth of 7TD1 cells. *Cancer Cell Int* **3**:1.
50. Jee SH, Chu CY, Chiu HC *et al.* (2004) Interleukin-6 induced basic fibroblast growth factor-dependent angiogenesis in basal cell carcinoma cell line via JAK/STAT3 and PI3-kinase/Akt pathways. *J Invest Dermatol* **123**:1169–75.
51. Akira S, Isshiki H, Sugita T *et al.* (1990) A nuclear factor for IL-6 expression (NF-IL6) is a member of a C/EBP family. *EMBO J* **9**:1897–906.
52. Shackel NA, McCaughan GW, Warner FJ. (2008) Hepatocellular carcinoma development requires hepatic stem cells with altered transforming growth factor and interleukin-6 signaling. *Hepatology* **47**:2134–6.
53. Mora LB, Buettner R, Seigne J *et al.* (2002) Constitutive activation of Stat3 in human prostate tumors and cell lines: Direct inhibition of Stat3 signaling induces apoptosis of prostate cancer cells. *Cancer Res* **62**:6659–66.
54. Bromberg JF, Wrzeszczynska MH, Devgan G *et al.* (1999) Stat3 as an oncogene. *Cell* **98**:295–303.

55. Wong VW, Yu J, Cheng AS *et al.* (2009) High serum interleukin-6 level predicts future hepatocellular carcinoma development in patients with chronic hepatitis B. *Int J Cancer* **124**:2766–70.
56. Tang Y, Kitisin K, Jogunoori W *et al.* (2008) Progenitor/stem cells give rise to liver cancer due to aberrant TGF-beta and IL-6 signaling. *Proc Natl Acad Sci USA* **105**:2445–50.
57. Iliopoulos D, Hirsch HA, Struhl K. (2009) An epigenetic switch involving NF-kappaB, Lin28, Let-7 MicroRNA, and IL6 links inflammation to cell transformation. *Cell* **139**:693–706.
58. Li J, Hu XF, Xing PX. (2005) CNTO-328 (Centocor). *Curr Opin Investig Drugs* **6**:639–45.
59. Zaki MH, Nemeth JA, Trikha M. (2004) CNTO 328, a monoclonal antibody to IL-6, inhibits human tumor-induced cachexia in nude mice. *Int J Cancer* **111**:592–5.
60. Voorhees PM, Chen Q, Kuhn DJ *et al.* (2007) Inhibition of interleukin-6 signaling with CNTO 328 enhances the activity of bortezomib in preclinical models of multiple myeloma. *Clin Cancer Res* **13**:6469–78.
61. Voorhees PM, Chen Q, Small GW *et al.* (2009) Targeted inhibition of interleukin-6 with CNTO 328 sensitizes pre-clinical models of multiple myeloma to dexamethasone-mediated cell death. *Br J Haematol* **145**:481–90.

Chapter 11

Role of Nuclear Factor-κB Pathway in Gastrointestinal Inflammation and Cancer

Muthu K. Shanmugam[1], Nadine Upton[1,3], Gautam Sethi[1] and WS Fred Wong[1,2,*]

[1]*Department of Pharmacology, Yong Loo Lin School of Medicine;*
[2]*Immunology Program, Life Science Institute,*
National University of Singapore, Singapore; and
[3]*Department of BioMedical Sciences, King's College London,*
United Kingdom

The link between inflammation and cancer development has been reported in numerous research publications and substantiates the involvement of nuclear factor-κB (NF-κB), a versatile transcription factor, in inflammatory bowel disease (IBD). NF-κB can be activated by a wide array of inducers including bacteria, fungi and viruses, cytokines and stress. NF-κB is identified as a key regulator in the immunopathogenesis of IBD and genetic polymorphisms in NF-κB have supported the connection between IBD and colorectal cancer progression. Importantly, the role of cytokines and chemokines secreted by the epithelial cells and infiltrating cells such as macrophages and neutrophils contributes to the sustained and constitutive activation of NF-κB in these cells. In addition, NF-κB hyperactivation has been observed in colorectal cancer and alters the expression of target genes such as TNF-α, IL-6, IL-23, COX-2, NOD2/CARD15 and matrix metalloproteases. In this chapter, we discuss our current understanding of the role of NF-κB in Crohn's disease, ulcerative colitis, Barrett's metaplasia

* Corresponding author. E-mail: phcwongf@nus.edu.sg

and colorectal cancer. Inhibiting NF-κB activity has been shown to suppress inflammation and slow down cancer progression. A number of genes and proteins are discussed in detail and their specific roles in various stages of the disease pathogenesis reveal the complexity of this intracellular signaling pathway. In this context, complete elucidation of the role of NF-κB signalling in gastrointestinal tract-associated inflammation and cancer may lead to identification of novel therapeutic strategies for IBD.

Introduction

David Baltimore and Ranjan Sen in 1986 characterized the protein nuclear factor-κB (NF-κB) and its functional role as a transcription factor that binds to enhancer sites on the genome and regulates the expression of immuno-globulin κ-light chain in B cells.[1,2] It can be agreed that our ever increasing knowledge of this vital signaling pathway in nearly all cell types, not just in B cells, has contributed substantially to our understanding of the pathophysiology of an endless list of human diseases. Activation of the NF-κB pathway leads to the expression of a wide array of genes essential for cellular differentiation, proliferation and survival.[3] Thus, dysregulation of this signalling pathway has been implicated in the development of diseases such as inflammatory bowel disease (IBD), chronic obstructive pulmonary disease, rheumatoid arthritis, cancers and many more.[4] Since the 1990's, an association of constitutive NF-κB activation with cancer development and progression has been established.[5] The first evidence for this proposed NF-κB-cancer-relationship stemmed from the structural similarities between the v-Rel oncogenic protein and the NF-κB *c*-Rel protein.[6] In fact, recent studies have shown a link between cancer and over-expression of the Rel proteins in cancer cell lines.[7,8] Future inflammation and cancer therapy is likely to be focused towards targeting the NF-κB pathway and its accompanying effects on other physiological processes and signalling pathways.

Structural components and organization of NF-κB pathway

There are currently five identified members in the NF-κB transcription factor family, namely p65/RelA, c-Rel, RelB, p52 and p50[9] (Figure 1).

NF-kB	Structure	Size (No. amino acids)	Main activating Phosphorylation sites
P65/RelA	NTD – DimD – L – TAD	551	Serines 276, 311, 529 & 536
c-Rel	NTD – DimD – L – TAD	619	Serines 267, 454, 460 & 471
RelB	LZ – NTD – DimD – L – TAD	557	Serines 368, 552
P52/p100	NTD – DimD – L – G – Ank – DD	447/899	Serines 99, 108, 115 & 123
P50/p105	NTD – DimD – L – G – Ank – DD	433/969	Serines 337, 903, 907, 927 & 932

<u>Key</u>

- NTD (amino terminal domain)
- DimD (dimerization domain)
- L 10 amino acid polypeptide linker to the NLS
- TAD (Transcription activation domain)
- G (Glycine-rich regions)
- LZ (Leucine-zipper)
- ANK (Ankyrin repeats)
- DD (Death domain)

Figure 1. Structure of Rel proteins.

They share similar structural domains such as the Rel Homology Domain (RHD) and transcription activation domain (TAD) (absent in p50 and p52), which enable them to dimerize and physically bind via promoter enhancer molecules to variations of specific DNA sequences, the κB sites: 5′-GGGRNYYYCC-3′, R being a purine, Y a pyrimidine, and N as any nucleotide.[10] They activate transcription in a stimulus-dependent manner of specific genes involved in processes such as inflammation, cell proliferation and survival.[3,9]

In resting cells, NF-κB subunits exist as homodimers or heterodimers (e.g. p52/52, p65/p50), out of 15 possible formations of dimers bound to the inhibitory κB proteins (IκBs) within the cytoplasm, which mask their nuclear localisation signals (NLS) and as such NF-κB dimers are unable to be translocated to the nucleus.(11) IκBs negatively regulate NF-κB activity by heterodimerizing with p65 in the cytosol and control NF-κB transcriptional activity. IκBs can be subdivided into the typical IκBs (IκBα, IκBβ and IκBε), the atypical IκBs (Bcl-3 and IκBζ), and the precursor IκBs (p100 & p105). They contain up to 7 of the 33-amino-acid consensus ankyrin repeats (ANK) in their C-terminals which can bind to Rel proteins and mask their NLS.[11] IκBα is the most extensively studied, especially for its activity with the p65/p50 heterodimers. Upon stimulation, IκBα can be phosphorylated at ser[32] and ser[36] residues by the upstream IκB kinase complex (IKK complex), and is recognised by the Skp1-Cull-F box protein-β-transducin repeat-containing protein ($SCF^{\beta TrCP}$), leading to rapid polyubiquitination by E3 ubiquitin-ligase and degradation in the 26S proteasome.[12] This effectively releases the bound NF-κB dimers for subsequent phosphorylation and acetylation, and promotes their nuclear translocation.

The IKK complex is composed of two catalytic kinases IKKα and IKKβ, and one non-catalytic adapter scaffold subunit IKKγ, also known as NF-κB essential modifier (NEMO). The main function of the IKK is to phosphorylate and remove the inhibitory effect of IκBs on NF-κB dimers. This heterotrimer complex formation is required to achieve optimal activation of kinase activity.[13] Recent gel filtration chromatography studies revealed a holocomplex of 700–900 kDa, far exceeding the predicted total molecular mass of 220 kDa for the heterotrimers, leading us to believe that there are additional components such as ELKS, Hsp90 and Cdc37 aggregated in the IKK complex.[14,15]

IKKα and IKKβ are not biochemically equivalent, but do share similar structures by having N-terminal kinase domains containing active T loop serine residues which are vital for activation, conserved leucine zippers allowing for dimerization, putative helix-loop-helix motifs and NEMO-binding domain in their C terminal.[16] The possession of an NLS in IKKα's kinase domain as compared to the critical ubiquitin-like domain located in IKKβ gives rise to potential IKK-independent function of the two kinases.[12,16]

NF-κB activation

There are two major pathways that eventually lead to nuclear translocation of specific NF-κB dimers: the canonical and the non-canonical pathways (Figures 2 and 3).

The canonical pathway

Activation of the canonical pathway is vital for both innate and adaptive immunity, in particular the inflammatory responses.[10,12] Thus, the majority of the resulting genes expressed are proteins involved in processes such

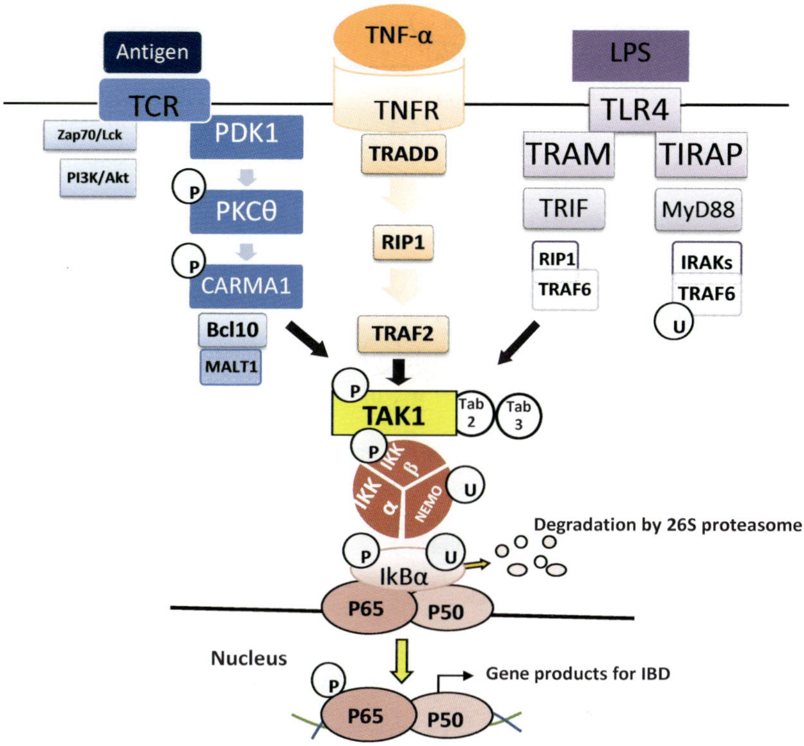

Figure 2. Canonical pathway — There are 3 proposed routes of activation which all converge to IKK activation following IKKβ phosphorylation. **TCR route**: Stimulation of TCR causes recruitment and activation of kinases Lck and ZAP70 as part of a cascade leading to PKCθ activation. The Akt kinase is activated and recruits PDK1. PDK1 can also phosphorylate and activate PKCθ enabling it to recruit and phosphorylate CARMA1. Bcl10 and MALT1 combined with CARMA1 to form a stable CBM complex. This CBM complex leads to NEMO ubiquitination and IKKβ phosphorylation via activation of TAK1. **TLR route**: LPS stimulates TLR4 receptor which leads to recruitment of Tab2/3 and TAK1 activation via two proposed pathways which converge to recruitment and activation of TRAF6 which lead to TAK1 activation: (A) MyD88-dependent pathway: TIRAP bridges MyD88 and the active receptor. MyD88 recruits members of the IRAK family which results in recruitment and self-ubiquitination of TRAF6. (B) TRIF-dependent pathway: TRAM bridges TRIF to TLR4 which directly interacts with Rip1-associated-TRAF6. **TNFR route**: TNFR1 stimulation recruits TRAF2 and Rip1 via TRADD. TRAF2 ubiquitinates Rip1 which binds to NEMO within the now stable IKK complex. IKK may be activated via autophosphorylation or by active Tab2/3 bound TAK-1. P, phosphorylation; U, ubiquitination.

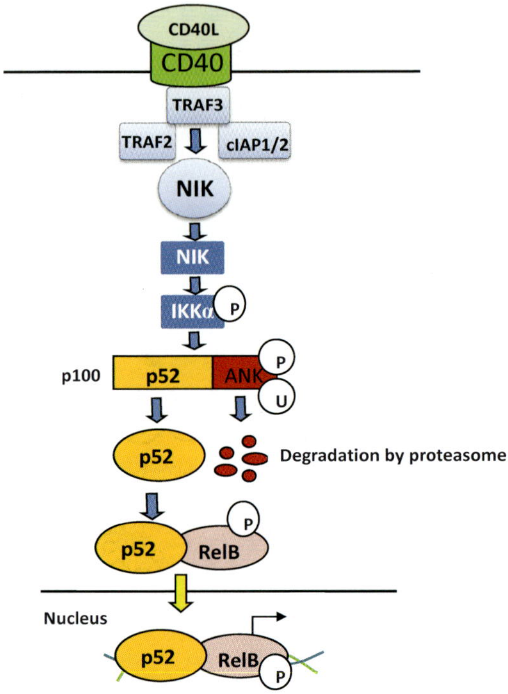

Figure 3. Non-canonical pathway — CD40 receptor stimulation results in recruitment of a complex containing TRAF2 and TRAF3 adapter molecules, cIAP1 and cIAP2, and NIK. Receptor stimulation triggers polyubiquitination and degradation of components of the complex which prevents binding of NIK. NIK is stabilised and released from the complex. NIK becomes activated by autophosphorylation prior to phosphorylating IKKα kinase. Active IKKα phosphorylates p100 Ankyrin repeats to yield the active p52 protein bound to RelB. The p52: RelB heterodimers is then able to translocate into the nucleus and bind to the DNA κB site and activate transcription. P, phosphorylation; U, ubiquitination.

as inflammatory cell recruitment and cytokine production. Therefore it does not come as a surprise that the canonical pathway is stimulated by a wide range of physiological and environmental stimuli including allergen, viral and bacterial products, ultraviolet radiation and cytokines (e.g. TNF-α), which converge to the activation of the common IKK complex. p65/p50 heterodimers are the most abundant NF-κB dimers in the canonical pathway. The activity of p65/p50 is tightly controlled by phosphorylation-induced activation of the IKK complex together with its downstream substrate inhibitory IκBα.

IKKβ plays a predominant role in the canonical pathway leading to pro-inflammatory responses[17] whereas IKKα is considered to have a more significant role in the non-canonical pathway.[18] Indeed, studies have shown that canonical pathway-mediated NF-κB activation is completely abolished in the absence of either IKKβ[17] or NEMO.[19] Upon activation of antigen receptors, toll-like receptors or TNF-α receptors, IKKβ is directly phosphorylated at the T loop ser[177] and ser[811] residues by TGF-β-activated kinase 1 (TAK1), leading to a conformational change in the IKK complex.[11] It is believed that NEMO is essential for mediating interactions of IKK via its N-terminus with the upstream signaling adapters.[11,19] Activated IKKβ with highest affinity for IκBα phosphorylates IκBα at Ser[32] and Ser[36,12,17] resulting in its rapid ubiquitin-induced degradation by the 26S proteasome, enhances NF-κB nuclear translocation and transcriptional activation.

The non-canonical pathway

In comparison to the canonical pathway, the range of activating stimuli is fairly limited to only a few of the TNF receptor family members such as B cell-activating factor (BAFF), B cell CD40, osteoclast membrane protein RANK (Receptor Activator of NF-κB) and lymphotoxin β on stromal cells. This pathway is associated with the generation and organisation of secondary lymphoid organs, B cell survival and maturation.[11] The main NF-κB involved is the p52/RelB heterodimers, which are derived from the p100/RelB inactive dimmers.[9,11]

Following receptor stimulation, NF-κB-inducing kinase (NIK) is activated by autophosphorylation, which in turn phosphorylates IKKα at its T-loop serine residues.[18,20] Activated IKKα phosphorylates p100 ankyrin repeats to yield the transcriptionally active p52 protein ("p100 processing").[18] As opposed to the canonical pathway whereby activation involves the IKK complex, only IKKα is required for p100 phosphorylation and processing to yield the active p52/RelB heterodimers.

Inflammatory bowel disease

IBD is an inflammatory disorder of the gastrointestinal tract and comprises of two major manifestations of the disease, Crohn's disease and ulcerative colitis. Crohn's disease and ulcerative colitis exhibit familial clustering and the risk factor of disease within close family members and relatives of IBD patients is increased by 15-fold in Crohn's disease and 10-fold in ulcerative colitis.[21] NF-κB is considered the principal transcription factor involved in diverse immune responses in the gastrointestinal tract[22] and activated NF-κB has been observed in IBD.[23] Crohn's disease-designated IBD1 locus is on chromosome 16q and contains CARD15/NOD2 susceptibility gene for IBD.[24] An additional linkage region maps to chromosome 4q. In this region NF-κB1 gene encodes 2 subunits of NF-κB, p50 and p105.[25,26] Polymorphism within NF-κB1 gene has been shown in ulcerative colitis and functional relevance of this polymorphism in the pathogenesis of IBD is also reported.[27] NF-κB family of proteins regulate the transcription of genes coding for cytokines, chemokines, cell adhesion molecules, metastatic genes, apoptosis, angiogenesis, chemoresistance and chemoprevention.[9,28,29] The important inflammatory mediators in IBD are summarised in Table 1. These molecules contribute to the initiation and progression of IBD and associated colorectal cancer.

Crohn's disease

Crohn's disease affects specifically terminal ileum, cecum, perianal area of the colon. It is characterized by dense infiltration of lymphocytes and macrophages and by the presence of granuloma fissuring ulceration and submucosal fibrosis. Crohn's disease affects 10–200 per 100,000 persons in North America and Europe with increased rate of disease occurrence in the last decade.[21,22] Activated NF-κB in mucosal macrophages and monocytes and up-regulated expression of TNF-α, IL-1β and IL-6 have been observed in Crohn's disease patients.[30] In lamina propria cells of the colon, CD40 and CD40L interaction activates NF-κB. The activation leads to increased expression of cytokines IL-6, IL-8 and monocyte chemoattractant protein (MCP).[31] NF-κB can also be activated via ligation of toll-like receptor (TLR) and NOD like receptors (NLR), with intracellular NLR signalling likely to be of particular significance in regulating intestinal immune tone in the gut. Crohn's disease is associated with NOD2 mutations which may impair NF-κB activation[32] and alter TLR/NLR cross-talk.[33]

Table 1. List of NF-κB-dependent genes up-regulated in IBD.

IBD	NF-κB signature genes up-regulated under various pathological settings	Target cells	References
Oesophagitis	IL-1β, IL-4, IL-6, IL-8, IL-10, IFNγ, TNFα, COX-2	Squamous oesophageal epithelium	37
Squamous oesophageal adenocarcinoma	IL-1β, IL-8, TNFα, COX-2	Squamous oesophageal epithelium	40
Barrett's Metaplasia	IL-1β, IL-4, IL-6, IL-8, IL-10, IFNγ, TNFα, COX-2, CDX2, CCR9, CCL25, NOD2/CARD15	Squamous oesophageal epithelium, columnar epithelium	37, 38, 41, 42
Crohn's disease	IL-1β, IL-4, IL-6, IL-8, IL-10, IL-12, IL12p40, IL-17, IL-22, IL-23, IL-23R, IL23p19, IFNγ, TNFα, COX-2, ATG16L1, MST1, PTGER4, SLC22A5, IRGM, ZNF365, NKX2-3, STAT3, PTPN2, SPAK, NOD2/CARD15, CX3CL1-CX3CR1, CCL20–CCR6, CCL25–CCR9, CXCL10–CXCR3	CD4+ T-lymphocytes, Th17 T cells macrophages, CD8+ T cells, lamina propria, dendritic, paneth, goblet, microfold and epithelial cells.	21, 22, 69–73
Ulcerative colitis	IL-1β, IL-4, IL- 5, IL-6, IL-8, IL-9, IL-10, IL-12, IL12p40, IL-13, IL-23, IL23R, IL23p19, IL-25, IFNγ, TNFα, COX-2, MST1, NKX2-3, STAT3, NOD2/CARD15, SPAK CCL20–CCR6, CCL25–CCR9, CXCL10–CXCR3,	Basophils, mast cells, eosinophils, B cells, epithelial cells, macrophages, neutrophils, mucosal cells and bacteria.	21, 22, 69–73
Colorectal cancer	IL-8, TIMP1, MMP1, Pai1, βCatenin, properidin, CDK1, Cyclin D1, Cyclin G2, FOS, ETS2, Serpine B5, Apaf1, VEGF, COX-2, EGFR, CD44	Epithelial cells	74–76
Pouchitis	IL-1β, TNFα, TLR2, TLR4, NOD2/CARD15	Mucosal cells and paneth cells.	76

Ulcerative colitis

Ulcerative colitis is characterized by chronic relapsing and crippling inflammation of the colonic mucosa, submucosa and epithelium. Inflammation in the rectum reaches caecum in a continuous fashion.[22] Chronic inflammation is widely recognized as a major source for DNA damage, reactive oxygen species generation and immune cell invasion and cancer development. Although the exact aetiology leading to ulcerative colitis remain unknown, it has been generally accepted that over-expression of pro-inflammatory cytokines play an important role in the pathogenesis of ulcerative colitis.[23] Immuno-histochemical analysis of mucosal tissues obtained from ulcerative colitis patients have shown increased activation of NF-κB in the macrophages, epithelial cells and in lamina propria cells of the colon.[30,34] Indeed, studies of the inflamed mucosa from patients with ulcerative colitis have shown increased expression of IL-1β, IL-6, and TNF-α.[35] IL-8 is a powerful chemotactic and neutrophil activating cytokine. It is produced by variety of cell types including monocytes, neutrophils, and epithelial cells following *in vitro* stimulation and increased expression of IL-8 is observed in ulcerative colitis.[36] Recent evidence suggests NF-κB induced activation of IL-8 leads to colorectal cancer.[35]

Barrett's metaplasia

Barrett's metaplasia occurs as a precursor lesion in the oesophagus that leads to oesophageal carcinoma. Barrett's metaplasia is defined as the replacement of squamous oesophageal epithelium with columnar epithelium.[37,38] Epithelial changes resulting in unpredictable neoplastic behaviour may be induced or potentiated as a consequence of interstitial inflammation. Inflammation is seen in both oesophageal carcinoma and Barrett's metaplasia as a result of long-term acid and bile reflux from the stomach back to the oesophagus. NF-κB and cyclooxygenase 2 (COX-2) are found in increased levels in Barrett's metaplasia,[39,40] thus forming the molecular basis for implicating chronic inflammation in cancer development. Besides, upregulation of caudal homeobox 2 (CDX2) expression by cytokines such as IL-1β, IL-6, IFNγ, TNFα, bile acids, LPS, and peptidoglycan (PGN) is associated with dysregulated intestinal development and Barrett's metaplasia.[41] CDX1 and CDX2 are NF-κB-regulated gene products and have been shown to regulate intestine development. Transgenic mouse models of CDX genes show development of Barrett's metaplasia. This significant publication provides for the first time evidence of the induction of CDX1 in oesophagitis before the development of intestinal metaplasia in a rat model of Barrett's metaplasia.[42]

Role of NF-κB in IBD and IBD-associated colorectal cancer

Constitutively high levels of NF-κB have been detected in epithelial cells, macrophages and lamina propria cells of IBD patients, thus providing strong evidence for constitutive NF-κB activation and that these patients have been identified to have increased risk of developing IBD associated colorectal cancer.[30]

TNF-α is an important cytokine for the pathogenesis of IBD. TNF-α induces phosphorylation of IκBα, p65 translocation to the nucleus and initiation of transcription leading to excessive production of cytokines and chemokines, expression of integrins on leukocytes for cell trafficking and of matrix metalloproteinase, resulting in severe inflammation and damage to extracellular matrix and mucosal layer. Anti-TNF-α therapy using monoclonal antibody has shown immediate relief to IBD patients.[43,44]

IL-6 has been shown to play a role in the pathogenesis of colorectal cancer.[45] IL-6 increases the expression of ICAM-1 involved in the recruitment of neutrophils and granulocytes to the site of inflammation.[46] In an animal model of colitis induced by azoxymethane and dextran sulfate sodium (DSS), inflammation of the gut mimics clinical manifestations of IBD in patients and is characterized by relapsing gut inflammation. Monoclonal antibody targeting at the IL-6Rα chain that blocks IL-6 trans-signalling reduced the number of tumor lesions.[45]

NF-κB-regulated gene product COX-2 is strongly induced in IBD.[47] The exact nature of COX-2 in cellular transformation to a malignant phenotype is not clear. In IBD and IBD-associated colorectal cancer, both non-selective non-steroidal anti-inflammatory drugs (NSAIDs) and COX-2 selective inhibitors have been used as first line treatment and proven effective in delaying colorectal cancer development.[47,48] In mouse model of colitis-induced colorectal cancer, oral nimesulide effectively suppressed azoxymethane/DSS-induced colon tumor.[49] These findings support the hypothesis that COX-2 might have a role in IBD-associated colorectal cancer.

TLR family of receptors plays a central role in the inflammatory process. In immune cells, bacterial and viral proteins bind to TLR and activate intracellular signaling that leads to activation of NF-κB gene products. Sustained TLR activation has been shown to induce tumor growth and progression.[50] Administration of various TLR antagonists has been shown to prevent DSS-induced colitis.[51] Toll like receptor 4 (TLR4) is activated by LPS. Two members of the nucleotide binding site/leucine rich repeat (NBS/LRR) family of proteins nucleotide-binding oligomerization domain (NOD) 1 and 2 are sensors for LPS and cell wall component peptidoglycan (PGN).[52] NOD1 binds to muropeptide which has a unique amino acid diaminopilemic acid (DAP) of PGN. This amino acid is especially present in gram negative bacteria. NOD2 binds to muramyl dipeptide (MDP) of PGN and acts as a general sensor of bacteria.[53] NOD2 is expressed in monocytes and a mediator of inflammation. NOD2 binds to MDP, activates IKK, oligomerizes and binds to caspase binding domain (CARD) and then activates serine/threonine kinase RICK. RICK phosphorylates and activates NEMO, phosphorylates IκBα, releases free NF-κB which subsequently translocates to the nucleus.[54] Crohn's disease is associated with mutation in NOD2/CARD15 on chromosome 16, rendering inability to activate NF-κB and reducing ability to fight invading bacteria in the gut.[55] The mechanism(s) by which the gut microbiota and NOD2 in innate and adaptive mucosal immune responses leading to chronic inflammatory disease and colorectal cancer is not completely understood.

Therapeutic strategy in IBD and IBD-associated colorectal cancer

Numerous therapeutic approaches have been developed to control IBD and IBD-associated colorectal cancer. Anti-inflammatory agents like sulphasalazine and mesalamine have been reported to inhibit NF-κB activity in the mucosa of patients with Crohn's disease and ulcerative colitis.[56,57] Besides, aspirin, methotrexate, immunosuppresants like corticosteroids, and anti-TNF-α antibodies have shown effectiveness in IBD partly mediated through inhibiting NF-κB.[58–60] Corticosteroids increase the expression of cytoplasmic IκBα and prevent activation of NF-κB. *Ex-vivo* cultures of cells extracted from patients with corticosteroid therapy showed lower levels of nuclear p65 compared to untreated patients with Crohn's disease.[61] New treatment options that target intracellular or secreted pro-inflammatory molecules in IBD such as IL-6, TNF-α, IL-17, IL-12p40 and IL-23p19 have been shown to be effective in inhibiting NF-κB activation.[46]

Treatment with anti-TNF-α antibodies (e.g. infliximab and adalimumab) has provided relief to patients afflicted with recurrent and relapsing Crohn's disease and is beneficial to patients who do not respond to standard anti-inflammatory therapy.[44] Anti-TNF-α antibody therapy has been shown to prevent downstream NF-κB activation. There is substantial evidence from both preclinical and clinical studies whereby direct inhibition of NF-κB can lead to suppression in cancer progression. The development of NF-κB inhibitors has focused mainly on selective IKK inhibitors, in particular the IKKβ inhibitors such as CHS 828 and RTA 402, which are in phase I clinical trials.[62] In addition, specific antisense NF-κB oligonucleotide has been developed to directly inhibit NF-κB activity.[63] In the trinitrobenzene sulphonic acid (TNBS)-induced colitis model, sequence specific decoy oligonucleotide that directly inhibits the binding of NF-κB protein on the κB sites on the genome, resulted in reduced cytokine secretion and diminished formation of fibrosis, and complete inhibition of TNBS-induced colitis.[64] NSAIDs have been shown to inhibit adenoma in patients with history of IBD and reduced susceptibility to colorectal cancer development.[65] In addition, COX-2-selective inhibitors have been effectively used to prevent recurrence of sporadic adenomatous polyps in patients with genetic predisposition to colorectal cancer.[47,48] Two polyphenolic compounds curcumin and rutin, have been shown to protect mdr1a-/- mice that spontaneously develop intestinal inflammation, predominantly in the colon, with pathology similar to IBD. This mouse model is relevant for studying diet-gene interactions and potential effects of foods on remission or development of IBD.[66,67] Kunnumakkara *et al.*[68] recently reported that curcumin can sensitize human colorectal cancer to capecitabine by modulation of cyclin D1,

COX-2, MMP-9, VEGF and CXCR4 expression in an orthotopic mouse model. All these studies indicate that blocking NF-κB activity would prevent the progression of IBD to colorectal cancer.

References

1. Sen R, Baltimore D. (1986) Multiple nuclear factors interact with the immunoglobulin enhancer sequences. *Cell* **46**:705–16.
2. Sen R, Baltimore D. (1986) Inducibility of kappa immunoglobulin enhancer-binding protein NF-κB by a posttranslational mechanism. *Cell* **47**:921–8.
3. Hayden MS, Ghosh S. (2008) Shared principles in NF-κB signaling. *Cell* **132**:344–62.
4. Courtois G, Gilmore TD. (2006) Mutations in the NF-κB signaling pathway: Implications for human disease. *Oncogene* **25**:6831–43.
5. Karin M. (2006) Nuclear factor-κB in cancer development and progression. *Nature* **441**:431–6.
6. Gilmore TD. (1999) Multiple mutations contribute to the oncogenicity of the retroviral oncoprotein v-Rel. *Oncogene* **18**:6925–37.
7. Gilmore TD, Starczynowski DT, Kalaitzidis D. (2004) RELevant gene amplification in B-cell lymphomas. *Blood* **103**:3243–44.
8. Bargou RC, Emmerich F, Krappmann D *et al.* (1997) Constitutive nuclear factor-κB-RelA activation is required for proliferation and survival of Hodgkin's disease tumor cells. *J Clin Invest* **100**:2961–69.
9. Oeckinghaus A, Ghosh S. (2009) The NF-κB family of transcription factors and its regulation. *Cold Spring Harb Perspect Biol* **1**:a000034.
10. Wan F, Lenardo MJ. (2009) Specification of DNA binding activity of NF-κB proteins. *Cold Spring Harb Perspect Biol* **1**:a000067.
11. Vallabhapurapu S, Karin M. (2009) Regulation and function of NF-κB transcription factors in the immune system. *Ann Rev Immunol* **27**: 693–733.
12. Hacker H, Karin M. (2006) Regulation and function of IKK and IKK-related kinases. *Sci STKE* **2006**:re13.
13. Scheidereit C. (2006) IκB kinase complexes: Gateways to NF-κB activation and transcription. *Oncogene* **25**:6685–705.
14. Chen G, Cao P, Goeddel DV *et al.* (2002) TNF-induced recruitment and activation of the IKK complex require Cdc37 and Hsp90. *Mol Cell* **9**: 401–10.

15. Ducat Sigala JL, Bottero V, Young DB *et al.* (2004) Activation of transcription factor NF-κB requires ELKS, an IκB kinase regulatory subunit. *Science* **304**:1963–7.
16. Huxford T, Ghosh G. (2009) A structural guide to proteins of the NF-κB signalling module. *Cold Spring Harb Perspect Biol* **1**:a000075.
17. Li ZW, Chu W, Hu Y *et al.* (1999) The IKKβ subunit of IκB kinase (IKK) is essential for nuclear factor κB activation and prevention of apoptosis. *J Exp Med* **189**:1839–45.
18. Senftleben U, Cao Y, Xiao G *et al.* (2001) Activation by IKKα of a second, evolutionary conserved, NF-κB signalling pathway. *Science* **293**:1495–9.
19. Rudolph D, Yeh WC, Wakeham A *et al.* (2000) Severe liver degeneration and lack of NF-κB activation in NEMO-deficient mice. *Genes Dev* **14**:854–62.
20. Vallabhapurapu S, Matsuzawa A, Zhang W *et al.* (2008) Nonredundant and complementary functions of TRAF2 and TRAF3 in an ubiquitination cascade that activates NIK-dependent alternative NF-κB signalling. *Nat. Immunol* **9**:1364–70.
21. Cho JH. (2008) The genetics and immunopathogenesis of inflammatory bowel disease. *Nature* **8**:458–6.
22. Abraham C and Cho JH. (2009) Inflammatory bowel disease. *N Engl J Med* **361**:2066–78.
23. Ghosh S, Hayden MS. (2008) New regulators of NF-κB in inflammation. *Nat Rev Immunol* **8**:837–48.
24. Hugot JP, Laurent-Puig P, Gower-Rousseau C *et al.* (1996) Mapping of a susceptibility locus for Crohn's disease on chromosome 16. *Nature* **379**:821–3.
25. Cho JH, Nicolae DL, Gold LH *et al.* (1998) Identification of novel susceptibility loci for inflammatory bowel disease on chromosomes 1p, 3q, and 4q: Evidence for epistasis between 1p and IBD1. *Proc Natl Acad Sci USA* **95**: 7502–7.
26. Le Beau MM, Ito C, Cogswell P *et al.* (1992) Chromosomal localization of the genes encoding the p50/p105 subunits of NF-κB (N-κB2) and the IκB/MAD-3 (NF-κB1) inhibitor of NF-κB to 4q24 and 14q13, respectively. *Genomics* **14**:529–31.
27. Glas J, Torok HP, Tonenchi L *et al.* (2006) Role of the NF-κB1-94ins/delATTG promoter polymorphism in IBD and potential interactions with polymorphisms in the CARD15/NOD2, IKBL, and IL-1RN genes. *Inflamm Bowel Dis* **12**:606–11.

28. Li F, Sethi G. (2010) Targeting transcription factor NF-κB to overcome chemoresistance and radioresistance in cancer therapy. *Biochim Biophys Acta* **1805**:167–80.
29. Karin M. (2009) NF-κB as a critical link between inflammation and cancer. *Cold Spring Harbor Perspect Biol* **1**:a000141.
30. Rogler G, Brand K, Vogl D *et al.* (1998) Nuclear factor-κB is activated in macrophages and epithelial cells of inflamed intestinal mucosa. *Gastroenterology* **115**:357-69.
31. Gelbmann CM, Leeb SN, Vogl D *et al.* (2003). Inducible CD40 expression mediates NF-κB activation and cytokine secretion in human colonic fibroblasts. *Gut* **52**:1448–56.
32. Ogura Y, Bonen DK, Inohara N *et al.* (2001) A frameshift mutation in NOD2 associated with susceptibility to Crohn's disease. *Nature* **411**:603–6.
33. van Heel DA, Ghosh S, Butler M *et al.* (2005) Muramyl dipeptide and toll-like receptor sensitivity in NOD2-associated Crohn's disease. *Lancet* **365**: 1794–6.
34. Schreiber S, Nikolaus S, Hampe J. (1998) Activation of nuclear factor kappa B inflammatory bowel disease. *Gut* **42**:477–84.
35. Karin M, Lawrence T, Nizet V. (2006) Innate immunity gone awry: Mechanisms linking microbial infections to chronic inflammatory disorders and cancer. *Cell* **124**:823–35.
36. Mahida YR, Ceska M, Effenberg F *et al.* (1992) Enhanced synthesis of neutrophil activating peptide-1/interleukin 8 in active ulcerative colitis. *Clin Sci* **82**:273–5.
37. Jenkins GJ, Mikhail J, Alhamdani A *et al.* (2007) Immunohistochemical study of nuclear factor-κB activity and interleukin-8 abundance in oesophageal adenocarcinoma; A useful strategy for monitoring these biomarkers. *J Clin Pathol* **60**:1232–7.
38. Jankowski JA, Harrison RF, Perry I *et al.* (2000) Barrett's metaplasia. *Lancet* **356**:2079–85.
39. Morris CD, Armstrong GR, Bigley G *et al.* (2001) Cyclooxygenase-2 expression in the Barrett's metaplasiadysplasia-adenocarcinoma sequence. *Am J Gastroenterol* **96**:990–6.
40. O'Riordan JM, Abdel-latif MM, Ravi N *et al.* (2005) Proinflammatory cytokine and nuclear factor-κB expression along the inflammation-metaplasia-dysplasia adenocarcinoma sequence in the esophagus. *Am J Gastroenterol* **100**:1257–64.

41. Souza RF, Krishnan K, Spechler SJ. (2008) Acid, bile and CDX: The ABCs of making Barrett's metaplasia. *Am J Physiol* **295**:G211–8.
42. Kazumori H, Ishihara S, Kinoshita Y. (2009) Roles of caudal-related homeobox gene Cdx1 in oesophageal epithelial cells in Barrett's epithelium development. *Gut* **58**:620–8.
43. Atreya R, Neurath MF. (2008) New therapeutic strategies for treatment of inflammatory bowel disease. *Mucosal Immunol* **1**:175–82.
44. Shale MJ, Seow CH, Coffin CS *et al.* (2009) Review article: Chronic viral infection in the anti-tumour necrosis factor therapy era in inflammatory bowel disease. *Aliment Pharmacol Ther* **31**:20–34.
45. Becker C, Fantini MC, Schramm C *et al.* (2004) TGF-beta suppresses tumor progression in colon cancer by inhibition of IL-6 trans-signaling. *Immunity* **21**:491–501.
46. Wang L, Walia B, Evans J *et al.* (2003) IL-6 induces NF-κB activation in the intestinal epithelia. *J Immunol* **171**:3194–201.
47. Singer II, Kawka DW, Schloemann S *et al.* (1998) Cyclooxygenase 2 is induced in colonic epithelial cells in inflammatory bowel disease. *Gastroenterology* **115**:297–306.
48. Wang D, DuBois RN. (2010) The role of COX-2 in intestinal inflammation and colorectal cancer. *Oncogene* **29**:781–8.
49. Kohno H, Suzuki R, Sugie S *et al.* (2005) Suppression of colitis-related mouse colon carcinogenesis by a COX-2 inhibitor and PPAR ligands. *BMC Cancer* **5**:46.
50. Fukata M, Abreu MT. (2008) Role of Toll-like receptors in gastrointestinal malignancies. *Oncogene* **27**:234–43.
51. Cario E. (2008) Therapeutic impact of toll-like receptors on inflammatory bowel diseases: A multiple-edged sword. *Inflamm Bowel Dis* **14**:411–21.
52. Inohara N, Nunez G. (2003) NODs: Intracellular proteins involved in inflammation and apoptosis. *Nat Rev Immunol* **3**:371–82.
53. Girardin SE, Boneca IG, Viala J *et al.* (2003) Nod2 is a general sensor of pepidoglycan through muramyl dipeptide (MDP) detection. *J Biol Chem* **278**:8869–72.
54. Abott DW, Wilkins A, Asara JM *et al.* (2004) The Crohn's disease protein, NOD2, requires RIP2 in order to induce ubiquitinylation of a novel site on NEMO. *Curr Biol* **14**:2217–27.
55. Yamamoto S, Ma X. (2009) Role of NOD2 in the development of Crohn's disease. *Microbes and infection* **11**:912–8.

56. Bantel H, Berg C, Vieth M *et al.* (2000) Mesalazine inhibits activation of transcription factor NF-κB in inflamed mucosa of patients with ulcerative colitis. *Am J Gastroenterol* **95**:3452–7.
57. Wahl C, Liptay S, Adler G *et al.* (1998) Sulfasalazine: A potent and specific inhibitor of nuclear factor kappa B. *J Clin Invest* **101**:1163–74.
58. Wang CY, Cusack JC Jr, Liu R *et al.* (1999) Control of inducible chemoresistance: Enhanced anti-tumor therapy through increased apoptosis by inhibition of NF-κB. *Nat Med* **5**:412–7.
59. Barnes PJ, Karin M. (1997) Nuclear factor-κB: A pivotal transcription factor in chronic inflammatory diseases. *N Engl J Med* **336**:1066–71.
60. De Bosscher K, Vanden Berghe W, Haegeman G. (2000) Mechanisms of anti-inflammatory action and of immunosuppression by glucocorticoids: Negative interference of activated glucocorticoid receptor with transcription factors. *J Neuroimmunol* **109**:16–22.
61. Thiele K, Bierhaus A, Autschbach F *et al.* (1999) Cell specific effects of glucocorticoid treatment on the NF-κBp65/IκBα system in patients with Crohn's disease. *Gut* **45**:693–704.
62. Sethi G, Tergaonkar V. (2009) Potential pharmacological control of the NF-κB pathway. *Trends in Pharm Sciences* **30**:313–21.
63. Neurath MF, Pettersson S, Meyer zum Buschenfelde KH *et al.* (1996) Local administration of antisense phosphorothioate oligonucleotides to the p65 subunit of NFκB abrogates established experimental colitis in mice. *Nat Med* **2**:998–1004.
64. Fichtner-Feigl S, Fuss IJ, Preiss JC *et al.* (2005) Treatment of murine Th1- and Th2-mediated inflammatory bowel disease with NF-κB decoy oligonucleotides. *J Clin Invest* **115**:3057–71.
65. Hoffmeister M, Chang-Claude J, Brenner H. (2006) Do older adults using NSAIDs have a reduced risk of colorectal cancer. *Drugs Aging* **23**:13–523.
66. Nones K, Dommels YE, Martell S *et al.* (2009) The effects of dietary curcumin and rutin on colonic inflammation and gene expression in multidrug resistance gene-deficient (mdr1a-/-) mice, a model of inflammatory bowel diseases. *Br J Nutr* **101**:169–81.
67. Hanai H, Sugimoto K. (2009) Curcumin has bright prospects for the treatment of inflammatory bowel disease. *Curr Pharm Des* **15**:2087–94.
68. Kunnumakkara AB, Diagaradjane P, Anand P *et al.* (2009) Curcumin sensitizes human colorectal cancer to capecitabine by modulation of cyclin D1,

COX-2, MMP-9, VEGF and CXCR4 expression in an orthotopic mouse model. *Int J Cancer* **125**:2187–97.
69. Hue S, Ahern P, Buonocore S *et al.* (2006) Interleukin-23 drives innate and T cell-mediated intestinal inflammation. *J Exp Med* **203**:2473–83.
70. Maloy KJ. (2007) Induction and regulation of inflammatory bowel disease in immunodeficient mice by distinct CD4+ T-cell subsets. *Methods Mol Bio* **380**:327–35.
71. Yan Y, Dalmasso G, Nguyen HT *et al.* (2008) Nuclear factor-kappaB is a critical mediator of Ste20-like proline-/alanine-rich kinase regulation in intestinal inflammation. *Am J Pathol* **173**:1013–28.
72. Yan Y, Merlin D. (2008) Ste20-related proline/alanine-rich kinase: A novel regulator of intestinal inflammation. *World J Gastroenterol* **14**:6115–21.
73. Nishimura M, Kuboi Y, Muramoto K *et al.* (2009) Chemokines as novel therapeutic targets for inflammatory bowel disease. *Ann N Y Acad Sci* **1173**:350–6.
74. Feagins LA, Souza RF, Spechler SJ. (2009) Carcinogenesis in IBD: Potential targets for the prevention of colorectal cancer. *Nat Rev Gastroenterol Hepatol* **6**:297–305.
75. Kraus S, Arber N. (2009) Inflammation and colorectal cancer. *Curr Opin Pharmacol* **9**:405–10.
76. Wu H, Shen B. (2009) Pouchitis: Lessons for inflammatory bowel disease. *Curr Opin Gastroenterol* **25**:314–22.

Chapter 12

Novel Mediators for Chronic Inflammation and Oncogenic Transformation: Tumor Necrosis Factor (TNF)-α

Naofumi Mukaida* and Boryana K. Popivanova

Division of Molecular Bioregulation, Cancer Research Institute, Kanazawa University, Kakuma, Kanazawa 920-1192, Japan

Tumor necrosis factor (TNF)-α was originally identified as a factor, which can induce hemorrhagic necrosis in tumor tissues in mouse. Subsequent studies have further revealed that its expression is under the control of an inflammation-induced transcription factor, NF-κB and that it can, in turn, activate NF-κB. Moreover, accumulating evidence indicates the crucial involvement of NF-κB in various types of carcinogenesis in mice, particularly one which develops after administration of azoxymethane (AOM) followed by repeated dextran sulfate sodium (DSS) ingestion. However, it remains elusive on which factor(s) is responsible for NF-κB activation in this process. Treating wild-type (WT) mice with AOM and DSS increased TNF-α expression and the number of infiltrating leukocytes expressing its major receptor, p55 (TNF-Rp55), in the lamina propria and submucosal regions of the colon. This was followed by the development of multiple colonic tumors. Mice lacking TNF-Rp55 and treated with AOM and DSS showed reduced mucosal damage, reduced leukocyte infiltration, and attenuated subsequent tumor formation. Furthermore, administration of Etanercept, a specific antagonist of TNF-α, to WT mice after treatment with AOM and DSS markedly reduced the number and size of tumors and reduced

* Corresponding author. E-mail: naofumim@kenroku.kanazawa-u.ac.jp

colonic infiltration by leukocytes. These observations identify TNF-α as a crucial mediator of the initiation and progression of colitis-associated colon carcinogenesis. Because evidence is accumulating to indicate that TNF-α can promote tumor development and progression, and metastasis formation in various mouse models, targeting TNF-α may be useful in treating various types of cancers, particularly chronic colitis-associated colon cancer.

Overview of tumor necrosis factor (TNF)-α

TNF-α is produced by numerous types of cells in response to a wide variety of activating stimuli.[1] The biosynthesis of TNF-α is tightly regulated at many different levels. TNF-α is expressed as an immediate early gene, and a variety of stimuli induce high levels of TNF-α mRNA rapidly within 30 min. Various stimuli activate Rac/Cdc42, and eventually Jun kinase (JNK) and p38 kinase pathways. These two pathways activate several distinct types of transcription factors including NF-κB, ATF-1, ATF-2, c-jun, CREB, and Elk-1, to induce the transcription of the TNF-*α* gene. p38 kinase pathway can stabilize TNF-α mRNA, thereby enhancing its translation.[1]

TNF-α is synthesized as a 26-kDa type II transmembrane precursor that is displayed on the plasma membrane, with the N-terminus in the cytoplasm and the C-terminus exposed to the extracellular space. The TNF-α precursor is proteolytically cleaved between alanine (−1) and valine (+1), mainly by the action of the TNF-α converting enzyme (TACE), a matrix metalloproteinase (MMP)-like enzyme. The proteolysis leads to the formation of biologically active 17-kDa mature TNF-α that forms a trimer in solution.[2]

TNF-α exerts its pleiotropic activities after binding two related but distinct receptors, TNF receptor (TNF-R)p55/TNFR1 and TNF-Rp75/TNFR2.[3] Both receptors are type I transmembrane glycoproteins and share sequence homologies within their extracellular domains, consisting of multiple cystine-rich repeats and exist as a trimer in the plasma membrane. TNF-Rp55 has a much wider distribution than TNF-Rp75.[3]

TNF-Rp55 activation leads to recruitment of intracellular adaptor proteins that activates multiple signal transduction pathways including

FAS-associated via death domain (FADD)/caspase 8/caspase 3, mitogen activated kinase (MAPK), JNK/activation protein (AP)-1, and NF-κB pathways.[4] TNF-Rp75 activation leads to the activation of MAPK, JNK/AP-1, and NF-κB but not FADD/caspase 8/caspase 3.[4] The activation of MAPK, JNK/AP-1, and NF-κB eventually induces the expression of various molecules including interleukin (IL)-1, IL-6, chemokines, adhesion molecules, cyclooxygenase (COX)-2, and matrix metalloproteinases (MMP) (Figure 1). The activation of FADD/caspase 8/caspase 3 pathway can induce apoptosis. However, unlike the rapid apoptosis that is induced by other members of TNF superfamily such as FAS ligand and TRAIL, apoptosis is a late response to TNF-α. Moreover, TNF-α-mediated NF-κB activation can counteract apoptosis by inducing negative regulators of apoptosis such as Bcl-2 and superoxide dismutase.[5]

TNF-α as a cancer treatment

TNF-α was initially identified as a factor, which can induce hemorrhagic necrosis in tumor tissues in mouse.[6] Subsequent characterization of the

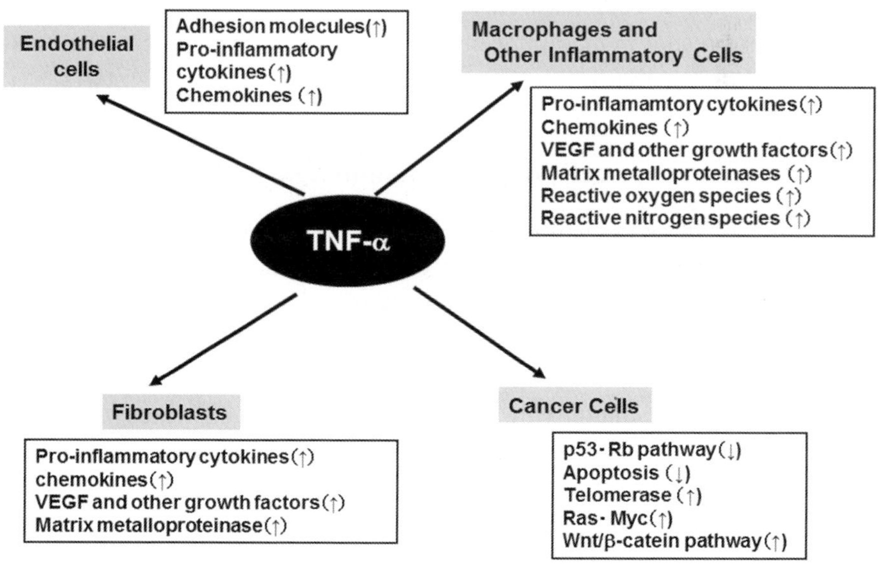

Figure 1. Biological actions of TNF-α.

factor revealed that this factor is identical to the factor, cachectin, which can cause cachexia.[7] TNF-α can exhibit cytotoxic actions against various tumor cells in the presence of RNA synthesis inhibitors or protein synthesis inhibitors.[6] TNF-α can inhibit the function of an adhesion molecule, αvβ3 integrin, expressed on tumor endothelial cells and concomitantly abrogate the support that endothelial cells receive from surrounding extracellular matrix. The loss of the support leads to the apoptosis of endothelial cells and hemorrhagic necrosis of tumor tissues.[8] These observations promote the application of TNF-α for cancer treatment.

Systemic administration of high dose of TNF-α induces necrosis of syngeneic and xenografted tumors in mice.[9] These encouraging preclinical results were obtained by the administration of human TNF to mice, because human TNF-α is less toxic to mice.[7] On the contrary, phase I and phase II clinical trials demonstrated that systemic administration of TNF-α was associated with severe toxicity including cytokine storm but did cause few tumor response.[10,11] For instance, at lower doses, TNF treatment was well tolerated with reversible flu-like symptoms, but at higher doses, hypotension and pulmonary edema developed.[12] Thus, it was proposed that local administration of TNF would have better clinical outcome than the systemic treatment. However, subsequent studies revealed that TNF-α was present in the tumor microenvironment of many cancers, raising the possibility that it might actually be enhancing cancer growth.[13]

Transcription factor activation in inflammation and tumorigenesis

The father of modern pathology, Virchow, pointed out an intimate relationship between inflammation and cancer, based on the presence of a large number of leukocytes in tumor tissues.[14] Inflammatory responses can promote tissue repair, together with leukocyte infiltration, neovascularization, and extracellular matrix protein production by fibroblasts. These pathological changes are also observed in cancer tissues. Moreover, Dvorak proposed that tumors are wounds that do not heal. This is based on the observations that solid tumor tissues always contain endothelial cells and fibroblasts as well as infiltrating leukocytes and that they exhibit similar histopathological features as tissue repair processed after inflammatory responses.[15] Several epidemiological studies further unraveled an essential contribution of chronic inflammation to tumorigenesis. Ulcerative colitis (UC), and silicosis and asbestosis, cause chronic inflammation and subsequently increase the frequency of tumorigenesis in colon and lung, respectively.[16,17] Nowadays, at least 20% of all cancer cases are presumed to arise from chronic inflammation.

Several molecular mechanisms are proposed to have a role in inflammation-associated tumorigenesis.[18] First, chronic inflammation accelerates cell cycles to repair damaged tissues and as a result, the numbers of replication errors are increased. Simultaneously, granulocytes and monocytes/macrophages massively infiltrate inflammatory sites and generate a massive amount of reactive oxygen species and reactive nitrogen species, the molecules which can cause mutations in chromosomal DNA and activate telomerase to immortalize cells.[19]

Inflammatory responses activate a limited set of transcription factors including NF-κB, STAT3, and hypoxia-inducible factor (HIF)-1α[18] (Figure 2). These transcription factors coordinately activate a selected set of genes such as pro-inflammatory cytokines, chemokines, and adhesion

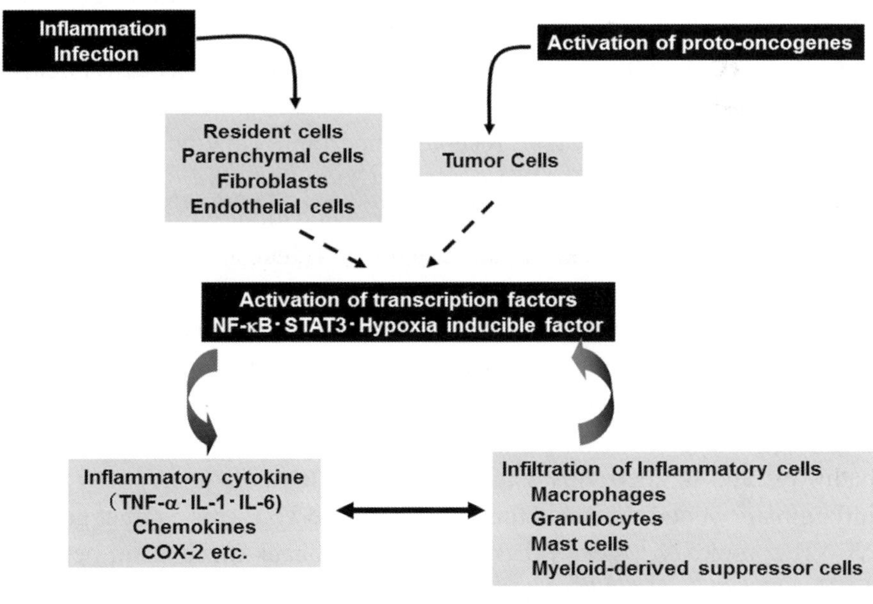

Figure 2. Inflammation- and oncogene-induced transcription factor activation.

molecules. Consequently, pro-inflammatory cytokine, chemokine, and adhesion molecule proteins are expressed and crucially contribute to the development of inflammatory responses. In carcinogenesis, which is induced by a number of proto-oncogenes, NF-κB, STAT3, and HIF-1α are also activated to induce the transcription and eventually the protein expression of the target genes. Thus, inflammatory responses and carcinogenesis can activate a similar set of transcription factors. They can eventually induce the protein expression of a similar set of the target genes.[18]

Among transcription factors activated in both inflammatory responses and carcinogenesis, NF-κB is the most frequently activated transcription gene.[20] In unstimulated cells, NF-κB proteins are sequestered in the cytoplasm by its inhibitory proteins, IκB. NF-κB can be activated through two pathways, canonical and noncanonical pathways.[21] The canonical pathway is activated by a large number of stimuli including TNF-α, IL-1 or lipopolysaccharide and stimulates the IκB kinase (IKK) complex consisting of IKKα, IKKβ, and NEMO to phosphorylate IκB and promotes its degradation mediated by proteasome. This leads to a nuclear translocation of NF-κB consisting of p50 and RelA[21] (Figure 3). The noncanonical NF-κB activation pathway involves stimulus-induced partial proteolysis of NF-κB2 p100, resulting in the formation of p52 and subsequent nuclear translocation of p52-RelB complexes. The noncanonical pathway is activated by a subset of TNF receptor superfamily members, including B cell-activating factor (BAFF) receptor, CD40, lymphotoxin β receptor, and RANK. Nevertheless, upon nuclear translocation, NF-κB complexes bind to the cis elements in the target gene and thereby induce their transcription.[21]

Several lines of evidence indicate the aberrant nuclear localization of p50-RelA NF-κB complexes in various types of cancers.[20] Nuclear localization of p50-RelA NF-κB complexes is initiated by the canonical NF-κB pathway. TNF-α is a potent activator of the canonical NF-κB pathway[4] and is aberrantly expressed with a high frequency in various inflammatory conditions and tumors.[13] Because TNF-α is a target gene of NF-κB complexes,[1] there exists a positive feedback mechanism between TNF-α and NF-κB. This assumption also promotes investigations on the roles of TNF-α in various tumorigenesis.

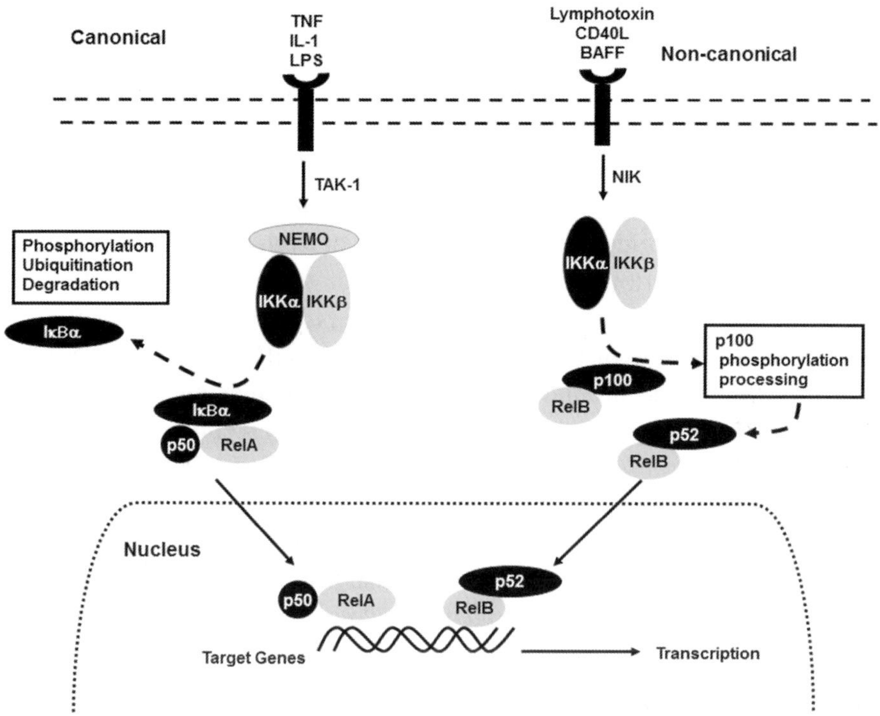

Figure 3. NF-κB activation pathway.

TNF-α as a tumor-promoting factor

Immediately after TNF-α cDNA cloning, accumulating evidence indicates that TNF-α mRNA and protein could be detected in malignant and stromal cells in human cancer tissues and that plasma TNF-α levels were increased in some cancer patients, especially those with poor prognosis.[13] Moreover, it became evident that TNF-α can induce angiogenesis,[22] an indispensable step for tumor growth and metastasis. TNF-α can induce various molecules involved in angiogenesis, including MMP, COX-2, IL-1, IL-6, stromal cell-derived factor (SDF-1/CXCL12), monocyte chemoattractant protein-1 (MCP-1/CCL2), and vascular endothelial growth factor (VEGF)[23] (Figure 1). This cytokine network can further induce the generation of tumor-associated macrophages, which are a rich source of various growth factors, particularly VEGF.[24] In addition,

TNF-α can cause the differentiation of myeloid progenitor cells into endothelial cells in the tumor microenvironment.[25]

TNF-α can directly contribute to oncogene activation and DNA damage, in addition to its effects on leukocyte infiltrate and endothelial cells (Figure 1). Long-term TNF-α treatment of immortalized mouse 3T3 cells rendered them capable of forming tumors in mice.[26] TNF-α stimulates JNK pathway in normal human epidermis to activate AP-1 and oncogenic Ras and the net result is the development of tumors indistinguishable from squamous cell carcinoma.[27] Moreover, TNF-α exposure results in increased production of reactive oxygen species (ROS), with a concomitant increase in the production of 8-oxo-deoxyguanosine, a marker for oxidative DNA damage, in human lung bronchial epithelial cells, by enhancing the expression of spermine oxidase (SMO/PAOh1), an enzyme which oxidizes spermine into spermidine, 3-aminopropanal, and H_2O_2.[28] Furthermore, TNF-α can induce the DNA and RNA editing enzyme, activation-induced cytidine deaminase (AID), in biliary cancer cells and aberrant expression of AID results in the generation of somatic mutations in tumor-related genes, including p53, c-myc, and the promoter region of the INK4A/p16 sequences.[29] Finally, TNF-α can induce the translocation to nucleus of the human telomerase catalytic subunit bound to NF-κB p65, thereby promoting elongation of telomere sequences, an essential step for immortalization of cells.[30]

Due to these pro-tumorigenic activities, TNF-α-deficient or TNF receptor-deficient mice are resistant to carcinogenic stimuli. 7,12-Dimethylbenz[a]anthracene (DMBA) and 12-O-tetradecanoylphorbol-13-acetate (TPA) are widely used as an initiator and a promoter of skin carcinogenesis, respectively. In this skin carcinogenesis process, TNF-α is extensively induced in the epidermis, but not the dermis only after the initiation with TPA. DMBA treatment induces DNA adduct formation and c-Ha-ras mutations with similar frequencies in both wild-type (WT) and TNF-α-deficient mice. TNF-α-deficient mice develop fewer numbers of tumors but exhibit similar rates of malignant progression, compared with WT mice.[31] Moreover, TNF-Rp55-deficient and to a lesser degree, TNF-Rp75-deficient mice develop fewer numbers of skin tumors than WT mice, when they are treated sequentially with DMBA and TPA.[32] These observations indicate that the TNF-α-TNF-Rp55 or TNF-α-TNF-Rp75 interactions are important to the early stages of tumor promotion in this skin carcinogenesis.

TNF-α can stabilize the protein Snail, the transcription factor that is capable of repressing E-cadherin expression. Reduced E-cadherin expression can induce epithelial-mesenchymal transition, the crucial step for metastasis.[33] This may account for the previous observations that treatment of tumor cells or mice with TNF-α increases the metastatic activity of transplantable tumor cells.[34] We also observed that intrasplenic injection of mouse colon cancer cells caused a massive liver metastasis, depending on the presence of a TNF-α-specific receptor, TNF-Rp55. We further demonstrated that endogenously produced TNF-α enhanced the expression of an adhesion molecule, vascular cell adhesion molecule (VCAM)-1, on sinusoidal endothelial cells and that the enhanced VCAM-1 expression could facilitate extravasation of cancer cells and subsequent metastasis focus formation in a TNF-Rp55-dependent manner.[35]

TNF-α in chronic inflammation-associated colon carcinogenesis in mice

In UC, dysplasia with nuclear atypia and loss of cytoplasmic differentiation can be present in multiple sites of colonic mucosa of UC patients, and is characterized by DNA damage with microsatellite instability. Carcinomas develop from these dysplasia.[16] Historically, the risk of cancer is the highest in patients with pancolitis of 10 or more years' duration, in whom it is 20- to 30-fold higher than in a control population. However, recent progress in the treatment of UC reduced the frequency of colon cancer complication in UC patients as it can effectively control the disease activities of UC.[36] These observations indicate the crucial roles of chronic inflammation in colon carcinogenesis.

Ingestion of dextran sulfate sodium (DSS) solution causes ulcer continually present in whole colons in mouse and rat,[37] mimicking the pathological changes observed in the acute phase of UC patients. Moreover, repeated oral DSS ingestion alone can cause colon carcinoma in a proportion of mice, when the ingestion is of 7 days' duration and is repeated 9 times.[38] These observations suggest that the inflammatory response alone can cause colon carcinoma. Azoxymethane (AOM) can induce the generation of O^6-methylguanine in chromosomal DNA and can cause abnormal crypt formation in colon when it is injected into rodents systemically.[39] A prior administration of AOM can accelerate and increase the incidence of DSS-induced colon carcinogenesis as evidenced by the very high incidence of nearly 100% of colon cancer after three subsequent rounds of DSS ingestion.[40] Hence, this model is frequently used as a model of chronic inflammation-associated colon carcinogenesis.

WT mice exhibited severe body weight loss and bloody diarrhea every time that they received DSS.[41] Moreover, in WT mice, edema and hyperemia of the middle to distal colon became evident after the first round of DSS intake and multiple tumors developed in the same region after the second round of DSS intake. Histological analysis consistently demonstrated massive infiltration of leukocytes into the mucosa and edema of the submucosa, with loss of entire crypts and surface epithelium after the first round of DSS intake, particularly in the middle to distal colon. Fourteen days after the start of the first series of DSS intake, mucosal inflammatory cell infiltration persisted and was accompanied by dysplastic glands with hyperchromatic nuclei, decreased mucin production and dystrophic goblet cells. By the end of the second round of DSS intake, macroscopically visible adenocarcinomatous lesions developed, and their sizes and numbers increased progressively, thereafter. Moreover, β-catenin accumulated in the nuclei of the tumor cells after the second round of DSS intake and the tumor cells were positive for cytokeratin-20, a marker of adenocarcinoma cells.[41]

Greten and colleagues examined the role of NF-κB activation in this mouse colon carcinogenesis model, by using the mice deficient in *IKKβ*, a serine/threonine kinase crucially involved in canonical NF-κB pathway activation.[42] Tumor incidence is markedly reduced by enterocyte-specific gene deletion of *IKKβ* and this is linked to increased epithelial apoptosis during tumor development. Moreover, these mice exhibit enhanced expression of proinflammatory cytokines including TNF-α, IL-1, IL-6, and CXC chemokines, which may serve as tumor growth factors. Deletion of *IKKβ* gene in myeloid cells results also in a significant decrease in tumor size, but this deletion attenuates inflammatory responses and diminishes expression of proinflammatory cytokines without affecting apoptosis. These observations would indicate that NF-κB activation can link inflammation to cancer, by regulating the functions of inflammatory cells.[42] However, Greten and colleagues did not identify the molecule(s), which is regulated by NF-κB and has an indispensable role in this colon carcinogenesis.

Accumulating evidence indicates that NF-κB activation can robustly induce TNF-α expression and that TNF-α is a potent activator of NF-κB.[1] Thus, there exists a positive feedback loop between TNF-α and NF-κB. These observations prompted us to investigate TNF-α expression in AOM+DSS-induced colon carcinogenesis process. TNF-α mRNA was faintly expressed in untreated mice, and AOM treatment alone did not enhance TNF-α mRNA expression, but subsequent DSS intake augmented TNF-α mRNA expression.[41] Moreover, TNF-α protein was detected by immunohistochemical analysis mainly in mononuclear cells present in lamina propria and submucosal region. This may mirror the observation that immunoreactive TNF-α protein was detected in the colons of patients with active ulcerative colitis and advanced colorectal cancer, but not in normal mucosa. Furthermore, immunohistochemical analysis detected the major receptor for TNF-α, TNF-Rp55, predominantly in leukocytes infiltrating the lamina propria and submucosal regions of the colon during the course of this colon carcinogenesis model.[41] These observations raise the possibility of the involvement of the TNF-α -TNF-Rp55 axis in this colon carcinogenesis process.

Indeed, TNF-Rp55-deficient mice had less body weight loss compared with WT mice, and did not exhibit bloody diarrhea even after DSS intake. Moreover, mucosal inflammatory cell infiltration and dysplastic changes of glands were attenuated in TNF-Rp55-deficient mice, during the whole course of this colon carcinogenesis, compared with WT mice. Even after the three rounds of DSS intake when WT mice developed multiple intracolonic adenocarcinomatous lesions with nuclear β-catenin accumulation, TNF-Rp55-deficient mice developed a remarkably fewer numbers of adenocarcinomatous lesions in colon.[41] These observations suggest a crucial role of TNF-Rp55-mediated signals in the development of chronic inflammation-associated colon carcinogenesis process.

Because TNF-Rp55 is expressed by both bone marrow-derived and non-bone marrow-derived cells,[3] we investigated the contribution of either type of cells to this colon carcinogenesis, by using bone marrow chimeric mice generated between WT and TNF-Rp55-deficient mice. The analysis using bone marrow chimeric mice revealed that TNF-Rp55-mediated signals acted mainly on bone marrow- but not non-bone marrow-derived cells in this carcinogenesis model. DSS intake induced the expression of COX-2, an enzyme crucially involved in colon carcinogenesis. COX-2 protein was mainly detected in infiltrating inflammatory cells and intracolonic COX-2-positive cell numbers were increased progressively in WT but not TNF-Rp55-deficient mice. Double-color immunofluorescence analysis detected COX-2 protein in F4/80-positive macrophages and to a lesser extent in Ly-6G-positive neutrophils.[41] Thus, the absence of TNF-Rp55 reduces the infiltration of bone marrow-derived cells, macrophages and neutrophils, which are a major source of COX-2 and eventually depressed colon carcinogenesis.

The role of the TNF-α-TNF-R axis in the progression phase of colon carcinogenesis was investigated by administering a TNF antagonist, Etanercept, to WT mice after the completion of AOM injection and three rounds of DSS ingestion, when mice developed multiple intracolonic adenocarcinomatous lesions with nuclear β-catenin accumulation. Etanercept treatment remarkably reduced the numbers and sizes of macroscopical tumors and attenuated intracolonic infiltration by inflammatory cells, particularly neutrophils and macrophages together with reduction in COX-2 mRNA expression and COX-2 expressing cell numbers [41] (Figure 4).

Etanercept decreased the intratumoral vascular density and the nuclear accumulation of β-catenin at the tumor sites.[41] Takahashi and colleagues observed that in these AOM-induced tumors, the β-*catenin* gene, particularly at its glycogen synthase kinase (GSK)-3β phosphorylation sites, mutated more frequently than *Adenomatous Poplyposis Coli* (*APC*) gene.[43] Consistently, we detected the mutations of the GSK-3β phosphorylation sites of the *β*-catenin gene, located in its exon 3 in all tumors derived from WT mice, but Etanercept treatment markedly reduced the mutation frequency. COX-2-derived prostaglandin E_2 can induce neovascularization[44] and activate Wnt/β-catenin pathway.[45] Moreover, Oguma and colleagues demonstrated that infiltrating macrophage-derived TNF-α can directly activate Wnt/β-catenin signaling pathway in murine gastric carcinogenesis models and human gastric cancer cell lines.[46] Thus,

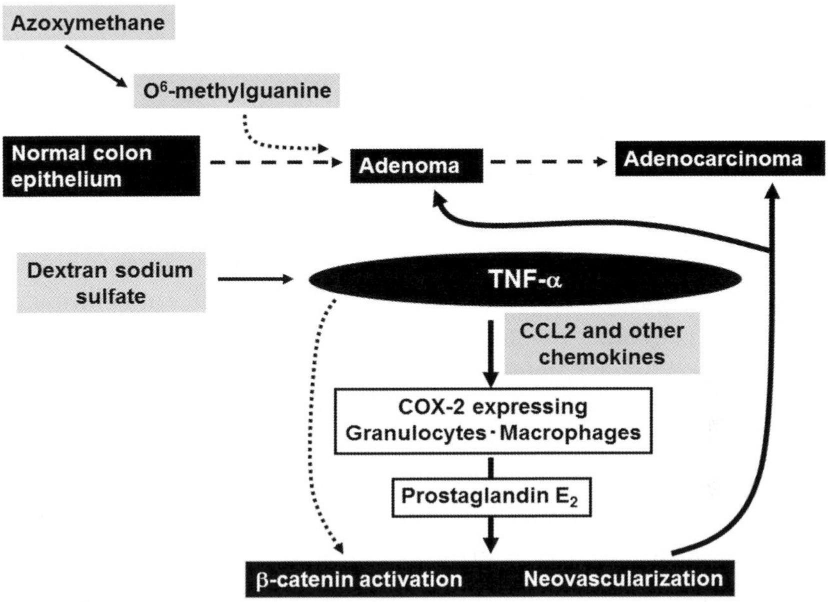

Figure 4. Presumed roles of TNF-α in chronic colitis-associated colonic carcinogenesis.

TNF-α can directly and/or indirectly through enhancing COX-2 expression, activate Wnt/β-catenin pathway, which is crucially involved in the whole steps of colon carcinogenesis process.

Failure of TNF-α to induce direct chemotaxis of macrophages, prompted us to investigate the role of a potent macrophage-tropic chemokine, CCL2, whose expression can robustly be enhanced by TNF-α.[1] In the course of this carcinogenesis process, the expression of CCL2, was enhanced together with intracolonic massive infiltration of macrophages. Mice deficient in CCL2-specific receptor, CCR2, exhibited less macrophage infiltration and lower tumor numbers with attenuated COX-2 expression. Moreover, CCL2 antagonists decreased intracolonic macrophage infiltration and COX-2 expression, attenuated neovascularization, and eventually reduced the numbers and sizes of colon tumors, even when given after multiple colon tumors have developed.[47] Thus, in collaboration with TNF-α, CCL2 can promote the initiation and progression of chronic colitis-associated colon carcinogenesis (Figure 4).

Perspective of TNF-α antagonists in cancer treatment

Oguma and colleagues demonstrated that macrophage-derived TNF-α can activate Wnt/β-catenin pathway directly in murine gastric carcinogenesis model.[46] Activation of Wnt/β-catenin pathway is frequently observed in carcinogenesis of various organs other than colon.[48] Moreover, accumulating evidence indicates aberrant expression of TNF-α in human cancer in various organs including colon, esophagus, ovary, breast, prostate, bladder, and kidney.[13] Thus, it is probable that TNF-α can contribute to carcinogenesis in other organs by activating Wnt/β-catenin pathway.

TNF-α expression is enhanced in various types of cancer and can exhibit pro-tumorigenic activities such as induction of angiogenesis.[13] These observations lead to phase I and/or phase II clinical trials using TNF-α antagonist as the treatment for breast, ovarian, and renal cancer.[49–52] These trials demonstrated that TNF-α antagonist treatment resulted in a period of disease stabilization or better in 20% of patients with advanced cancer. The anti-TNF-α antibody treatment suggested that low or absent plasma TNF-α can predict a good response, but the reason for this is not clear.

Since TNF-α-producing cancer cells frequently gained resistance to cisplastin,[53] the combined treatment of TNF-α antagonist and cisplatin may enhance the action of the chemotherapeutic agent. Moreover, radioresistance requires TNF-α produced by tumor-associated macrophages and blockade of TNF-α can improve the efficacy of radiotherapy.[24] Furthermore, TNF-α antagonist treatment in chronic inflammatory diseases demonstrated that angiogenesis was markedly inhibited.[54] Thus, radiotherapy and anti-angiogenic agents such as bevacizumab can be good candidates to combine with TNF-α antagonists. Nevertheless, in order to further advance TNF-α antagonist treatment as cancer therapy, it is mandatory to have a greater understanding of the malignant and stromal cell-derived TNF-α in human cancers and its relative importance in early and late cancers.

References

1. Wang H, Czura CJ, and Tracey KJ (2003) Tumor necrosis factor, *The Cytokine Handbook 4th Edition*, Elsevier Science Ltd., pp.837–70.
2. Black RA. (2002) Tumor necrosis factor-α converting enzyme. *Int J Biochem Cell Biol* **34**:1–5.

3. Hohmann HP, Brockhaus M, Bauerler PA *et al.* (1990) Expression of types A and B tumour necrosis factor (TNF) receptors is independently regulated, and both receptors mediate activation of transcription factor NF-κB. TNF-α is not needed for induction of a biological effect via TNF receptors. *J Biol Chem* **265**:22409–17.
4. Liu ZG. (2005) Molecular mechanism of TNF signaling and beyond. *Cell Res* **15**:24–7.
5. Aggarwal BB. (2003) Signalling pathways of the TNF superfamily: A double-edged sword. *Nature Rev Immunol* **3**:745–56.
6. Pennica D, Nedwin GE, Hayflick JS *et al.* (1984) Human tumour necrosis factor: precursor structure, expression and homology to lymphotoxin. *Nature* **312**:724–9.
7. Beutler B and Cerami A. (1986) Cachectin and tumour necrosis factor as two sides of the same biological coin. *Nature* **320**:584–8.
8. Rüegg C, Yilmaz A, Bieler G *et al.* (1998) Evidence for the involvement of endothelial cell integrin αvβ3 in the disruption of the tumor vasculature induced by TNF and IFN-α . *Nat Med* **4**:408–14.
9. Talmadge JE, Phillips H, Schneider M *et al.* (1988) Immunomodulatory properties of recombinant murine and human tumor necrosis factor. *Cancer Res* **48**:544–50.
10. Selby P, Hobbs S, Viner C, *et al.* (1987). Tumour necrosis factor in man: Clinical and biological observations. *Br J Cancer* **56**:803–8.
11. Feldman ER, Creagan ET, Schaid DJ *et al.* (1992) Phase II trial of recombinant tumor necrosis factor in disseminated malignant melanoma. *Am J Clin Oncol* **15**:256–9.
12. Blick M, Sherwin SA, Rosenblum M *et al.* (1987). Phase I study of recombinant tumor necrosis factor in cancer patients. *Cancer Res* **47**:2986–9.
13. Balkwill F. (2009) Tumour necrosis factor and cancer. *Nature Rev Cancer* **9**:361–71.
14. Balkwill F and Mantovani A. (2001) Inflammation and cancer: Back to Virchow. *Lancet* **357**:539–45.
15. Dvorak HF. (1986) Tumors: wounds that do not heal. Similarities between tumor stroma generation and wound healing. *N Engl J Med* **315**:1650–9.
16. Fiocchi C. (1998). Inflammatory bowel disease: Etiology and pathogenesis. *Gastroenterology* **115**:182–205.
17. Mossman BT and Churg, A. (1998) Mechanisms in the pathogenesis of asbestosis and silicosis *Am J Respir Crit Care Med* **157**:1666–80.

18. Mantovani A, Allavena P, Sica A *et al.* (2008) Cancer-related inflammation. *Nature* **454**:436–44.
19. Szlosarek P, Charles KA, Balkwill FR. (2006) Tumour necrosis factor-α as a tumour promoter. *Eur J Cancer* **42**:745–50.
20. Naugler WE, Karin M. (2008) NF-κB and cancer — identifying targets and mechanisms. *Curr Opinion Genetics Deveop* **18**:19–26.
21. Pasparakis M. (2009) Regulation of tissue homeostasis by NF-κB signaling: Implications for inflammatory diseases. *Nature Rev Immunol* **9**:778–88.
22. Leibovich SJ, Polverini PJ, Shepard HM *et al.* (1987) Macrophage-induced angiogenesis is mediated by tumour necrosis factor-α. *Nature* **329**:630–2.
23. Kulbe H, Thompson R, Wilson JL *et al.* (2007) The inflammatory cytokine tumor necrosis factor-alpha generates an autocrine tumor-promoting network in epithelial ovarian cancer cells. *Cancer Res* **67**:585–92.
24. Meng Y, Beckett MA, Liang H *et al.* (2010) Blockade of tumor necrosis factor α signaling in tumor-associated macrophages as a radiosensitizing strategy. *Cancer Res* **70**:1534–43.
25. Li B, Vincent A, Cates J *et al.* (2009) Low levels of tumor necrosis factor α increase tumor growth by inducing an endothelial phenotype of monocytes recruited to the tumor site. *Cancer Res* **69**:338–48.
26. Komori A, Yatsunami J, Suganuma M *et al.* (1993) Tumor necrosis factor acts as a tumor promoter in BALB/3T3 cell transformation. *Cancer Res* **53**:1982–5.
27. Zhang, JY, Adams AE, Ridky TW *et al.* (2007) Tumor necrosis factor receptor 1/c-Jun-NH2-kinase signaling promotes human neoplasia. *Cancer Res* **67**:3827–34.
28. Babbar N and Casero RA. (2006) Tumor necrosis factor-α increases reactive oxygen species by inducing spermine oxidase in human lung epithelial cells: A potential mechanism for inflammation-induced carcinogenesis. *Cancer Res* **66**:11125–30.
29. Komori J, Marusawa H, Machimoto T *et al.* (2008) Activation-induced cytidine deaminase links bile duct inflammation to human cholangiocarcinoma. *Hepatol* **47**:888–96.
30. Akiyama M, Hideshima T, Hayashi T *et al.* (2003) Nuclear factor-κB p65 mediates tumor necrosis factor**α** -induced nuclear translocation of telomerase reverse transcriptase protein. *Cancer Res* **63**:18–21.
31. Moore RJ, Owens DM, Stamp G *et al.* (1999). Mice deficient in tumor necrosis factor-α are resistant to skin carcinogenesis. *Nature Med* **6**:828–31.

32. Arnott CH, Scott KA, Moore RJ *et al.* (2004). Expression of both TNF-α receptor subtypes is essential for optimal skin tumour development. *Oncogene* **23**:1902–10.
33. Wu Y, Deng J, Rychhou PG *et al.* (2009) Stabilization of Snail by NF-κB is required for inflammation-induced cell migration and invasion. *Cancer Cell* **15**:416–28.
34. Orosz P, Echtenacher B, Falk W *et al.* (1993) Enhancement of experimental metastasis by tumor necrosis factor. *J Exp Med* **177**:1391–8.
35. Kitakata H, Nemoto-Sasaki Y, Takahashi Y *et al.* (2002). Essential roles of tumor necrosis factor receptor p55 in liver metastasis of intrasplenic administration of colon 26 cells. *Cancer Res* **62**:6682–7.
36. Abraham C, Cho JH. (2009) Inflammatory bowel disease. *N Engl J Med* **361**:2066–78.
37. Okayasu I, Hatakeyama S, Yamada M *et al.* (1990) A novel method in the induction of reliable experimental acute and chronic ulcerative colitis in mice. *Gastroenterology* **98**:694–702.
38. Okayasu I, Yamada M, Mikami T *et al.* (2002) Dysplasia and carcinoma development in a repeated dextran sulfate sodium-induced colitis model. *J Gastroenterol Hepatol* **17**:1078–83.
39. Boivin GP, Washington K, Yang K *et al.* (2003) Pathology of mouse models of intestinal cancer: Consensus report and recommendations. *Gastroenterology* **124**:762–77.
40. Okayasu I, Ohkusa T, Kajiura K *et al.* (1996) Promotion of colorectal neoplasia in experimental murine ulcerative colitis. *Gut* **39**:87–92.
41. Popivanova BK, Kitamura K, Wu Y *et al.* (2008). Blocking TNF-α in mice reduces colorectal carcinogenesis associated with chronic colitis. *J Clin Invest* **118**:560–70.
42. Greten FR, Eckmann L, Greten TF *et al.* (2004). IKKβ links inflammation and tumorigenesis in a mouse model of colitis-associated cancer. *Cell* **118**:285–96.
43. Takahashi M, Wakabayashi K. (2004) Gene mutations and altered gene expression in azoxymethane-induced colon carcinogenesis. *Cancer Sci* **95**:475–80.
44. Sonoshita M, Takaku K, Sasaki N *et al.* (2001) Acceleration of intestinal polyposis through prostaglandin receptor EP2 in Apc(δ716) knockout mice. *Nat Med* **7**:1048–51.

45. Castellone MD, Teramoto H, Williams BO *et al.* (2005) Prostaglandin E2 promotes colon cancer cell growth through a Gs-axin-beta-catenin signaling axis. *Science* **310**:1504–10.
46. Oguma K, Oshima H, Aoki M *et al.* (2008) Activated macrophages promote Wnt signalling through tumour necrosis factor-α in gastric tumour cells. *EMBO J* **27**:1671–81.
47. Popivanova BK, Kostadinova FI, Furuichi K *et al.* (2009) Blockade of a chemokine, CCL2, reduces chronic colitis-associated carcinogenesis in mice. *Cancer Res* **69**:7884–92.
48. Markowitz SD, Bertagnolli MM. (2009) Molecular Basis of colorectal cancer. *N Engl J Med* **361**:2449–60.
49. Madhusudan S, Foster M, Muthuramalingam SR *et al.* (2004) A phase II study of etanercept (Enbrel), a tumor necrosis factor alpha inhibitor in patients with metastatic breast cancer. *Clin Cancer Res* **10**:6528–34.
50. Madhusudan S, Muthuramalingam SR, Braybrooke JP *et al.* (2005) Study of etanercept, a tumor necrosis factor-alpha inhibitor, in recurrent ovarian cancer. *J Clin Oncol* **23**:5950–9.
51. Harrison ML, Obermueller E, Maisey NR *et al.* (2007) Tumor necrosis factor alpha as a new target for renal cell carcinoma: Two sequential phase II trials of infliximab at standard and high dose. *J Clin Onocl* **25**:4242–9.
52. Brown ER, Charles KA, Hoare SA *et al.* (2008) A clinical study assessing the tolerability and biological effects of infliximab, a TNF-alpha inhibitor, in patients with advanced cancer. *Ann Oncol* **19**:1340–6.
53. Gordon GJ, Mani M, Mukhopadhyay L *et al.* (2007) Inhibitor of apoptosis proteins are regulated by tumour necrosis factor-α in malignant pleural mesothelioma. *J Pathol* **211**:439–46.
54. Charles P, Elliott MJ, Davis D *et al.* (1999) Regulation of cytokines, cytokine inhibitors, and acute-phase proteins following anti-TNF-α therapy in rheumatoid arthritis. *J Immunol* **163**:1521–8.

Chapter 13

Peroxisome Proliferator Activated Receptor-γ (PPARγ): Roles in Chronic Inflammation and Intestinal Oncogenic Transformation

Ioannis A. Voutsadakis*

Department of Medical Oncology, University Hospital of Larissa, Larissa, Greece

PPARγ is a nuclear receptor transcription factor involved in both carcinogenesis and inflammation. It displays a high expression in adipose tissue controlling adipogenesis and fat metabolism but is also expressed in equivalent levels in colorectal tissue where it plays a role in metabolism but also in signal transduction, proliferation and motility. PPARγ roles in inflammatory bowel disease and in colorectal cancer have been studied and some of their aspects have been elucidated. An inflammation-suppressing effect of PPARγ seems to emerge in most experimental models. Additionally, PPARγ has anti-tumor effects in most models of inflammation-induced but also sporadic carcinogenesis. The current knowledge on PPARγ in these processes and perspectives on therapeutic opportunities will be the subject of this paper.

Introduction

An association of chronic inflammation with cancer is well established and chronically inflamed tissues due to either microbial pathogens or chemical irritants are prone to carcinogenesis. An example in the gastrointestinal

* E-mail: ivoutsadakis@yahoo.com

tract is the increased risk of patients with inflammatory bowel diseases (IBDs), Crohn's disease and ulcerative colitis to develop cancer, mainly colorectal but also small bowel cancer and cholangiocarcinoma.[1]

Peroxisome Proliferator Activated Receptor-γ (PPARγ) is a transcription factor belonging to the nuclear receptor family that has its higher expression in adipose tissue and plays a significant role in adipogenesis and fat metabolism. It is also highly expressed in large bowel wall and has been found to be involved in both inflammation and carcinogenesis.[2,3]

In this paper, I will discuss the pathogenic association of chronic inflammation with carcinogenesis generally and in colon specifically and the role of PPARγ in these processes. I will conclude with therapeutic opportunities from pharmacologic manipulations of this transcription factor.

Peroxisome proliferator activated receptor γ (PPARγ) and ligands

PPARγ together with PPARα and PPARβ/δ are the three PPARs making up a sub-family of the nuclear hormone receptor super-family. PPARγ is expressed mainly in adipose tissue but also in equivalent levels in colonic epithelium.[4] PPARγ is also expressed at lower levels in beta cells of the pancreas, vascular endothelium, macrophages and other tissues (Table 1). PPARγ expression begins during embryogenesis in humans.[5] The two other PPARs, PPARα and PPARβ/δ are expressed mainly in liver, heart, muscle and vascular wall the former, and in skin, brain and adipose tissue the latter.[6]

Table 1. Profile of PPARγ molecule.

• Function	Transcription factor
• Family	Nuclear transcription factors
• Chromosome location	3p25
• Tissue expression	adipose tissue, colon, vascular wall, macrophages
• Domain organization	Similar to other nuclear transcription factors
• Examples of ligands	Lipids, thiazolidinediones, NSAIDs, CDDO, c-DIMs
• Examples of target genes	Cytokeratins, CEA, p21, p27, PTEN, PPARγ

The PPARγ gene is located in the human chromosome 3p25[7] while PPARα and PPARβ/δ genes are located in human chromosomes 22 and 6 respectively.[8] Two isoforms are transcribed from the PPARγ locus. PPARγ2 is fat tissue restricted and PPARγ1 displays a more ubiquitous expression.[9] In the aminoterminal end of PPARγ molecule it is situated a domain called A/B domain which is responsible for ligand-independent transcriptional regulation through phosphorylation and SUMOylation.[10–12]

DNA-binding or C domain of PPARγ contains two zinc finger-like and α-helical DNA binding motifs typical of transcription factors and lays carboxy-terminal to A/B domain. The C domain binds PPRE (Peroxisome Proliferator Response Element) sequences. These sequences have a DR1 pattern, a direct repeat sequence with a single nucleotide base spacer between the two repeats. PPARγ recognizes the PPRE with the sequence TGACCTxTGACCT (where x is the spacer nucleotide). DNA binding takes place in a heterodimerized form with the 9-cis retinoic acid receptor or retinoic X receptor (RXR). More carboxy-terminal to DNA-binding domain in the PPARγ molecule there is a hinge domain (domain D) which allows independent movement of the next and last domain of the PPARγ molecule, domain E/F. This is the ligand binding domain. After ligation it facilitates PPARγ dimerization with RXR and recruitment of co-activators for transcription. The three dimensional structure of this domain dimerized with RXR both bound to respective ligands and two peptides from the transcription co-activator SRC1 (Steroid Receptor Co-activator 1) displays similarities to co-activator interactions with other nuclear receptors.[13]

PPARγ is the receptor for the anti-diabetic class of drugs thiazolidinediones or glitazones. Drugs of the Non-Steroidal Anti-Inflammatory Drugs (NSAIDs) class such as indomethacin, ibuprofen, and flufenamic acid display PPARγ activation activity in concentrations 2–3 orders of magnitude higher than that required for their COX (cyclooxygenase) inhibiting activity.[14] This is not a class effect given that other NSAIDs such as piroxicam, salicylic acid and acetaminophen are not PPARγ agonists.

Another synthetic PPARγ ligand is the oleanane triterpenoid 2-cyano-3,12-dioxoolean-1,9-dien-28-oic acid (CDDO).[15] CDDO is a weaker inducer of PPARγ transcription than rosiglitazone, a fact correlating with a weaker ability of CDDO to recruit co-activators.

Natural ligands for PPARγ were initially obscure. A naturally occurring metabolite of prostaglandin D (PGD_2), 15-deoxy-$\Delta^{12,14}$-PGJ_2 (15d-PGJ_2) has been shown to activate PPARγ in micromolar concentrations but these exceed the endogenously occurring concentrations of this metabolite by orders of magnitude and thus it remains questionable whether it can fulfill this function *in vivo*.[16] Linoleic acid derivative nitrolinoleic acid is an endogenous PPARγ ligand that activates the receptor in concentrations found in physiologic conditions and is able to induce target genes transcription.[17] Dietary conjugated linoleic acid derivatives found in dairy products and meat can also activate PPARγ.[18] Other fatty acids such as eicosapentaenoic and arachidonic acid, 9-hydroxyoctadecadienoic acid (9-HODE), 13-HODE, 15-hydroxyeicosatetraenoic acid (15-HETE) and 13-oxooctadecadienoic acid are additional activators of PPARγ.[19–21]

The natural phytochemicals curcumin (diferuloylmethane) and methylene-substituted di-indolylmethanes (c-DIMs) are PPARγ activators but probably not through direct ligation but through promoting phosphorylation by MAPKs.[22,23]

Studies using thiazolidinediones and concentrations of 15-deoxy-$\Delta^{12,14}$-PGJ_2 above those endogenously achieved, have helped in elucidating the role of PPARγ activation. This transcription factor has been characterized as critical for adipose tissue differentiation and fatty acid homeostasis. Activation of PPARγ drives the differentiation of preadipocytes to adipocytes[24] and increases the oxidation and storage of fatty acids. On the contrary, in liver and muscle, PPARγ activation decreases fatty acid oxidation and hepatic glyconeogenesis, resulting in the hypoglycemic effects of PPARγ. PPARγ/RXR dimers bound to DNA recruit co-activators such as Steroid Receptor Co-activator-1 (SRC1), Peroxisome Proliferator Receptor-γ Coactivator 1α (PGC-1α),[25] AP220/PPARγ binding protein (PBP),[26] and p300/CBP (CREB Binding Protein).[27] Finally the general transcription machinery is recruited to the complex for the initiation of target gene transcription. As there are no known negative PPARγ response elements, trans-repression observed in some genes may be mediated by competition with other transcription factors or by recruitment of co-repressors that has been observed after PPARγ SUMOylation.

PPARγ activation after ligands binding leads, concomitantly, to its ubiquitination and proteasome degradation,[28] a regulatory mechanism common to both membrane associated receptors and other nuclear hormone receptors including PPARγ's transcriptional partner RXRα.[29] Transcriptional activity of PPARγ is not required for ubiquitination and proteasome degradation,[28] but ligand binding is required.

Inflammation and cancer

Inflammation is a cancer-promoting condition that favors both cancer initiation and progression. Many pathogens are associated with cancers, some examples being *Helicobacter pylori* and gastric carcinoma, EBV and nasopharyngeal carcinoma and Burkitt lymphoma, HBV and HCV and hepatoma and schistosoma and bladder carcinoma.[30] In addition exogenous irritating agents causing chronic inflammation such as tobacco smoke, alcohol, asbestos and coal tar are strongly associated with diverse carcinomas.

Both pathogens and physical agents induce the accumulation of inflammatory cells such as macrophages, T cells, NK cells and dendritic cells in damaged tissues. These cells are activated to secrete various cytokines and chemokines that regulate the inflammatory response. They also have effects on cancer cells mostly promoting their survival and proliferation.

Main inflammatory cytokines that promote tumor formation include TNF-α, Interleukin-6 (IL-6) and IL-17. TNF-α signals after ligation of its cell surface receptor TNFR to activate transcription factor NF-κB, a significant factor for inflammation and tumor promotion. IL-17 signaling, through its surface receptor IL-17R also culminates in NF-κB activation. IL-17 is secreted by a sub-set of T cells called Th17 cells that has been characterized as an important component of chronic inflammation.[31] Th17 cells respond to IL-23 secreted by APC (Antigen Presenting) cells to secrete IL-17 which in turn activates NF-κB in cells expressing IL-17R. NF-κB activation resulting from both TNF-α and IL-17 signaling favors both inflammation and carcinogenesis through transcription regulation of genes including cytokines and chemokines such as IL-1, IL-2, IL-6, IL-8, GM-CSF and TNF-α, adhesion molecules such as ICAM and E-selectin, inflammation promoting enzymes such as COX-2, anti-apoptotic proteins such as bcl-xl, cIAP1 and cIAP2 and proliferation promoting proteins such as cyclin D and c-myc.[32] IL-23, in addition to promoting IL-17 production by Th17 cells, has pro-inflammatoty effects by inducing TNF-α production by macrophages in an autocrine manner.[33]

IL-6 is a target of NF-κB and ligates its heterodimeric cell surface receptor consisting of IL-6Rα and gp130 (glucoprotein 130).[34] Signal transduction takes place through activation of JAK1 (Janus kinase 1) and STAT1 and 3 (Signal Transducer and Activator of Transcription 1 and 3), finally resulting in transcription of growth promoting and apoptosis inhibiting molecules.[35]

In contrast to the above cytokines, other cytokines suppress inflammation. Two important such molecules are IL-10 and TGF-β. IL-10 suppresses NF-κB activation and thus leads to anti-inflammatory effects. Homozygous knock out mice for IL-10 have been found to develop an enterocolitis resembling ulcerative colitis and colitis-associated cancer.[36] These effects were reversed by treatment of the animals with exogenous IL-10. TGF-β is also a cytokine that suppresses inflammation. It acts through ligation of its surface receptors TβRI and TβRII which activate intracellular signal transducers Smads2/3 and 4.[37] TGF-β signaling possesses also tumor suppressive effects in most occasions and inhibits epithelial to mesenchymal transition. In many cases of colorectal cancer TGF-β signalling is defective due to disabling mutations of either the receptor or of Smad4.

It is evident from this discussion that there is an interplay between inflammation and cancer with cytokines as mediators. Both pro-inflammatory and anti-inflammatory cytokines have a role in this interplay and, in most instances, when the balance is shifted towards inflammation, cancer is concomitantly promoted.

Chemokines and their receptors are another category of ligands-receptors molecular pairs that play a role in inflammation but also cancer. Their primary physiologic role is in the regulation of leukocyte motility and trafficking to sites of active inflammation.[38] Chemokines are divided in four sub-families called CXC, CC, C and CX3C depending on the number of conserved cysteine residues that their molecules have and the number of in-between amino-acids. Their receptors are of the type of seven trans-membrane domain receptors producing their effects through the activation of various intracellular pathways. An example of chemokine ligand-receptor pair that plays a role in both inflammation and cancer is CXCL12 (also known as SDF-1 [Stem cell-Derived Factor 1]) and CXCR4. CXCR4 is expressed in leukocytes but also in endothelial, vascular smooth muscle, epithelial cells of the intestine and neural cells. Together with CXCL12, CXCR4 is important in development of the hematopoietic system and homing of hematopoietic progenitors in the bone marrow but also in chemo-attraction of inflammatory cells to sites of inflammation.[39] In carcinogenesis, CXCL12 and CXCR4 are involved in tissue invasion and metastasis. CXCR4 is expressed by cancer cells of gastrointestinal, geniturinary, breast and other origins[40,41] and the ligand CXCL12 is expressed in several occasions in favored metastatic sites. CXCR4 ligation in these sites leads to matrix metalloproteinases up-regulation on metastatic cancer cells further facilitating tissue invasion.[42] Thus, cancer cells mimic physiologically migratory cells and, as this example illustrates, take advantage of physiologically existent mechanisms to effectuate their migration to metastatic sites.

PPARγ and inflammation

PPARγ is linked with the inflammatory proccess through diverse mechanisms. In general PPARγ activation has anti-inflammatory effects although pro-inflammatory influences have been found in some experimental systems. Nevertheless these effects may be related to PPARγ-independent mechanisms of exogenous PPARγ activators used.[43]

A first mechanism of PPARγ interference with inflammation is by inhibiting transcription factors involved in it such as NF-κB, AP-1 (Activating Protein 1) and NFAT (Nuclear Factor of Activated T Cells) and, as a result, decreasing expression of target genes of these transcription factors involved in inflammatory cells activation, tissue invasion and adhesion. The function of several types of cells involved in inflammation is perturbed (Table 2). Lymphocyte proliferation and migration is decreased due to attenuation of IL-2 and IFN-γ production. Platelet aggregation ability is decreased and adhesion molecules, such as ICAM-1 expression in the endothelial cells surface is also decreased. Extra-cellular

Table 2. Important mechanisms of inflammation suppression by PPARγ.

- Interference with inflammation promoting transcription factors NF-κB, AP-1 and NFAT
- Decreased proliferation and migration of lymphocytes
- Decreased platelet aggregation
- Inhibition of NO-mediated vasodilation

matrix metalloproteinases such as MMP-9 levels fall, leading to decreased ability for tissue invasion.[44] iNOS (inducible Nitric Oxide Synthase), the enzyme responsible for production of NO in inflamed tissues is decreased by PPARγ action.[45] NO, a potent vasodilator, contributes to vasodilation which is a hallmark component and clinical sign of inflammation.[46]

Another mechanism of PPARγ mediation of anti-inflammatory responses is a direct repression of inflammatory genes. This repression is taking place after PPARγ sumoylation [covalent link with SUMO (Small Ubiquitin-like Modifier)] at lysine 365 that promotes recruitment of co-repressor complexes.[47] PPARγ expression has been found to be decreased in inflammatory states[44] further supporting a role of the nuclear receptor in suppressing inflammation. A key mediator of PPARγ expression decrease is TNF-α through activation of NF-κB.[48] NF-κB interferes with PPARγ activity in at least three ways. It decreases PPARγ gene transcription by inhibiting transcription factor C/EBPδ. It directly inhibits PPARγ and it recruits Histone deacetylase 3 in PPARγ transcription sites. Evidently there is a reciprocal relationship of NF-κB and PPARγ in inflammation, the former promoting while the latter suppressing it.[49]

PPARγ role in carcinogenesis

PPARγ has tumor suppressing effects through transcriptional induction of tumor suppressor genes. The tumor suppressor PTEN (Phosphatase and Tensin homolog at chromosome Ten) possesses PPARγ response elements on its promoter and is a PPARγ target gene.[50] PTEN encodes for a phosphatase that dephosphorylates and inactivates kinase PI3K (Phospho-Inositol-3-Kinase). PI3K through activation of akt kinase (also known as Protein Kinase B) inhibits apoptosis. In colon cancer cells and cells from other cancers, activation of PPARγ induces PTEN an effect that results in inhibition of akt phosphorylation and decreased cell survival.[51] Moreover PPARγ antisense oligonucleotide treatment resulted in significant decrease of caspase 9 activity, further witnessing for a pro-apoptotic action of PPARγ through a PTEN/caspase mechanism. In conditionally K-ras transformed rat intestinal epithelial cells, activation of PPARγ by rosiglitazone inhibited the phosphorylation of akt down-stream of K-ras and inhibited cell proliferation.[52] In these conditions, akt inhibition was not mediated by PTEN induction. Cyclin D was suppressed by PPARγ activation, a fact associated with a growth arrest in G1 phase of the cell cycle.[52] In breast cancer cells PPARγ activation suppresses cyclin D by a proteasome degradation mechanism.[53]

PPARγ was found to interact with Rb protein, a target of cyclin D.[54] The PPARγ/Rb complex recruits histone deacetylase 3 (HDAC3) and causes cell cycle arrest at the G1 phase of the cell cycle in mouse embryo fibroblasts. Thus, PPARγ interferes with the cyclin D/CDK4/Rb pathway in two ways both culminating in G1 arrest. In contrast, in Rb negative cells, PPARγ activation results in G2/M arrest, endo-reduplication and finally apoptosis.[54] G2/M arrest is accompanied by up-regulation of cyclin B1 and down-regulation of its inhibitor protein cdc25c.[55] Cdk inhibitors p21, p18 and p27 are induced by PPARγ and contribute further to cell cycle arrest.[56,57]

β-catenin, a protein with multiple functions and particular interest in the pathogenesis of colorectal cancer as a target of the APC (Adenomatous Polyposis Coli) protein, is down-regulated by PPARγ. The decrease of β-catenin after PPARγ activation involves a post-translational degradation mechanism which is proteasome-dependent but is distinct from the two APC-dependent degradation pathways that involve the kinase GSK3β and E3 ligase βTrCP the former and p53 and its target E3 ligase Siah-1 the latter.[58]

COX-2 is the inducible form of the enzyme that converts arachidonic acid to prostaglandin precursor PGH_2. An important role of COX-2 and prostaglandins in colon carcinogenesis has been suggested by the fact that COX inhibiting NSAIDs reduce the frequency of colon polyps and inhibit colorectal cancer cells *in vitro*.[59] Moreover double negative Min/COX-2 mice exhibit reduced number of polyps in comparison with Min mice.[60]

COX-2 expression was shown to be reduced in colorectal cancer HT-29 cells treated with PPARγ inhibitors, a result that may contribute to the induction of apoptosis seen after ciglitazone treatment.[59]

PPARγ in inflammatory diseases and carcinogenesis in colon

Inflammatory bowel diseases (IBDs), ulcerative colitis and Crohn's disease, predispose to colorectal cancer and represent a link between inflammation and carcinogenesis. IBDs are together with the two hereditary cancer syndromes, familial adenomatous polyposis and hereditary non-polyposis colorectal cancer, the three most high risk predisposing conditions for colorectal cancer. The true incidence of colorectal cancer in ulcerative colitis seems to be around 3.5 to 5.5%[61] and the risk in Crohn's disease patients with anatomically substantial colitis is similar.[62]

IBDs establishment requires in general an environmental trigger and an altered immune response in individuals with genetic predisposition (Fig. 1). Genetic predisposition in the form of polymorphisms in susceptibility genes which have products involved in innate immunity and gut wall barrier maintenance such as NOD2/CARD15 and IL23R is most probably playing a significant role in the pathogenesis of IBDs[63,64] but clearly the environment has also a saying as witnessed by the fact that concordance in the presence of disease between monozygotic twins is

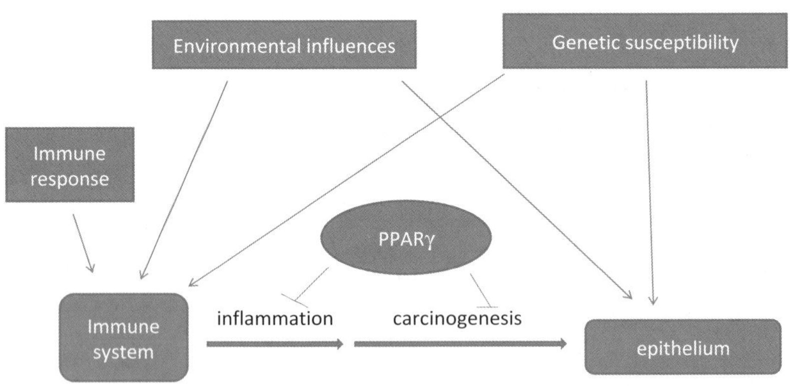

Figure 1. The interplay between environment and heredity in the pathogenesis of inflammation and cancer in bowel. Arrows denote positive effect, ⊥ sign denotes inhibition.

only about 50%.[65] Environment in the form of enteric bacteria (mainly commensal but also pathogenic), drugs, dietary components and smoking acts on a permissive genetic background and skews immune response towards an inappropriate inflammation perpetuation. Different subsets of T-cells interact with other inflammatory cells and activate each other through cytokines and chemokines in a vicious cycle that damages epithelium and produces further inflammatory responses due to defective epithelial barrier.[66]

Colon is one of the tissues where PPARγ has a high expression. Colonic flora up-regulates PPARγ through ligation of Toll-like receptor 4 (TLR4) by lipopolysaccharide which activates intra-cellular signaling culminating in PPARγ expression[67] and through production of butyrate. Butyrate is a PPARγ ligand and, as a result, up-regulated PPARγ is concomitantly activated completing a negative feed-back loop and counter-balancing high NF-κB pro-inflammatory activity. In patients with ulcerative colitis, there is impaired expression of PPARγ.[68] Moreover, mice with decreased expression of PPARγ due to heterozygous gene deletion display a propensity for colitis development.[69] Although the specific molecular pathogenesis event or events that mediate PPARγ's anti-inflammatory effects in colitis are not completely elucidated,[70] it is experimentally suggested that the nuclear receptor has salutary influence in preventing and decreasing bowel inflammation,[71] a fact that also correlates with the general effects of PPARγ in inflammation derived from various experimental systems.

PPARγ role in colorectal carcinogenesis has been investigated in various pre-clinical *in vivo* models to correlate with *in vitro* results. Various animal models have been used to study PPARγ activation in colon cancer. In most occasions PPARγ activation suppresses colorectal carcinogenesis as seen also *in vitro*.[72–74] One exemption is models that use mice with APC mutations where, in most occasions, PPARγ activation leads to increased tumor formation.[75,76] Thus it seems that PPARγ activation may need β-catenin degradation mechanism to be intact in order to suppress carcinogenesis. An alternative explanation would be that the genetic background of mice in which PPARγ-dependent promotion of carcinogenesis has been observed (C57BL/6J mice) is playing a crucial role in this result. This hypothesis would corroborate also the fact that in this mouse strain thiazolidinediones treatment has been found to aggravate DDS-induced colitis.[77]

IBD-related colorectal cancer pathogenesis shares in general the same molecular lesions with sporadic colorectal cancer but the sequence of events is different.[1] The classic sequence of events in most sporadic colorectal cancers is described as a process in which the normal epithelium acquires step-wise molecular lesions that transform it to anatomic lesions of increasing malignant potential such as Aberrant Crypt Foci (ACF), polyps and finally carcinoma. The most common initial molecular lesion in sporadic carcinomas is a mutation in APC, a protein that takes part in a complex that facilitates phosphorylation of transcription factor β-catenin, an event leading to β-catenin's ubiquitination and proteasome degradation, keeping this transcription factor that has proliferation promoting effects in colon, under control.[78] Disabling mutations of APC leaves β-catenin activity unregulated and produces the initial microscopically detectable neoplastic lesion in colon called Aberrant Crypt Focus. Other genetic lesions accumulate in turn such as k-ras oncogene activating mutations and, in more advanced stages leading to polyp/carcinoma transition, disabling mutations of p53 and of DPC4 (Deleted in Pancreatic Cancer 4).

In colitis-associated colorectal cancer the precursor lesion is dysplasia of increasing grade (Fig. 2). Similar molecular events to those happening in sporadic colorectal cancer development lead to colitis-associated carcinogenesis, albeit with a different sequence.[79] In this instance, p53 mutations occur in an earlier phase of cancer development and are usually followed by loss of heterozygosity (LOH) in the remaining normal allele, completely disabling this tumor suppressor. Indeed p53 LOH happens with increasing frequency as the neoplastic lesion progresses from mild dysplasia to severe dysplasia to cancer. In contrast APC and k-ras mutations are later and rarer events in colitis-associated carcinogenesis.[80,81] This is of particular importance for PPARγ-targeted interventions given the fact that PPARγ activation has produced unequivocal anti-carcinogenic effects in APC wild type models but not in APC mutant models where its effects is less homogeneous (see the above discussion).

In view of these differences in molecular events between sporadic and colitis-associated colorectal cancer, PPARγ-targeted interventions may be

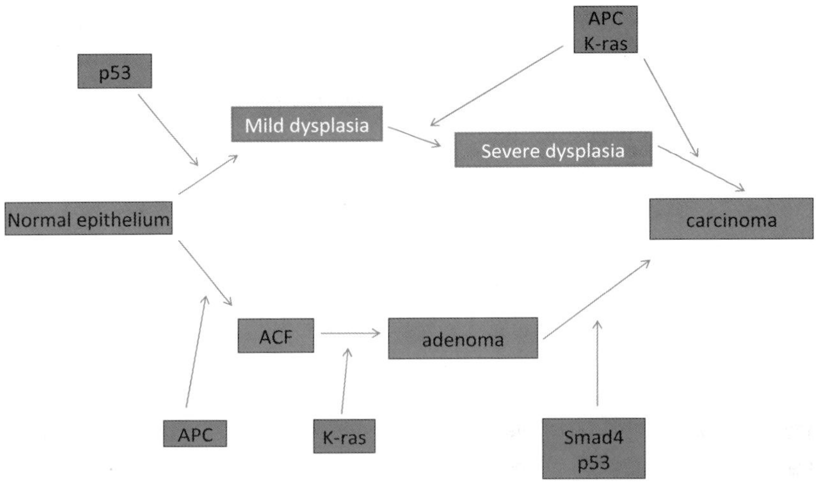

Figure 2. Simplified schematic representation of proposed sequence of events in inflammation-induced (upper sequence) and inflammation-independent (lower sequence) molecular carcinogenesis in colon.

of particular relevance in the latter. Chronic inflammation in the form of ulcerative colitis can be viewed as a precursor lesion and has also been investigated in PPARγ-targeted therapies. Using a DSS (Dextran Sodium Sulfate) mouse model of colitis,[82] it was shown that activation of PPARγ by conjugated linoleic acid-containing feeding suppressed colitis indexes compared with mice fed with a control diet or a diet rich in a lipid that is not PPARγ ligand.[18] Mice that had PPARγ gene deleted in their colon could not benefit from conjugated linoleic acid feeding. In a related mouse model that associates DSS treatment to azoxymethane (AOM) administered intraperitoneally and produces a high rate of invasive cancer on a background of colitis, PPARγ activation by troglitazone treatment was effective in reducing adenocarcinoma incidence by 60%[83] in a manner similar to that of non-colitis associated cancer models.

In clinical practice, the class of 5-aminosalicylic acid derivatives (5-ASAs) used in relapse prevention and remission induction in IBDs has been found to up-regulate PPARγ expression and thus to suppress inflammation and maintain mucosal integrity.[84] This mechanism of action of 5-ASAs together with other proposed mechanisms including NF-κB inhibition and modulation of inflammatory cytokines production may all act on the interplay between pro-inflammatory NF-κB and anti-inflammatory PPARγ and push the balance towards inflammation suppression.[85] Inflammation suppression mediates both therapeutic effects of 5-ASAs in IBDs and colorectal cancer incidence decrease obtained in IBDs patients treated with these drugs. In addition PPARγ activation may have additional anti-neoplastic effects independent of inflammation suppression as witnessed by its effectiveness in many models of sporadic colorectal cancer. In future studies it remains to be seen if combination of 5-ASAs with other PPARγ activators such as thiazolidinediones or other targeted therapies will further ameliorate treatment results in patients with IBDs and further decrease the incidence of cancer, a dreaded complication in this population of patients.

References

1. Xie X, Itzkowitz SH (2008). Cancer in inflammatory bowel disease. *World J Gastroenterol* **14**:378–89.
2. Voutsadakis IA (2007). PPARγ and colorectal carcinogenesis. *J Cancer Res Clin Oncol* **133**:917–28.
3. Necela BM, Thompson EA. (2008) Pathophysiological roles of PPARγ in gastrointestinal epithelial cells. *PPAR Res* **2008**: Article ID 148687.
4. Bull AW (2003). The role of peroxisome proliferator-activated receptor-γ in colon cancer and inflammatory bowel disease. *Arch Pathol Lab Med* **127**:1121–3.
5. Huin C, Corriveau L, Bianchi A *et al.* (2000). Differential expression of Peroxisome Proliferator-activated Receptors (PPARs) in the developing human fetal digestive tract. *J Histochem Cytochem* **48**:603–11.
6. Yki-Järvinen H (2004). Thiazolidinediones. *N Engl J Med* **351**:1106–18.
7. Vigouroux C, Fajas L, Khallouf E *et al.* (1998). Human peroxisome proliferator-activated receptor-γ_2 Genetic mapping, identification of a variant in the coding sequence, and exclusion as the gene responsible for lipoatrophic diabetes. *Diabetes* **47**:490–2.
8. Devergne B, Wahli W (1999). Peroxisome Proliferator-activated Receptors: nuclear control of metabolism. *Endocr Rev* **20**:649–88.
9. Cock T-A, Houten SM, Auwerx J (2004). Peroxisome proliferators-activated receptor-γ: too much of a good thing causes harm. *EMBO Rep* **5**:142–7.

10. Adams M, Reginato MJ, Shao D *et al.* (1997) Transcriptional activation by peroxisome proliferators-activated receptor γ is inhibited by phosphorylation at a consensus mitogen-activated protein kinase site. *J Biol Chem* **272**:5128–32.
11. Ohshima T, Koga H, Shimotohno K. (2004) Transcriptional activity of Peroxisome Proliferator-activated Receptor γ is modulated by SUMO-1 modification. *J Biol Chem* **279**:29551–7.
12. Diradourian C, Girard J, Pégorier J-P. (2005) Phosphorylation of PPARs: from molecular characterization to physiological relevance. *Biochim* **87**:33–8.
13. Nolte RT, Wisely GB, Westin S *et al.* (1998) Ligand binding and co-activator assembly of the peroxisome proliferators-activated receptor-γ. *Nature* **395**:137–43.
14. Lehmann JM, Lenhard JM, Oliver BB *et al.* (1997) Peroxisome Proliferator-activated Receptors α and γ are activated by indomethacin and other non-steroidal anti-inflammatory drugs. *J Biol Chem* **272**:3406–10.
15. Wang Y, Porter WW, Suh N *et al.* (2000) A synthetic triterpenoid, 2-cyano-3, 12-dioxooleana-1,9-dien-28-oic acid (CDDO), is a ligand for the Peroxisome Proliferator-activated Receptor γ. *Mol Endocrinol* **14**:1550–6.
16. Bell-Parikh LC, Ide T, Lawson JA *et al.* (2003) Biosynthesis of 15-deoxy-$\Delta^{12,14}$-PGJ_2 and the ligation of PPARγ. *J Clin Invest* **112**:945–55.
17. Schopfer FJ, Lin Y, Baker PRS *et al.* (2005) Nitrolinoleic acid: An endogenous peroxisome proliferator-activated receptor γ ligand. *Proc Natl Acad Sci USA*. **102**:2340–5.
18. Bassaganya-Riera J, Reynolds K, Martino-Catt S *et al.* (2004) Activation of PPARγ and δ by conjugated linoleic acid mediates protection from experimental inflammatory bowel disease. *Gastroenterol* **127**:777–91.
19. Bull AW, Steffensen KR, Leers J, Rafter JJ. (2003) Activation of PPARγ in colon tumor cell lines by oxidized metabolites of linoleic acid, endogenous ligands for PPARγ. *Carcinogenesis* **24**:1717–22.
20. Sasaki T, Yoshida K, Shimura H *et al.* (2006) Inhibitory effect of linoleic acid on transformation of IEC6 intestinal cells by *in vitro* azoxymethane treatment. *Int J Cancer* **118**:593–9.
21. Schild RL, Schaiff WT, Carlson MG *et al.* (2002) The activity of PPARγ in primary human trophoblasts is enhanced by oxidized lipids. *J Clin Endocrinol Metab* **87**:1105–10.
22. Chen A, Xu J. (2005) Activation of PPARγ by curcumin inhibits Moser cell growth and mediates suppression of cyclin D1 and EGFR. *Am J Physiol Gastrointest Liver Physiol* **288**:G447–56.

23. Chintharlapalli S, Smith III R, Samudio I *et al.* (2004) 1,1-Bis(3'-indolyl)-1-(p-substitutedphenyl)methanes induce Peroxisome Proliferator-Activated Receptor γ-mediated growth inhibition, transactivation, and differentiation markers in colon cancer cells. *Cancer Res* **64**:5994–6001.
24. Hiragun A, Sato M, Matsui H. (1988) Preadipocyte differentiation *in vitro*: Identification of a highly active adipogenic agent. *J Cell Phys* **134**:124–30.
25. Puigserver P, Spiegelman BM. (2003) Peroxisome proliferators-activated receptor-γ coactivator 1α (PGC-1α): Transcriptional coactivator and metabolic regulator. *Endocrine Rev* **24**:78–90.
26. Ge H, Guermah M, Yuan CX *et al.* (2002) The TRAP220 subunit of the TRAP/ mediator is required for PPARγ2-stimulated adipogenesis. *Nature* **417**:563–7.
27. Gelman L, Zhou G, Fajas L *et al.* (1999) p300 interacts with the N-and C-terminal part of PPARγ2 in a ligand-independent and — dependent manner, respectively. *J Biol Chem* **274**:7681–8.
28. Hauser S, Adelmant G, Sarraf P *et al.* (2000) Degradation of the Peroxisome Proliferator-activated Receptor γ is linked to ligand-dependent activation. *J Biol Chem* **275**:18527–33.
29. Boudjelal M, Wang Z, Voorhees JJ *et al.* (2000) Ubiquitin/proteasome pathway regulates levels of retinoic acid receptor γ and retinoid X receptor α in human keratinocytes. *Cancer Res* **60**:2247–52.
30. Lin W-W, Karin M. (2007) A cytokine-mediated link between innate immunity, inflammation, and cancer. *J Clin Invest* **117**:1175–83.
31. Moseley TA, Haudenschild DR, Rose L, Reddi AH. (2003) Interleukin-17 family and IL-17 receptors. *Cytokine Growth Factor Rev* **14**:155–74.
32. Ghosh S, Karin M. (2002) Missing pieces in the NF-κB puzzle. *Cell* **109**:S81–S96
33. Hao JS, Shan BE. (2006) Immune enhancement and anti-tumour activity of IL-23. *Cancer Immunol Immunother* **55**:1426–31.
34. Hodge DR, Hurt EM, Farrar WL. (2005) The role of IL-6 and STAT3 in inflammation and cancer. *Eur J Cancer* **41**:2502–12.
35. Ishihara K, Hirano T. (2002) IL-6 in autoimmune disease and chronic inflammatory proliferative disease. *Cytokine Growth Factor Rev* **13**:357–68.
36. Berg DJ, Davidson N, Kühn R *et al.* (1996) Enterocolitis and colon cancer in interleukin-10-deficient mice are associated with aberrant cytokine production and $CD4^{+}$TH1-like responses. *J Clin Invest* **98**:1010–20.

37. Attisano L, Lee-Hoeflich ST. (2001) The Smads. *Genome Biol* **2**: reviews 3010.1–3010.8.
38. Mellado M, Rodríguez- Frade JM, Mañes S, Martínez-A C. (2001) Chemokine signalling and functional responses: The role of receptor dimerization and TK pathway activation. *Annual Rev Immunol* **19**:397–421.
39. Richard CL, Blay J. (2008) CXCR4 in cancer and its regulation by PPARγ. *PPAR Res* 2008: Artcle ID 769413.
40. Balkwill F. (2004) The significance of cancer cell expression of the chemokine receptor CXCR4. *Sem Cancer Biol* **14**:171–9.
41. Zeelenberg IS, Ruuls-Van Stalle L, Roos E. (2003) The chemokine receptor CXCR4 is required for outgrowth of colon carcinoma micrometastases. *Cancer Res* **63**:3833–9.
42. Scotton CJ, Wilson JL, Milliken D *et al.* (2001) Epithelial cancer cell migration: a role for chemokine receptors? *Cancer Res* **61**:4961–5.
43. Delerive P, Fruchart JC, Staels B. (2001) Peroxisome Proliferator-activated Receptors in inflammation control. *J Endocrinol* **169**:453–9.
44. Moraes LA, Piqueras L, Bishop- Bailey D. (2006) Peroxisome Proliferator-activated Receptors and inflammation. *Pharmacol Ther* **110**:371–85.
45. Heneka M, Klockgether T, Feinstein D. (2002) Peroxisome Proliferator-activated Receptor-gamma ligands reduce neuronal inducible nitric oxide synthase expression and cell death in vivo. *J Neurosci* **20**:6862–7.
46. Youssef J, Badr M. (2004) Role of Peroxisome Proliferator-activated Receptors in inflammation control. *J Biomed Biotechnol* **3**:156–66.
47. Pascual G, Fong AL, Ogawa S *et al.* (2005) A SUMOylation-dependent pathway mediates transrepression of inflammatory response genes by PPAR-gamma. *Nature* **437**:759–63.
48. Ye J. (2008) Regulation of PPARγ function by TNF-α. *Biochem Biophys Res Commun* **374**:405–8.
49. Carter AB, Misyak SA, Hontecillas R, Bassaganya-Riera J. (2009) Dietary modulation of inflammation-induced colorectal cancer through PPARγ. *PPAR Res* **2009**, Article ID 498352
50. Patel L, Pass I, Coxon P *et al.* (2001) Tumor suppressor and anti-inflammatory actions of PPARγ agonists are mediated via upregulation of PTEN. *Curr Biol* **11**:764–8.
51. Chen GG, Lee JF, Wang SH *et al.* (2002) Apoptosis induced by activation of peroxisome-proliferator activated receptor-gamma is associated with Bcl-2 and NF-kappa B in human colon cancer. *Life Sci* **70**:2631–46.

52. Shao J, Sheng H, DuBois RN. (2002) Peroxisome Proliferator-activated receptors modulate K-Ras-mediated transformation of intestinal epithelial cells. *Cancer Res* **62**:3282–8.
53. Qin C, Burghardt R, Smith R *et al.* (2003) Peroxisome proliferators-activated receptor γ agonists induce proteasome-dependent degradation of cyclin D1 and estrogen receptor α in MCF-7 breast cancer cells. *Cancer Res* **63**:958–64.
54. Fajas L, Egler V, Reiter R *et al.* (2003) PPARγ controls cell proliferation and apoptosis in an RB-dependent manner. *Oncogene* **22**:4186–93.
55. Kim EJ, Park KS, Chung SY *et al.* (2003) Peroxisome proliferator-activated receptor-γ activator 15-deoxy-$\Delta^{12,14}$-Prostaglandin J_2 inhibits neuroblastoma cell growth through induction of apoptosis: Association with extracellular signal-regulated kinase signal pathway. *J Pharmacol Exper Therapeutics* **307**:505–17.
56. Morrison RF, Farmer SR. (1999) Role of PPARγ in regulating a cascade expression of cyclin-dependent kinase inhibitors, p18 (INK4c) and p21 (Waf1/Cip1), during adipogenesis. *J Biol Chem* **274**:17088–97.
57. Chen F, Harrison LE. (2005) Ciglitazone-induced cellular anti-proliferation oncreases $p27^{kip1}$ protein levels through both increased transcriptional activity and inhibition of proteasome degradation *Cell Signaling* **17**:809–16.
58. Sharma C, Pradeep A, Wong L *et al.* (2004) Peroxisome proliferators-activated receptor γ activation can regulate β-catenin levels via a proteasome-mediated and adenomatous polyposis coli-independent pathway. *J Biol Chem* **279**:35583–94.
59. Gupta RA, DuBois RN. (2001) Colorectal cancer prevention and treatment by inhibition of cyclooxygenase-2. *Nat Rev Cancer* **1**:11–21.
60. Oshima M, Dinchuk JE, Kargman SL *et al.* (1996) Suppression of intestinal polyposis in Apc delta716 knockout mice by inhibition of cyclooxygenase 2(Cox-2). *Cell* **87**:803–9.
61. Eaden JA, Abrams KR, Mayberry JF. (2001) The risk of colorectal cancer in ulcerative colitis: a meta-analysis. *Gut* **48**:526–35.
62. Sachar DB. (1994) Cancer in Crohn´s disease: dispelling the myths. *Gut* **35**:1507–8.
63. Ogura Y, Bonen DK, Inohara N *et al.* (2001) A frameshift mutation in NOD2 associated with susceptibility to Crohn' s disease. *Nature* **411**:603–6.
64. Duerr RH, Taylor KD, Brant SR *et al.* (2006) A genome-wide association study adentifies IL23R as an inflammatory bowel disease gene. *Science* **314**:1461–3.

65. Halme L, Paavola-Sakki P, Turunen U *et al.* (2006) Family and twin studies in inflammatory bowel disease. *World J Gastroenterol* **12**:3668–72.
66. Mayer L. (2010) Evolving paradigms in the pathogenesis of IBD. *J Gastroenterol* **45**:9–16.
67. Dubuquoy L, Rousseaux C, Thuru X *et al.* (2006) PPARγ as a new therapeutic target in inflammatory bowel diseases. *Gut* **55**:1341–9.
68. Dubuquoy L, Jansson EÅ, Deeb S *et al.* (2003) Impaired expression of Peroxisome Proliferator-Activated Receptor γ in ulcerative colitis. *Gastroenterol* **124**:1265–76.
69. Desreumaux P, Dubuquoy L, Nutten S *et al.* (2001) Attenuation of colon inflammation through activators oft he retinoid X receptor (RXR)/Peroxisome Proliferator-Activated Receptor gamma (PPARgamma) heterodimer. A basis for new therapeutic strategies. *J Exp Med* **193**:827–38.
70. Wu GD. (2003) Is there a role for PPAR γ in IBD? Yes, No, Maybe. Gastroenterol **124**:1538–42.
71. Adachi M, Kurotani R, Morimura K *et al.* (2006) Peroxisome proliferator activated receptor γ in colonic epithelial cells protects against experimental inflammatory bowel disease. *Gut* **55**:1104–13.
72. Sarraf P, Mueller E, Jones D *et al.* (1998) Differentiation and reversal of malignant changes in colon cancer through PPARγ. *Nat Med* **4**:1046–52.
73. Tanaka T, Kohno H, Yoshitani S *et al.* (2001) Ligands for Peroxisome Proliferator-activated Receptors α and γ inhibit chemically induced colitis and formation of aberrant crypt foci in rats. *Cancer Res* **61**:2424–8.
74. Kohno H, Yoshitani S, Takashima S *et al.* (2001) Troglitazone, a ligand for peroxisome proliferators-activated receptor γ, inhibits chemically-induced aberrant crypt foci in rats. *Jpn J Cancer Res* **92**:396–403.
75. Lefebvre A-M, Chen I, Desreumaux P *et al.* (1998)Activation of the peroxisome proliferator-activated receptor γ promotes the development of colon tumors in C57BL/6J-APC^{Min}/+ mice. *Nat Med* **4**:1053–7.
76. Saez E, Tontonoz P, Nelson MC *et al.* (1998) Activators of the nuclear receptor PPARγ enhance colon polyp formation. *Nat Med* **4**:1058–61.
77. Ramakers JD, Verstege MI, Thuijls G *et al.* (2007) The PPARγ agonist rosiglitazone impairs colonic inflammation in mice with experimental colitis. *J Clin Immunol* **27**:275–83.
78. Voutsadakis IA. (2008) The ubiquitin- proteasome system in colorectal cancer. *Biophys Biochim Acta* **1782**:800–8.

79. Itzkowitz SH, Yio X. (2004) Colorectal cancer in inflammatory bowel disease: the role of inflammation. *Am J Physiol Gastrointest Liver Phys* **287**:G7–17.
80. Umetani N, Sasaki S, Watanabe T *et al.* (1999) Genetic alterations in ulcerative colitis-associated neoplasia focusing on APC, K-ras gene and microsattelite instability. *Jpn J Cancer Res* **90**:1081–7.
81. Yashiro M, Carethers JM, Laghi L *et al.* (2001) Genetic pathways in the evolution of morphologically distinct colorectal neoplasm. *Cancer Res* **61**:2676–83.
82. Clapper ML, Cooper HS, Chang W-CL. (2007) Dextran sulfate sodium-induced colitis-associated neoplasia: a promising model for the development of chemopreventive interventions. *Acta Pharmacol Sin* **28**:1450–9.
83. Kohno H, Suzuki R, Sugie S, Tanaka T. (2005) Suppression of colitis-related mouse colon carcinogenesis by a COX-2 inhibitor and PPAR ligands. *BMC Cancer* **5**:46.
84. Rousseaux C, Lefebvre B, Dubuquoy L *et al.* (2005) Intestinal anti-inflammatory effect of 5-aminosalicylic acid is dependent on peroxisome proliferator-activated receptor-gamma. *J Exp Med* **201**:1205–15.
85. Butterworth JR. (2009) Chemoprevention of colorectal cancer in inflammatory bowel disease. *Dig Liver Dis* **41**:338–9.

Chapter 14

Proteinase-Activated Receptors

Hongying Wang*

*State Key Laboratory of Molecular Oncology,
Cancer Institute and Cancer Hospital,
Chinese Academy of Medical Sciences, Beijing, China*

Proteinase-activated receptors (PARs) are G-protein-coupled receptors that are activated by a unique proteolytic mechanism. PARs are widely expressed in the gastrointestinal tract, which is replete with proteinases that participate in digestion and host defense, as well as those produced by the bacterial flora of the gut. Mounting evidence indicates that PARs take active part in the pathophysiology of inflammatory diseases and cancer. As a signal transducer of extracellular proteinase activity, PARs regulate inflammation and promote tumorigenesis through a variety of mechanisms. It is emerging that PARs may be novel therapeutic targets for a variety of settings including inflammation and cancer. In this chapter, we discuss the general characteristics of the PAR family and the important roles of PARs in the processes of inflammation and tumor development.

Introduction

With the completion of human genome project, a total of 553 genes have been identified to encode proteinases.[1] Identification of proteinase-activated receptors (PARs) reveals a key role for proteinases, not only as protein-degrading enzymes, but also as potential activators that transmit extracellular stimuli into intracellular signaling events. Extensive studies demonstrate that PARs are widely expressed in the human body and

* E-mail: hongyingwang@cicams.ac.cn

play important physiological and pathophysiological roles in a wide range of biological systems, including the cardiovascular system, the gastrointestinal system, skin function, the respiratory system, and the peripheral nerves.[2] Of all the body systems, the gastrointestinal (GI) tract is the most exposed to proteinases from digestive secretions, bacterial flora, and cells involved with host defense. PARs, especially PAR_2, are expressed in every region of the GI tract including the stomach, intestine, pancreas and liver.[3] The exploration of the function of PARs reveals that proteinases and PARs have important roles in both inflammation and carcinogenesis.

The PAR family

Proteinase-activated receptors (PARs) are seven transmembrane domain G-protein coupled receptors (GPCRs) which are activated by the action of extracellular proteinases (Fig. 1(a)). After the identification of PAR_1 two decades ago, to date, four PAR family members have been identified, PAR_1 to PAR_4 (Table 1). All four members share similarities with respect to their chromosome location, protein structure, and also the activation mechanisms.

Regulation of PAR activity

Activation of PARs

As their name indicates, the activation of PARs is dependent upon the proteolytic activity of proteinases to initiate cell signaling. The intrinsic ligands of PARs preexist within their extracellular N-terminus, and are exposed by proteolytic cleavage. The newly created N-terminus serves as a tethered ligand for the receptors, binding to the extracellular domain of the receptor to trigger a conformational change in the receptor. This in turn leads to guanine nucleotide exchange on associated G proteins and initiates intracellular signaling (Fig. 1(b)). Besides proteinases, activating peptides (AP) can also activate PARs specifically (Table 1). Synthetic 6-amino-acid peptides with sequences matching those of the exposed tethered ligand can

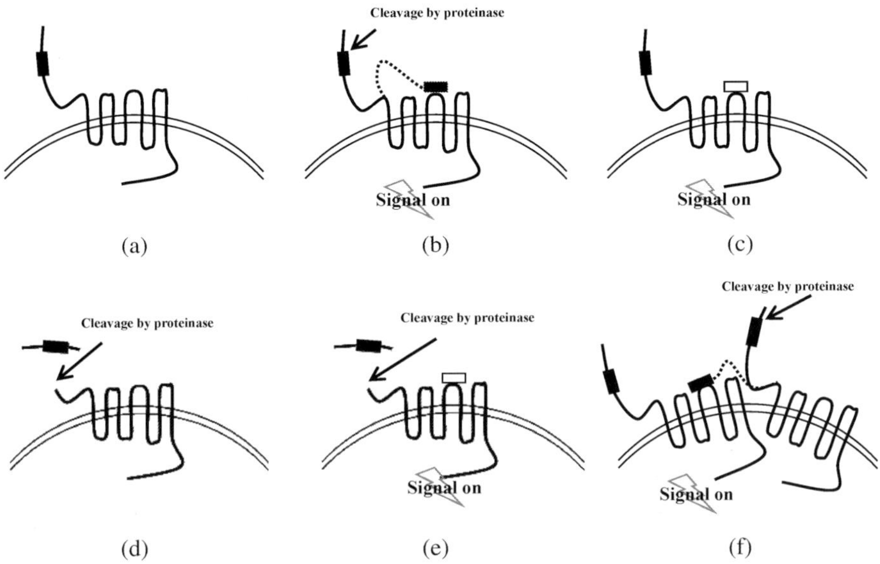

Figure 1. Mechanisms of activation of PARs (a) PAR is a G-protein coupled receptor with 7 transmembrane domains. The extracellular N terminus of the receptor contains the intrinsic ligand sequence (black rectangle). (b) Proteinase cleaves the N terminus upstream from the ligand sequence and exposes the tethered ligand, which in turn binds to the second extracellular loop of the receptor and to initiate intracellular signaling. (c) Synthetic activating peptide (white rectangle), mimics the PAR's tether ligand sequence by binding to the extracellular loop and triggering the signaling cascade. (d) Some proteinases cleave the receptor at sites downstream from the tethered ligand. This disarming disassociates the tethered ligand from the receptor to prevent signal transduction. (e) Disarmed receptor can still be activated by activating peptide, which binds to the receptor directly. (f) In some cases, intact PAR can be activated by a neighboring PAR with exposed tethered ligand. The figure is modified from reference 18.

bind to the second extracellular loop of the receptor and activate the receptor in the absence of proteolysis[9] (Fig. 1(c)). These peptides have been very useful in assessing PAR function experimentally.

Endogenous agonist for PARs

Without any evidence of endogenous peptide activators, the main roles of PARs appear to be in the detection and response to extracellular

Table 1. The current PAR family members.

	PAR_1	PAR_2	PAR_3	PAR_4
Chromosome	(h) 5q13 (m) 13d2	(h) 5q13 (m) 13d2	(h) 5q13 (m) 13d2	(h) 19p12 (m) 8b3
Cleavage site (h)	R^{41}-S	R^{34}-S	K^{38}-T	R^{47}-G
Tethered ligand sequence[4]	(h) SFLLRN (r,m) SFFLRN	(h) SLIGKV (r,m) SLIGRL	(h) TFRGAP (m) SFNGGP	(h) GYPGQV (m) GYPGKF (r) GFPGKP
Standard AP[5]	TFLLR-NH2	SLIGRL-NH2	Unknown	AYPGKF-NH2
Activating proteinases[6]	Thrombin Factor Xa Granzyme A Plasmin MMP-1	Trypsin Tryptase Factor Xa TF/factor VIIa Matriptase	Thrombin	Thrombin Trypsin Cathepsin G
Inactivating proteinases[6]	Cathepsin G Elastase Proteinase 3			
G protein coupling[7]	Gq/11, G_i, G12/13, G0	Gq, G_0, Gq/11	Unknown	Unknown
Gene deletion in mice[6]	Partial embryonic lethality; no hemostatic abnormalities in surviving knock out mice.	Mild impairment of leukocyte migration; no embryonic loss.	Loss of thrombin signaling in platelets at low thrombin concentration; no embryonic loss.	Prolonged bleeding time. Deficient response to thrombin.[8]

Abbreviations: AP, activating peptide; h, human; m, mouse; r, rat.

proteinases *in vivo*. To date, many serine proteinases have been found to activate PARs, including coagulation-derived factors (such as thrombin, FXa, FVIIa), immune cell derived factors (such as tryptase), tumor-derived factors (such as trypsin, MT-SP1/matriptase) (Table 1). The discovery of matrix metalloproteinase-1 (MMP-1) as an endogenous activator for PAR_1[10] strongly implies that there must be undiscovered proteinases which can activate PARs *in vivo*. Moreover, since the well-known cleavage sites in PAR_{1-4} (Table 1) are not favored by MMP-1, new cleavage sites or even novel activation mechanisms may remain to be discovered.

Inactivation of PARs by proteinase

Although proteinase can activate PARs using tethered-ligand mechanism, in some cases, proteinases can "disarm" or inactivate PARs by cleavage of a PAR N-terminal sequence downstream of the tethered ligand (Fig. 1(d)). For example, the elastase released by the neutrophil can cleave and remove the tethered ligand from PAR_2, thereby silencing the receptor on the epithelial cells.[11] Most interestingly, some proteinases such as Cathepsin G have two-faced role in the regulation of PAR activities: it activates PAR_4 by releasing the tethered ligand, while it inactivates PAR_1 by disarming (Table 1). However, receptors that have been inactivated by disarming still can be activated by AP (Fig. 1(e)).

Transactivation of PARs

Although intramolecular activation by cleavage is the predominant mechanism for PAR activation, it has been shown in some cases that intact PAR can be activated by cleaved PAR located in close proximity in the cell membrane (Fig. 1(f)). Examples include the transactivation of PAR_1 by PAR_1, transactivation of PAR_2 by cleaved PAR_1,[12] and activation of PAR_4 by PAR_3.[13] Although this transactivation event is not the main activation mechanism for PARs, it provides alternative mechanism to explain the limitations of the use of synthetic PAR peptide antagonists experimentally.[6] Taken together, PARs have a variety of circulating agonists and also circulating functional antagonists to stimulate or silence the receptors.

PAR-induced signaling

Once activated by their tethered ligands, the PARs (except for PAR_3) couple to distinct G proteins (Table 1) and induce the activation of various signaling pathways. PARs induce the mobilization of intracellular Ca^{2+}, activation of mitogen-activated protein kinases (MAPK), protein kinase C (PKC), PI3K/Akt, Rho, and Rac signaling.[14,15] Like most GPCRs, activated PARs are rapidly desensitized. However, unlike most GPCRs, which are internalized and then recycled, activated PARs are internalized, sorted directly to lysosomes, and rapidly degraded either dependently or independently of arrestins.[16] In the case of PAR_2, arrestin can mediate the activation of ERK1/2 signaling induced by PAR_2 activation.[17]

PARs in the gastrointestinal system

Considering the array of proteinases existing in GI tract, it is not surprising that all four PARs can be detected in GI tract, from the stomach to the colon.[18] Both PAR_1 and PAR_2 are present on endothelial cells, epithelial cells, smooth muscle cells, myofibroblast cells, and neurons. There is evidence that indicates the presence of PAR_3 and PAR_4 in stomach and intestine. However, the cellular source of PAR_3 and PAR_4 is still unknown. In addition, PARs are also widely expressed on immune cells. PAR_1 and PAR_2 have been detected on monocytes, macrophages, and mast cells. Although the function of PARs on immune cells is not clear, substantial evidence shows that PAR_2 plays an important role to regulate neutrophil function, including changing shape, presenting antigen, and increasing cell motility.[19] In addition, PARs widely expressed in GI tract play important roles in the regulation of inflammation and tumorigenesis through a variety of mechanisms.

PAR and inflammation

After two decades of study, it is emerging that PARs function as important inflammatory mediators. When localized on endothelial and blood cells, PAR_1 modulates platelet aggregation, increases adhesion molecule expression, and facilitates rolling and transmigration of neutrophils and other cells to sites of vessel damage.[15] Concomitant with these effects, PAR_1 also stimulates aggregation of neutrophils and chemotaxis of neutrophils and monocytes.[15] In addition to cardiovascular functions, PAR_2 mediates numerous GI functions, such as chloride secretion, prostaglandin release, smooth muscle contraction or relaxation.[3] Activation of either PAR_1 or PAR_2 stimulates the release of cytokines such as IL-8 and IL-6.[20–25] Since PAR_2 is identified on 50–60% of the enteric neurons, PAR_2 not only is related to inflammatory pain but also mediates neurogenic inflammation.[26] Taken together, PARs mediate inflammatory process through effects on epithelial, immune, neuronal and blood vessel cells.

Substantial evidence suggests that PARs play important roles in chronic inflammation, such as inflammatory bowel disease (IBD). Both PAR_1 and PAR_2 are upregulated in IBD patient samples compared with normal tissues.[27,28] Administration of PAR_1 or PAR_2-activating peptides can induce colitis in animal models directly.[27] Using PAR_2-deficient mice, research clearly demonstrates important roles of PAR_2 in intestinal inflammation.[29] Therefore, PARs are important proinflammatory mediators in the gut and may emerge as potential therapeutic targets for GI diseases, as discussed below.

PAR and carcinogenesis

PARs not only are actively involved in inflammatory process, but also mediate carcinogenesis. Tumors are replete with proteinases, such as urokinase-plasminogen activator (uPA)/plasmin, MMPs, tissue factors[16] and tissue-kallikreins.[30] The activation of the proteinase cascade generates abundance of proteinases, e.g. plasmin, FXa, FVIIa, thrombin, MMP1, which all can activate PARs directly. Abnormal expression of PAR_1 and PAR_2 is found in different cancers and cancer cell lines, including GI tract cancers.[31–33] Ectopic expression of PAR_1 sufficiently induces transformation via the Rho pathway.[34] Moreover, deregulation of matriptase, an activator of PAR_2, initiates oncogenic transformation *in vivo*.[35] Thus, PARs are not only highly correlated with malignant behavior of tumor cells, but are also involved in the initiation of carcinogenesis.

Both PAR_1 and PAR_2 interact with multiple key genes in oncogenesis. Wild-type p53 can bind to the PAR_1 promoter and downregulate PAR_1 expression at the transcriptional level. Moreover, mutated p53 directly correlated with PAR_1 overexpression.[36] This may explain the phenomena that the expression of PAR_1 is low in normal epithelial cells, while it is much higher in cancer cells. Different lines of evidence indicate that the activation of PARs upregulates the expression of cyclooxygenase-2,[37–41] which plays a key role in spontaneous and inflammation-associated GI carcinogenesis.[42] Moreover, PAR_2 inactivates GSK-3b and transcriptionally activates beta-catenin pathway,[41] which has critical roles in GI development and carcinogenesis.[43] Although PAR_1 cannot activate beta-catenin directly,[41] it stabilizes beta-catenin through the upregulation of

Wnt-4.[44] All of these observations provide intriguing molecular mechanisms by which PARs are involved in carcinogenesis.

PAR and cell proliferation

PARs can promote tumor progression through a variety of mechanisms, including cell proliferation, invasion, and metastasis. The importance of trypsin, a potent activator of PAR_2, has been shown recently in many cancers including GI tract tumors. Extra-pancreatic cellular expression of trypsin has been shown in gastric and colonic cancers.[45,46] Overexpression of trypsinogen dramatically increases the tumorigenicity of gastric cancer cells in nude mice.[45] Trypsin, acting on PAR_2, is a very potent growth factor for human colon cancer cells.[47] In addition, the transactivation of EGFR mediates PAR_2-induced MAPK activation and cell proliferation.[48]

PAR and invasion and metastasis

As the sensor for extracellular proteinase activity, PARs have been highly correlated with the invasion and metastasis of malignant cells. Thrombin, a potent agonist for PAR_1, PAR_3, and PAR_4, contributes to a more malignant behavior of cancer cells by enhancing the adhesion of tumor cells to platelets, endothelial cells and subendothelial matrix proteins, increasing metastasis.[49] Although the activation of PAR_1 cannot completely explain the role of thrombin, treatment of cell lines with PAR_1 activating peptide enhances metastasis by hundreds-fold.[49] Therefore, it is likely that activation of PAR_1 plays a critical role during metastasis.

The discovery of the MMP-PAR pathway provides a new way to interpret the role of PARs in the tumor metastasis process. Although it is well established that MMPs are associated with tumor invasion and metastasis, the mechanisms by which MMPs mediate tumor progression are still debatable. In 2005, Boire and colleagues showed that MMP-1 secreted by tumor stromal cells can cleave and activate PAR_1 on tumor cell surface and then trigger tumor cell invasion and metastasis.[10] Although the mechanism by which MMP-1 induces the activation of PAR_1 is still unknown,[50] the MMP-PAR pathway represents an intriguing new direction for both PAR and MMP fields.

PAR and inflammation-associated carcinogenesis

Functioning as both inflammatory and oncogenic factors, PARs have been shown to be correlated with inflammation-associated cancer. In primary tumors, the higher expression of PAR_2 is closely associated with chronic pancreatitis with severe fibrosis,[31] strongly suggesting the involvement of PAR_2 activation in chronic inflammation-induced pancreatic cancer and induction of fibrosis. As a key transcriptional factor for inflammation, NF-κB has been shown to link inflammation and tumorigenesis in colitis-associated colon cancer *in vivo*.[51] Different groups have shown that activation of PARs increases the transcriptional activity of NF-κB.[52–54] Most recently, our studies show that both PAR_1 and PAR_2 induce the epigenetic modification of NF-κB activity through p300 and histone deacetylase 2 (HDAC2) in colon epithelial cells.[25] However, more studies are required to elucidate the mechanisms by which PARs mediate in inflammation-associated cancer.

PAR-related therapy for gastrointestinal diseases

As evidence mounts to implicate PARs in both inflammation and carcinogenesis, the blockage of PAR-mediated signaling has been considered as a new strategy for human diseases, such as thrombosis, arthritis, and inflammatory bowel diseases. As a therapeutic approach, receptor inhibitors are more specific and have taken priority compared with the development of inhibitors of the activating proteinases. To date, the development of antagonists of PAR_1 activation has been partially successful. A number of peptide and peptidomimetic PAR_1 antagonists for both experimental studies and pharmaceutical use in humans are currently available, such as Trans-cinnamoyl-parafluoro-F-paraguanidino-FLLR-NH_2.[5] Moreover, selective and potent non-peptide PAR_1 antagonists have been successfully developed by different groups, e.g. RWJ compounds by the Johnson & Johnson team and the Schering group and SCH-205831 by Schering.[5] The development of potent and selective PAR_2 antagonist has been more challenging. Some peptides derived from PAR_2 activating peptides, FSLLRY-NH_2 and LSIGRL-NH_2, have been claimed to antagonize trypsin-induced PAR_2 activation.[55] However, these peptides fail to block activating peptide induced PAR_2 activation. Although ENMD-1068 can antagonize the activation of PAR_2 induced by both trypsin and peptide, its potency is too low to administrate systemically.[56]

Conclusion

PARs are unique and critical receptors that sense extracellular proteinase activity, transduce signaling, and modulate various cell functions. Of most importance is the function of PARs as both inflammatory mediators and oncogenic factors. PARs are activated by coagulation-derived and immune cell-derived proteinases in response to vascular injury, thrombosis, and host defense, and then initiate and modulate the inflammation process. In tumor settings, PARs have potential as excellent drug targets. Therefore, dissection of the molecular mechanisms of proteinases produced by tumor cells and immune cells promotes tumor progression through the activation of PARs on target cells. Although PARs are implicated in tumor development, the precise mechanisms by which PARs contribute to tumorigenesis are still not clear. The failure of proteinase inhibitor treatment in cancer is, at least in part, due to lack of specificity. The properties of PARs indicate how proteinases and PARs regulate carcinogenesis and inflammation; they will be crucial for identifying more specific treatment for these diseases.

Acknowledgments

I would like to thank Dr. Wallace K. MacNaughton of University of Calgary for valuable comments on the drafts.

References

1. Puente XS, Sanchez LM, Overall CM *et al.* (2003) Human and mouse proteases: A comparative genomic approach. *Nat Rev Genet* **4**:544–58.
2. Kanke T, Takizawa T, Kabeya M *et al.* (2005) Physiology and Pathophysiology of Proteinase-Activated Receptors (PARs): PAR-2 as a Potential Therapeutic Target. *Pharmacol Sci* **97**:38–42.

3. MacNaughton WK. (2005) Epithelial effects of proteinase-activated receptors in the gastrointestinal tract. *Mem Inst Oswaldo Cruz* **100** (Suppl 1):211–5.
4. Hansen KK, Oikonomopoulou K, Li Y *et al.* (2008) Proteinases, proteinase-activated receptors (PARs) and the pathophysiology of cancer and diseases of the cardiovascular, musculoskeletal, nervous and gastrointestinal systems. *Naunyn Schmiedebergs Arch Pharmacol* **377**:377–92.
5. Ramachandran R, Hollenberg MD. (2008) Proteinases and signalling: Pathophysiological and therapeutic implications via PARs and more. *Br J Pharmacol* **153**(Suppl 1):S263–82.
6. O'Brien PJ, Molino M, Kahn M *et al.* (2001) Protease activated receptors: Theme and variations. *Oncogene* **20**:1570–81.
7. Cocks TM, Moffatt JD. (2000) Protease-activated receptors: Sentries for inflammation? *Trends Pharmacol Sci* **21**:103–8.
8. Sambrano GR, Weiss EJ, Zheng YW *et al.* (2001) Role of thrombin signalling in platelets in haemostasis and thrombosis. *Nature* **413**:74–8.
9. Vu TK, Hung DT, Wheaton VI *et al.* (1991) Molecular cloning of a functional thrombin receptor reveals a novel proteolytic mechanism of receptor activation. *Cell* **64**:1057–68.
10. Boire A, Covic L, Agarwal A *et al.* (2005) PAR1 is a matrix metalloprotease-1 receptor that promotes invasion and tumorigenesis of breast cancer cells. *Cell* **120**:303–13.
11. Dulon S, Cande C, Bunnett NW *et al.* (2003) Proteinase-activated receptor-2 and human lung epithelial cells: Disarming by neutrophil serine proteinases. *Am J Respir Cell Mol Biol* **28**:339–46.
12. Chen J, Ishii M, Wang L *et al.* (1994) Thrombin receptor activation. Confirmation of the intramolecular tethered liganding hypothesis and discovery of an alternative intermolecular liganding mode. *J Biol Chem* **269**:16041–5.
13. Nakanishi-Matsui M, Zheng YW, Sulciner DJ *et al.* (2000) PAR3 is a cofactor for PAR4 activation by thrombin. *Nature* **404**:609–13.
14. Coughlin SR. (2000) Thrombin signalling and protease-activated receptors. *Nature* **407**:258–64.
15. Macfarlane SR, Seatter MJ, Kanke T *et al.* (2001) Proteinase-activated receptors. *Pharmacol Rev* **53**:245–282.
16. Arora P, Ricks TK, Trejo J. (2007) Protease-activated receptor signalling, endocytic sorting and dysregulation in cancer. *J Cell Sci* **120**:921–8.

17. DeFea KA, Zalevsky J, Thoma MS *et al.* (2000) beta-arrestin-dependent endocytosis of proteinase-activated receptor 2 is required for intracellular targeting of activated ERK1/2. *J Cell Biol* **148**:1267–81.
18. Hollenberg MD, Compton SJ. (2002) International Union of Pharmacology. XXVIII. Proteinase-activated receptors. *Pharmacol Rev* **54**:203–17.
19. Howells GL, Macey MG, Chinni C *et al.* (1997) Proteinase-activated receptor-2: Expression by human neutrophils. *J Cell Sci* **110**(Pt 7):881–7.
20. Asokananthan N, Graham PT, Fink J *et al.* (2002) Activation of protease-activated receptor (PAR)-1, PAR-2, and PAR-4 stimulates IL-6, IL-8, and prostaglandin E2 release from human respiratory epithelial cells. *J Immunol* **168**:3577–85.
21. Page K, Strunk VS, Hershenson MB. (2003) Cockroach proteases increase IL-8 expression in human bronchial epithelial cells via activation of protease-activated receptor (PAR)-2 and extracellular-signal-regulated kinase. *J Allergy Clin Immunol* **112**:1112–8.
22. Chi L, Li Y, Stehno-Bittel L *et al.* (2001) Interleukin-6 production by endothelial cells via stimulation of protease-activated receptors is amplified by endotoxin and tumor necrosis factor-alpha. *J Interferon Cytokine Res* **21**:231–40.
23. Shpacovitch VM, Brzoska T, Buddenkotte J *et al.* (2002) Agonists of proteinase-activated receptor 2 induce cytokine release and activation of nuclear transcription factor kappaB in human dermal microvascular endothelial cells. *J Invest Dermatol* **118**:380–5.
24. Chiu YC, Fong YC, Lai CH *et al.* (2008) Thrombin-induced IL-6 production in human synovial fibroblasts is mediated by PAR1, phospholipase C, protein kinase C alpha, c-Src, NF-kappa B and p300 pathway. *Mol Immunol* **45**:1587–99.
25. Wang H, Moreau F, Hirota CL *et al.* (2010) Proteinase-activated receptors induce interleukin-8 expression by intestinal epithelial cells through ERK/RSK90 activation and histone acetylation. *FASEB J* **24**:1971–80.
26. Vergnolle N, Wallace JL, Bunnett NW *et al.* (2001) Protease-activated receptors in inflammation, neuronal signaling and pain. *Trends Pharmacol Sci* **22**:146–152.

27. Vergnolle N, Cellars L, Mencarelli A *et al.* (2004) A role for proteinase-activated receptor-1 in inflammatory bowel diseases. *J Clin Invest* **114**: 1444–56.
28. Kim JA, Choi SC, Yun KJ *et al.* (2003) Expression of protease-activated receptor 2 in ulcerative colitis. *Inflamm Bowel Dis* **9**:224–9.
29. Cenac N, Coelho AM, Nguyen C *et al.* (2002) Induction of intestinal inflammation in mouse by activation of proteinase-activated receptor-2. *Am J Pathol* **161**:1903–15.
30. Borgono CA, Diamandis EP. (2004) The emerging roles of human tissue kallikreins in cancer. *Nat Rev Cancer* **4**:876–90.
31. Ikeda O, Egami H, Ishiko T *et al.* (2003) Expression of proteinase-activated receptor-2 in human pancreatic cancer: A possible relation to cancer invasion and induction of fibrosis. *Int J Oncol* **22**:295–300.
32. Bohm SK, Kong W, Bromme D *et al.* (1996) Molecular cloning, expression and potential functions of the human proteinase-activated receptor-2. *Biochem J* **314**(Pt 3):1009–16.
33. Ribeiro FS, Simao TA, Amoedo ND *et al.* (2009) Evidence for increased expression of tissue factor and protease-activated receptor-1 in human esophageal cancer. *Oncol Rep* **21**:1599–604.
34. Martin CB, Mahon GM, Klinger MB *et al.* (2001) The thrombin receptor, PAR-1, causes transformation by activation of Rho-mediated signaling pathways. *Oncogene* **20**:1953–63.
35. List K, Szabo R, Molinolo A *et al.* (2005) Deregulated matriptase causes ras-independent multistage carcinogenesis and promotes ras-mediated malignant transformation. *Genes Dev* **19**:1934–50.
36. Salah Z, Haupt S, Maoz M *et al.* (2008) p53 controls hPar1 function and expression. *Oncogene* 27:6866–74.
37. Seymour ML, Binion DG, Compton SJ *et al.* (2005) Expression of proteinase-activated receptor 2 on human primary gastrointestinal myofibroblasts and stimulation of prostaglandin synthesis. *Can J Physiol Pharmacol* **83**:605–16.
38. Yada K, Shibata K, Matsumoto T *et al.* (2005) Protease-activated receptor-2 regulates cell proliferation and enhances cyclooxygenase-2 mRNA expression in human pancreatic cancer cells. *J Surg Oncol* **89**:79–85.

39. Sekiguchi F, Saito S, Takaoka K *et al.* (2007) Mechanisms for prostaglandin E2 formation caused by proteinase-activated receptor-1 activation in rat gastric mucosal epithelial cells. *Biochem Pharmacol* **73**:103–14.
40. Seo JH, Kim KH, Kim H. (2007) Role of proteinase-activated receptor-2 on cyclooxygenase-2 expression in H. pylori-infected gastric epithelial cells. *Ann N Y Acad Sci* **1096**:29–36.
41. Wang H, Wen S, Bunnett NW *et al.* (2008) Proteinase-activated Receptor-2 Induces Cyclooxygenase-2 Expression through beta-Catenin and Cyclic AMP-response Element-binding Protein. *J Biol Chem* **283**:809–15.
42. Gupta RA, DuBois RN. (2001) Colorectal cancer prevention and treatment by inhibition of cyclooxygenase-2. *Nat Rev Cancer* **1**:11–21.
43. Su LK, Vogelstein B, Kinzler KW. (1993) Association of the APC tumor suppressor protein with catenins. *Science* **262**:1734–7.
44. Yin YJ, Katz V, Salah Z *et al.* (2006) Mammary gland tissue targeted overexpression of human protease-activated receptor 1 reveals a novel link to beta-catenin stabilization. *Cancer Res* **66**:5224–33.
45. Miyata S, Miyagi Y, Koshikawa N *et al.* (1998) Stimulation of cellular growth and adhesion to fibronectin and vitronectin in culture and tumorigenicity in nude mice by overexpression of trypsinogen in human gastric cancer cells. *Clin Exp Metastasis* **16**:613–22.
46. Williams SJ, Gotley DC, Antalis TM. (2001) Human trypsinogen in colorectal cancer. *Int J Cancer* **93**:67–73.
47. Darmoul D, Marie JC, Devaud H *et al.* (2001) Initiation of human colon cancer cell proliferation by trypsin acting at protease-activated receptor-2. *Br J Cancer* **85**:772–9.
48. Darmoul D, Gratio V, Devaud H *et al.* (2004) Protease-activated receptor 2 in colon cancer: Trypsin-induced MAPK phosphorylation and cell proliferation are mediated by epidermal growth factor receptor transactivation. *J Biol Chem* **279**:20927–34.
49. Nierodzik ML and Karpatkin S. (2006) Thrombin induces tumor growth, metastasis, and angiogenesis: Evidence for a thrombin-regulated dormant tumor phenotype. *Cancer Cell* **10**:355–62.
50. Pei D. (2005) Matrix metalloproteinases target protease-activated receptors on the tumor cell surface. *Cancer Cell* **7**:207–8.

51. Greten FR, Eckmann L, Greten TF *et al.* (2004) IKKbeta links inflammation and tumorigenesis in a mouse model of colitis-associated cancer. *Cell* **118**: 285–96.
52. Rahman A, Anwar KN, True AL *et al.* (1999) Thrombin-induced p65 homodimer binding to downstream NF-kappa B site of the promoter mediates endothelial ICAM-1 expression and neutrophil adhesion. *J Immunol* **162**: 5466–76.
53. Ryu J, Pyo H, Jou I *et al.* (2000) Thrombin induces NO release from cultured rat microglia via protein kinase C, mitogen-activated protein kinase, and NF-kappa B. *J Biol Chem* **275**:29955–9.
54. Page K, Hughes VS, Odoms KK *et al.* (2005) German cockroach proteases regulate interleukin-8 expression via nuclear factor for interleukin-6 in human bronchial epithelial cells. *Am J Respir Cell Mol Biol* **32**:225–31.
55. Al-Ani B, Saifeddine M, Wijesuriya SJ *et al.* (2002) Modified proteinase-activated receptor-1 and -2 derived peptides inhibit proteinase-activated receptor-2 activation by trypsin. *J Pharmacol Exp Ther* **300**:702–8.
56. Kelso EB, Lockhart JC, Hembrough T *et al.* (2006) Therapeutic promise of proteinase-activated receptor-2 antagonism in joint inflammation. *J Pharmacol Exp Ther* **316**:1017–24.

Section IV

Molecular Markers of Cancers and Their Clinical Implications

Chapter 15

Use of Tumor Markers in the Detection and Management of Patients with Colorectal Cancer

Michael J. Duffy*

Department of Pathology and Laboratory Medicine,
St Vincent's University Hospital, Dublin 4,
UCD School of Medicine and Medical Science,
Conway Institute of Biomolecular and Biomedical Research,
University College Dublin, Dublin 4, Ireland

Tumor markers are currently playing an important role in colorectal cancer (CRC) detection and management. Fecal occult blood testing with either a guaiac or preferably an immunochemical test may be used to screen for early CRC. Following curative surgery for CRC, regular measurements of serum CEA is recommended, especially for patients that may be candidates for liver resection or systemic therapy, should recurrences develop. For patients with advanced CRC under consideration for treatment with the anti-EGFR antibodies, panitumumab or cetuximab, the mutational status of k-ras should be determined. K-ras-positive patients should not receive these treatments. Finally, regular measurement of CEA is recommended in patients with advanced CRC undergoing treatment for CRC.

Introduction

Colorectal cancer (CRC) is the third most common cancer, worldwide with an estimated one million new cases and half a million deaths each

* E-mail: Michael.J.Duffy@ucd.ie

year.[1] In the Western world, CRC is the second most common cancer in women, after breast cancer and the third most common cancer in men, after lung and prostate cancers.[2,3] Its incidence is increasing in parts of the world, especially in some economically transitioning countries in Eastern Europe, Asia and South America.[4] This increased incidence in some of these countries may be due to the adoption of Western lifestyles and behaviors such as the consumption of a Western diet and decreased physical activity.[4] In contrast, the incidence has stabilized or decreased in certain Western countries.[4]

In recent years, tumor markers have begun to play an increasingly important role in the detection and management of patients with CRC. Thus, fecal occult blood testing (FOBT) may be used in screening for early CRC. Following a diagnosis of CRC, CEA may be combined with histological parameters in assessing prognosis. Similarly, CEA may be used in postoperative surveillance following curative surgery and monitoring therapy in patients with advanced disease. A new therapy predictive marker for CRC is the use of k-ras mutation testing for identifying patients with advanced malignancy likely to benefit from the therapeutic monoclonal antibodies, cetuximab or panitumumab. The aim of this Chapter is to discuss the utility of these and other markers in patients with CRC.

Use of markers in screening for CRC

The aim of screening is to reduce mortality through a reduction in the incidence of advanced disease.[5] Screening for CRC can achieve this by the detection of early stage CRC and the detection and removal of adenomatous polyps that increase the risk of invasive disease. Although several screening tests are available for CRC,[5–9] this Chapter will focus on markers that are measured in stools. Stools tests for screening for CRC involve either fecal occult blood testing (FOBT)) or the measurement of a panel of DNA markers. Both these tests are briefly discussed below.

Fecal occult blood tests in screening for CRC

Two main types of fecal occult blood tests (FOBT) are available, i.e., the guaiac test (GT) and the fecal immunochemical test (FIT).[5,8,9] The guaiac test measures the pseudoperoxidase activity of haem in haemoglobin while the immunochemical test detects human globin protein levels. Although the GT has been more widely used in screening than the FIT, it is now generally agreed that the immunochemical method is the superior test. The advantages of the immunochemical test over the GT include the following (for review, see refs. [5, 8–12]).

- FITs generally have better sensitivity and specificity for CRC.
- FITs are not affected by certain dietary components or medications that may interfere in the GT.
- Some FITs can be automated, thus increasing throughput.
- Evidence suggests that the use of FITs increases patient participation in screening for CRC and
- FITs can be quantitated, enabling adjustment of sensitivity, specificity and positivity rates.

A disadvantage of FITs compared to GTs is their increased costs. Furthermore, FITs have not yet been shown to reduce mortality for CRC in large prospective randomized control trials, although based on available evidence, this is highly likely.

In order to address the effectiveness of FOBT in reducing mortality for CRC, Hewitson *et al.*[13] carried out a systematic review of the literature published over the period 1989 to February 2006. The authors identified 9 articles describing 4 randomized controlled trials. In excess of 320,000 subjects participated in the trials and follow-up ranged from 8 to 18 years. The primary analysis used intention to screen as end point. A secondary analysis adjusted for non-attendance. All trials used a GT in screening for CRC.

Although the individual trials varied with respect to population selection, age of subjects studied, screening interval, specific FOBT used, length of follow-up and attendance for screening, the relative reduction in mortality in the screened group was consistent across the trials. Combined analysis showed that screening reduced the relative risk (RR) of death from CRC by 16% (RR, 0.84; 95% CI, 0.78–0.90). When adjusted for attendance at screening, the relative risk reduction was 25% (RR, 0.75; 95% CI, 0.66–0.84) for those attending at least one round of screening.

No difference in all cause mortality however, was found between the screened and the non-screened subjects.[13] As might be expected, all trials investigated found a greater proportion of early stage (stage I/Dukes'A and stage II/Dukes' B) cancers and fewer late stage (stages III/Dukes' C and IV/Dukes' D) in the screened than in the control population.

Although GT have been more frequently used in the past and extensively validated for reducing mortality from CRC, new centers embarking on screening for this malignancy should use an appropriate FIT. This is because of the numerous advantages of FIT over GTs, see above.

DNA Markers

In attempt to enhance the accuracy of FOBT in screening for CRC, a considerable amount of research in recent years has focused on other fecal markers. One of the most promising non-occult blood tests to emerge involves measurement of specific DNA profiles. These tests detect mutant forms of c-oncogenes and tumor suppressor genes that are involved in the pathogenesis of CRC and are subsequently shed into the lumen and excreted in stools. Amongst the most widely investigated DNA markers, are mutant k-ras, mutant p53, mutant APC, specific methylated genes, microsatellite instability (MSI) genes and long DNA.[14–16]

Recently, a specific DNA panel was investigated as a screening test for CRC in a large asymptomatic population, involving in excess of 4000 subjects.[17] Of the 31 invasive CRCs detected, the DNA panel diagnosed 16, whereas FOBT detected only 4 (51.6% vs 12.9%, $p = 0.003$). Of the 71 invasive cancers and adenomas with high-grade dysplasia, the DNA panel diagnosed 29, while FOBT detected only ten ($p < 0.001$). Clearly, in this study, the DNA panel displayed a higher sensitivity than the specific FOBT investigated. However, in another large population-based study, Ahlquist *et al.*[18] found that a stools-based DNA test provided no significant improvement over FOBT in the detection of screen-relevant neoplasms (i.e., curable stage cancer, high grade dysplasia or adenomas >1 cm).

Arguments against the use of DNA-based tests in screening for CRC include their relatively high costs, the technically demanding nature of their measurement and lack of validation in a prospective randomized trial. Stools DNA tests are continually evolving and at present, it is not clear which combination of DNA markers provides the optimum balance of sensitivity and specificity. Despite these drawbacks, joint guidelines published by the American Cancer Society, the US Multi-Society Task Force and the American College of Radiology concluded that there is now sufficient data to include fecal DNA markers "as an acceptable option for CRC screening".[5]

Use of markers in determining prognosis in patients with colorectal cancer

Cancer stage at initial diagnosis is universally used for evaluation of prognosis in patients with CRC. In predicting outcome, tumor stage is most useful at its extremes, i.e., for patients with stage I and stage IV disease. Thus, 5-year survival rates for patients with stage 1 disease is >90% but <10% for those with stage IV malignancy.[3] For patients with intermediate stages, stage II and III, additional prognostic factors are urgently required. New prognostic factors/markers are particularly required in order to identify patients with aggressive stage II disease that might benefit from adjuvant chemotherapy. Consequently, in recent years, several serum and tissue-based markers have been investigated for potential independent prognostic impact in patients with newly diagnosed CRC, especially in those with stage II disease.

The most widely investigated serum marker for assessing prognosis is CEA.[19,20] Studies carried out in the 1980s and 1990s concluded that patients with high preoperative levels of this marker (e.g., >5 μg/L) had a worse outcome that those with low levels.[20] Indeed, in some of these studies, CEA was reported to supply prognostic information in patients with stage II disease.[20] Thus, for newly diagnosed patients with CRC, a number of expert panels state that preoperative CEA levels might be used in combination with other factors in assessing prognosis and planning surgical treatment.[11,21–27] According to the American Society of Clinical Oncology (ASCO) [21–23] and the European Group on Tumor Markers (EGTM)[25,26] however, preoperative CEA concentrations should not be used at present in selecting CRC patients for adjuvant therapy. The European Society for Medical Oncology (ESMO), on the other hand, state that adjuvant chemotherapy may be considered in selected node-negative (stage II) patients, especially if high risk factors for recurrence are present.[27] Amongst the high risk factors mentioned were elevated preoperative levels of CEA.[27]

Many of the studies reporting a prognostic value for CEA were carried out prior to the widespread use of adjuvant chemotherapy (i.e., for patients with stage III disease). A recent study suggested that the prognostic impact of CEA in stage III patients may have been diminished due to the improvement in outcome in these patients as a result of treatment with adjuvant chemotherapy.[28] Further studies are required to confirm this observation.

As well as CEA, other serum markers such as CA 19–9, CA 242, and cytokeratins have been investigated for potential prognostic value in patients with CRC.[25,26] Although elevated preoperative levels of these markers also predict adverse outcome, their routine measurement is not currently recommended.[26] Similarly, no tissue-based prognostic marker is currently recommended for clinical use.[26]

Use of therapy predictive markers in patients with colorectal cancer

The traditional systemic therapy for patients with CRC was 5-fluorouracil (5-FU) and folinic acid in combination. In the mid 1990s, 3 new cytotoxic agents were introduced, capecitabine (an oral fluoropyrimidine), oxaliplatin and irinotecan. The use of these drugs in combination has increased median survival for patients with advanced CRC from approximately 10–12 months with 5-FU to >20 months.[29,30,31] More recently, 3 monoclonal antibodies have been approved for the treatment of advanced CRC, i.e., bevacizumab, cetuximab and panitumumab.[29,30,31] As all of these treatments may cause considerable toxicity and only a proportion of patients (usually a minority) benefit from their administration, predictive markers are required in order to make rationale therapy decisions.

The best validated therapy predictive marker in CRC is *k-ras* for predicting response to the monoclonal antibodies, cetuximab and panitumumab.[32] Cetuximab is a chimeric human-mouse monoclonal antibody that acts by binding to EGFR, thus blocking downstream signaling.

Panitumumab is a fully human monoclonal antibody that also acts by binding to the EGFR. Since these 2 monoclonal antibodies target EGFR, it was expected that its levels in CRC tumor tissue would predict response to therapy. However, studies to date have failed to find a significant association between levels of EGFR as determined by immunohistochemistry and benefit from the antibodies. Indeed, cetuximab appeared to induce tumor regression in patients with apparent EGFR-negative tumors.[33]

While levels of EGFR protein as determined by immunohistochemistry do not appear to predict response to cetuximab or panitumumab, retrospective studies from several randomized trials have shown that CRC patients harboring specific mutations in the k-ras gene rarely benefit from treatment with these antibodies. Following a review of the literature, Peeters *et al.*[34] identified 7 retrospective studies in which the mutational status of k-ras was related to response to anti-EGFR therapy. *K-ras* mutations were found in 35–45% of the patients investigated. Of the patients with tumors containing mutant k-*ras*, objective response was found in only 2. In contrast objective response was observed in 9–28% of patients with wild-type k-ras.

Because of the consistency of these findings, an ASCO Provisional Clinical Opinion published in 2009 stated that "all patients with metastatic colorectal carcinoma who are candidates for anti-EGFR antibody therapy should have their tumor tested for *k-ras* mutations. If a *k-ras* mutation in codon 12 or 13 is detected, then patients with metastatic colorectal carcinoma should not receive anti-EGFR antibody therapy as part of their treatment".[35] The European Medicines Agency has also restricted the administration of cetuximab and panitumumab to CRC patients expressing the wild-type *k-ras* gene. As well as k-ras, the mutational status of other genes such as *BRAF* and *PI3KCA* may also be of value in predicting sensitivity/resistance to anti-EGFR antibodies.[36,37]

A number of studies have also been carried out in an attempt to identify predictive markers for the cytotoxic drugs used to treat CRC.[38] These include dihydropyrimidine dehydrogenease, thymidine phosphorylase, thymidylate synthase and microsatellite instability (MSI) status for predicting benefit from fluoropyrimidines; topoisomerase for predicting benefit from irinotecan and excision cross complementing gene expression for predicting benefit from oxaliplatin.[38] Of these, the marker subjected to most detailed investigation is the use of microsatellite instability for predicting the efficacy of adjuvant chemotherapy, especially 5-FU based therapy. Following a meta-analysis of published studies, Guetz *et al*[39] concluded that there was less benefit from adjuvant chemotherapy for MSI-high patients compared to those with microsatellite-stable disease. For patients with advanced disease however, MSI status did not predict the efficacy of chemotherapy.[40] Measurement of microsatellite instability status is not currently recommended for routinely predicting response to chemotherapy in patients with CRC.

Use of markers in surveillance following curative resection of colorectal cancer

Routine surveillance is now common practice following curative resection for CRC. The aim of this surveillance is to detect locoregional recurrences, distant metastasis and metachronus cancers as early as possible, thus offering "salvage" surgery and chemotherapy as soon as possible.[42] Early detection is particularly important for liver metastasis. The most widely used tumor marker in postoperative surveillance following curative surgery for CRC is CEA.[20]

In order to determine the diagnostic accuracy of CEA in detecting recurrent disease following curative surgery for CRC, Tan *et al.*[41] carried out a review of the literature on this topic. Twenty eligible studies containing 4,285 patients were identified and used for analysis. CEA was regarded as being positive for recurrence at cut-off values ranging from 3–15 μg/L. The overall sensitivity and specificity of CEA for detecting recurrence was 64% (95% CI, 0.61–0.67) and 90% (95% CI, 0.89–0.91), respectively. Using meta-regression analysis, the optimum cut-off point for CEA that gave the optimum combination of sensitivity and specificity was 2.2 μg/L.[41] It should be added that this cut-off value is lower that that used in clinical practice which is 3.5–5 μg/L.

CEA is rarely used alone in the surveillance of patients undergoing curative surgery for CRC. Rather, it is usually combined with other diagnostic modalities such as imaging and colonoscopy. This combined use of multiple diagnostic procedures is sometimes referred to as intensive follow-up.

Several randomized controlled trials have compared intensive vs less intensive/minimal follow-up strategies following curative surgery for CRC. Tjandra *et al.*[42] carried out a systematic review of the literature on these trials in an attempt to identify the optimal follow-up strategy. Overall 8 eligible trials involving 2,923 patients were evaluated. Following analysis of the combined data, the key conclusions were as follows:[42]

- Patients with intensive follow-up had a significant reduction in overall mortality compared to those with minimal follow-up
- Intensive follow-up detected asymptomatic recurrences more frequently than less intensive follow-up regimes (18.9% vs 6.3%, $p < 0.00001$)
- Intensive follow-up detected asymptomatic recurrences earlier than less intensive follow-up regimes (5.9 months, $p < 0.00001$)
- Regular surveillance with serial CEA levels ($p = 0.0002$) and colonoscopy ($p = 0.04$) reduced overall mortality
- Cancer-related mortality did not differ significantly between those followed-up with intensive vs less intensive approaches.

As mentioned above, intensive follow-up involves multiple diagnostic modalities that may include CT scanning, chest X-ray, colonoscopy, physical examination as well as CEA. The question therefore arises as to whether the regular measurements of CEA are necessary for the improved outcome. Two independent meta-analyses have addressed this issue. In both,[43,44] it was shown that intensive follow-up improved outcome, only when serial CEA measurements were performed.

The importance of CEA in follow-up was also shown in a recent large randomized prospective trial comparing laparoscopic-assisted colectomy with open colectomy for curable colon cancer patients. In this study, serial CEA measurements outperformed other modalities for patients with both early stage disease (stage I and IIa) and late stage (stage IIb and III). For the 537 patients with early stage disease, CEA detected 29.1% of the first recurrences compared with 23.6% for CT scan, 12.7% for colonoscopy and 7.3% for chest X-ray. For the 254 patients with late stage disease, CEA detected 37.4% of the first recurrences, CT scan 26.4%, chest x-ray 12.1% and colonoscopy 8.8%.[45]

Clearly, therefore regular measurement of CEA is necessary for optimum surveillance following curative resection for CRC. Several expert panels including ASCO,[21–23] NCCN,[29] EGTM[24–26] and NACB[11] thus now recommend that CEA should be measured approximately every 3 months in patients with Stage II or III CRC for at least 3 years following diagnosis, if the patient is a candidate for surgery or systemic therapy for metastatic disease.

Although serial measurements of CEA are widely recommended as part of a surveillance regime, agreement is lacking as to the extent of concentration change that constitutes a clinically significant increase in marker levels. According to the EGTM Panel,[25] a significant increase in CEA occurs if the elevation is at least 30% over that of the previous level. Prior to any intervention, this increase must be confirmed by a second sample taken within approximately one month. If the second sample is also increased, the patient should undergo further investigations.[25] This definition of CEA increase however, has not been clinically validated. Furthermore, it should not be regarded as exclusive. For example, small increases in CEA (e.g., 15–20%, maintained over at least three successive assays) may also prompt intervention.[25]

Increasing CEA levels following curative surgery for CRC does not however, also denote recurrent/metastatic disease. Benign lesions that may be associated with CEA increase include lung nodules, liver lesions, ovarian masses and mediastinal lymphadenopathy[4] It should also be remembered that low concentrations of CEA concentrations do not necessarily exclude progression, and in patients with clinical symptoms of disease recurrence, additional tests such as CT-scan, X-rays, and colonoscopy are required, irrespective of the CEA concentration.[25]

Use of markers in monitoring therapy in patients with advanced colorectal cancer

The rationale for the use of serum markers in monitoring therapy in patients with advanced malignancy is based on the assumption that increasing levels indicate tumor progression while decreasing levels reflect tumor regression. Factors other that tumor response may however, effect marker levels, see below. For monitoring therapy in patients with advanced CRC, the only recommended marker is CEA. According to ASCO guidelines,[21–23] "CEA should be measured at the start of treatment for metastatic disease and every 1–3 months during active treatment. Persistently rising values above baseline should prompt restaging but suggest progressive disease even in the absence of corroborating radiographs. Caution should be used when interpreting a rising CEA level during the first 4–6 weeks of a new therapy, since spurious early rises may occur especially after oxaliplatin". Similar recommendations have been published by EGTM[24–26] and NACB.[11]

Conclusion

It is clear from above that tumor markers are playing an increasingly important role in the detection and management of patients with CRC. Although multiple screening tests are available for this malignancy, the use of FOBT is a validated and accepted population screening test. Following curative resection, especially in patients with stages II and III disease, surveillance using CEA is now recommended by multiple expert panels. For patients with advanced disease undergoing systemic therapy, measurement of CEA is a minimally invasive and inexpensive method for assessing disease response or progression. Finally, in patients with advanced disease being considered for treatment with cetuximab or panitumumab, the mutational status of k-ras should be determined. Clearly, the use of tumor markers is paving the way towards personalized treatment in patients with CRC.

References

1. Parkin DM, Bray F, Ferlay J *et al.* (2005) Global cancer statistics, 2002. *CA Cancer J Clin* **55**:74–108.
2. Jemal A, Siegel R, Ward E *et al.* (2007) Cancer statistics, 2007. *CA Cancer J Clin* **57**:43–66.
3. Ballinger AB, Anggianah C. (2007) Colorectal cancer. *Br Med J* **235**:715–8.
4. Center MM, Jemal A, Ward E. (2009) International trends in colorectal cancer incidence rates. *Cancer Epidemiol Biomarkers Prev* **18**:1688–94.
5. Levin B, Lieberman DA, McFarland B *et al.* (2008) Screening and surveillance for the early detection of colorectal cancer and adenomatous polyps, a joint guideline from the American Cancer Society, the US Multi-Society

Task Force on Colorectal Cancer, and the American College of Radiology. *CA Cancer J Clin* **58**:130–60.

6. Huang CS, Lal SK, Farraye FA. (2005) Colorectal cancer screening in average risk individuals. *Cancer Causes Control* **16**:171–88.
7. Kahi CJ, Rex DK, Imperiale TF. (2008) Screening, surveillance, and primary prevention for colorectal cancer: A review of the recent literature. *Gastroenterol* **135**:380–99.
8. Mandel JS. (2007) Which colorectal cancer screening test is best? *J Natl Cancer Inst* **99**:1424–5
9. Allison JE, Lawson M. (2006) Screening tests for colorectal cancer: A menu of options remains relevant. *Curr Oncol Rep* **8**:492–8.
10. Allison JE, Tekawa IS, Ransom LJ *et al.* (1996) A comparison of fecal occult-blood tests for colorectal-cancer screening. *N Engl J Med* **334**:155–9.
11. Sturgeon CM, Duffy MJ, Stenman UH *et al.* (2008) National academy of clinical biochemistry laboratory medicine practice guidelines for use of tumor markers in testicular, prostate, colorectal, breast, and ovarian cancers. *Clin Chem* **54**:e11–e79.
12. Imperiale TF, Jemal A, Siegel R *et al.* (2007) Quantitative immunochemical fecal occult blood tests: Is it time to go back to the future? *Ann Intern Med* **146**:309–11.
13. Hewitson P, Glasziou P, Watson E *et al.* (2008) Cochrane systematic review of colorectal cancer screening using the fecal occult blood test (hemoccult): an update. *Am J Gastroenterol* **103**:1541–9.
14. Davies RJ, Miller R, Coleman N. (2005) Colorectal cancer screening: Prospects for molecular stool analysis. *Nat Rev Cancer* **5**:199–209.
15. Brenner DE, Rennert G. (2005) Fecal DNA biomarkers for the detection of colorectal neoplasia: Attractive, but is it feasible? *J Natl Cancer Inst* **97**:1107–9.
16. Haug U, Brenner H. (2005) New stool test for colorectal cancer screening: A systematic review focusing on performance characteristics and practicalness. *Int J Cancer* **117**:169–76.
17. Imperiale T, Ransohoff D, Itzkowitz SH *et al.* (2004) Fecal DNA versus fecal occult blood for colorectal-cancer screening in an average risk population. *N Engl J Med* **351**:2704–14.
18. Ahlquist DA, Sargent DJ, Loprinzi CL *et al.* (2008) Stool DNA and occult blood testing for screen detection of colorectal neoplasia. *Ann Int Med* **149**:441–50.

19. Fletcher RH. (1986) Carcinoembryonic antigen. *Ann Intern Med* **104**:66–73.
20. Duffy MJ. (2001) Carcinoembryonic antigen as a marker for colorectal cancer: Is it clinically useful? *Clin Chem* **47**:624–30.
21. Clinical practice guidelines for the use of tumor markers in breast and colorectal cancer. Adopted on May 17, 1996 by the American Society of Clinical Oncology. *J Clin Oncol* **14**:2843–77.
22. Bast RC Jr, Ravdin P, Hayes DF *et al.* (2001) 2000 update of recommendations for the use of tumor markers in breast and colorectal cancer: Clinical practice guidelines of the American Society of Clinical Oncology. *J Clin Oncol* **19**:1865–78.
23. Locker GY, Hamilton S, Harris J *et al.* (2006) ASCO 2006 update of recommendations for the use of tumor markers in gastrointestinal cancer. *J Clin Oncol* **24**:5313–27.
24. Klapdor R, Aronsson AC, Duffy MJ *et al.* (1999) Tumor markers in gastro-intestinal cancers: EGTM recommendations. *Anticancer Res* **119**:2811–5.
25. Duffy MJ, van Dalen A, Haglund C *et al.* (2003) Clinical utility of biochemical markers in colorectal cancer: European Group on Tumour Markers (EGTM) guidelines. *Eur J Cancer* **39**:718–27.
26. Duffy MJ, van Dalen A, Haglund C *et al.* (2007) Tumor Markers in Colorectal Cancer: European Group on Tumor Markers (EGTM) Guidelines for Clinical Use. *Eur J Cancer* **43**:1348–60.
27. Van Cutsem E, Oliveira J. (2009) Primary colon cancer: ESMO clinical recommendations for diagnosis, adjuvant treatment and follow-up. *Ann Oncol* **20** (Suppl 4): iv49–50.
28. Katoh H, Yamashita K, Kokuba Y *et al.* (2008) Diminishing impact of preoperative carcinoembryonic antigen (CEA) in prognosis of Dukes' C colorectal cancer. *Anticancer Res* **28**:1933–41.
29. National Comprehensive Cancer Network Clinical Practice Guidelines in Oncology, Colorectal Cancer Screening. Version 2.2009. Available at http://www.nccn.org/physician_gls?PDF/colorectal_screening.pdf Accessed, July 30, 2009.
30. Segal NH, Saltz LB. (2009) Evolving treatment of advanced colon cancer. *Ann Rev Med* **60**:207–19.
31. De Dosso S, Sessa C, Saletti P. (2009) Adjuvant therapy for colon cancer: Present and perspectives. *Cancer Treat Rev* **35**:160–6.

32. Jimeno A, Messersmith WA, Hirsch FR *et al.* (2009) KRAS mutations and susceptibility to cetuximab and panitumumab in colorectal cancer. *Cancer J* **15**:110–3.
33. Chung KY, Shia J, Kemeny NE *et al.* (2005) Cetuximab shows activity in colorectal cancer patients with tumors that do not express the epidermal growth factor receptor by immunohistochemistry. *J Clin Oncol* **23**:1803–10.
34. Peeters M, Price T, Van Laethem JL. (2009) Anti-epidermal growth factor receptor monotherapy in the treatment of metastatic colorectal cancer: Where are we today? *Oncologist* **14**:29–39.
35. Allegra CJ, Jessup JM, Somerfield MR *et al.* (2009) American Society of Clinical Oncology provisional clinical opinion: Testing for KRAS gene mutations in patients with metastatic colorectal carcinoma to predict response to anti-epidermal growth factor receptor monoclonal antibody therapy. *J Clin Oncol* **27**:2091–6.
36. Di Nicolantonio F, Martini M, Molinari F *et al.* (2008) Wild-type BRAF is required for response to panitumumab or cetuximab in metastatic colorectal cancer. *J Clin Oncol* **26**:5705–12.
37. Sartore-Bianchi A, Martini M, Molinari F *et al.* (2009) PIK3CA mutations in colorectal cancer are associated with clinical resistance to EGFR-targeted monoclonal antibodies. *Cancer Res* **69**:1851–7.
38. Koppman M, Venderbosch S, Nagtegaal ID *et al.* (2009) A review on the use of molecular markers of cytotoxic therapy for colorectal cancer, what have we learned? *Eur J Cancer* **45**:1935–49.
39. Des Guetz G, Schischmanoff O, Nicolas P *et al.* (2009) Does microsatellite instability predict the efficacy of adjuvant chemotherapy in colorectal cancer? A systematic review with meta-analysis. *Eur J Cancer* **45**:1890–6.
40. Des Guetz G, Uzzan B, Nicolas P *et al.* (2009) Microsatellite Instability does not predict the efficacy of chemotherapy in metastatic colorectal cancer. a systematic review and meta-analysis. *Anticancer Res* **29**:1515–20.
41. Tan E, Gouvas N, Nicholls RJ *et al.* (2009) Diagnostic precision of carcinoembryonic antigen in the detection of recurrence of colorectal cancer. *Surgical Oncol* **18**:15–24.
42. Tjandra JJ, Chan MK. (2007) Follow-up after curative resection of colorectal cancer: A meta-analysis. *Dis Colon Rectum* **50**:1783–99.
43. Bruinvels DJ, Stiggelbout AM, Kievit J *et al.* (1994) Follow-up of patients with colorectal cancer. A meta-analysis. *Ann Surg* **219**:174–82.

44. Figueredo A, Rumble RB, Maroun J *et al*. (2003) Follow-up of patients with curatively resected colorectal cancer: A practice guideline. *BMC Cancer* **3**:26–38.
45. Tsikitis VL, Malireddy K, Green EA *et al*. (2009) Postoperative surveillance recommendations for early stage colon cancer based on results from the clinical outcomes of surgical therapy trial. *J Clin Oncol* **27**:371–6.
46. Chao M, Gibbs P. (2009) Caution is required before recommending routine CEA and imaging follow-up for patients with early-stage colorectal cancer. *J Clin Oncol* **27**:e279–e80.

Chapter 16

Genetic Biomarkers for the Diagnosis and Prognosis of Hepatocellular Carcinoma

John M. Luk[1,2,3,4,*], Angela M. Liu[1,4], Kwong-Fai Wong[3], and Ronnie T. P. Poon[4]

[1]*Department of Pharmacology,* [2]*Department of Surgery,* [3]*Cancer Science Institute, National University of Singapore, Singapore and* [4]*Department of Surgery, Queen Mary Hospital, Pokfulam, Hong Kong, China*

Identification of genetic biomarkers is a highly active area of research. With the development of microarray technology, researchers could characterize tumors at the genomic level, and this catalyzed a shift toward the discovery of genetic biomarkers for cancer. Genetic biomarkers could be used to identify the presence of a tumor at an early stage and to predict the natural course of an individual tumor, both of which are key factors in improving survival rate of patients. For hepatocellular carcinoma (HCC), the 5-year survival rate is only about 5%, the identification of novel biomarkers would clearly be beneficial. Physicians could use biomarkers to determine the best treatment option for patients with a particular tumor characteristic. This is especially important given the heterogeneity of HCC. To date, serum α-fetoprotein (AFP) level measurement is a standard means for detecting HCC, but its sensitivity and specificity are limited. Novel biomarkers are therefore being developed in order to improve the diagnosis and prognosis of HCC. In this chapter,

*Corresponding author. E-mail: luk_john_moonching@nuhs.edu.sg

the potential genetic biomarkers that could be used for detection, subtype classification, and estimation of prognosis are discussed.

Introduction

Treatment of hepatocellular carcinoma (HCC) has long been challenging. Although surgical resection of the tumor can be curative, many patients with late-stage HCC are not eligible for surgery, and those who are operated on have a high risk of tumor recurrence.[1] The limitations of surgical treatment have prompted clinical trials on various novel therapeutic agents such as monoclonal antibodies and small-molecule inhibitors. Despite some satisfactory results, the clinical benefits afforded by such therapeutics remain to be established.[2]

The heterogeneity of HCC makes the development of new drug treatments a very difficult task. Clinically, HCC can result from a wide spectrum of etiologies (e.g. hepatitis, alcohol, and aflatoxin, etc). Genetically, tumors in different individuals show diverse backgrounds of genomic alterations (e.g. DNA copy number), mRNA and microRNA expressions, and proteomes.[3–5] A systemic approach for characterizing genetic and proteomic networks that are essential to the processes of hepatocarcinogenesis should therefore reveal promising biomarkers or targets for the treatment of HCC (Figure 1).

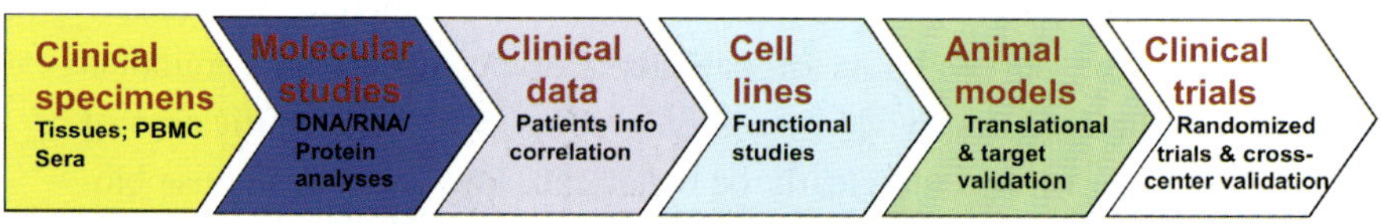

Figure 1. Systematic approach to HCC biomarkers and targets discovery. A systematic approach to HCC biomarkers and targets discovery involves six main components. (1) Clinical specimens such as tumor tissues, peripheral blood mononuclear cells (PBMC), and serum samples are collected from HCC patients. (2) In order to understand how HCC can be differentiated at molecular levels, various profiling methods are used to detect changes in DNA copy number, mRNA, microRNA, and protein expressions. (3) Associations between the molecular changes and clinical data of patients are analyzed. (4) A target's biological activities are being studied in cell lines. (5) Animal models are used for target validation. (6) Finally, the biomarkers or targets are tested in clinical trials before their uses in clinical settings.

Many research groups worldwide have put much effort to investigate the relationship between molecular changes and clinical features. Ours is one such group. Through combined analyses on HCC proteomes and clinicopathological data obtained from biobank (Figure 2), we have identified vimentin[6] and lamin B1[6] for detecting early HCC, Yes-associated protein (YAP) for predicting patients' survival times,[7] and mortalin for identifying tumors at risk for metastasis and resurrence.[8] On the basis of these findings, our group has also explored the potential usefulness of monoclonal antibodies[9,10] and inhibitory peptides[11] in the diagnosis and treatment of HCC.

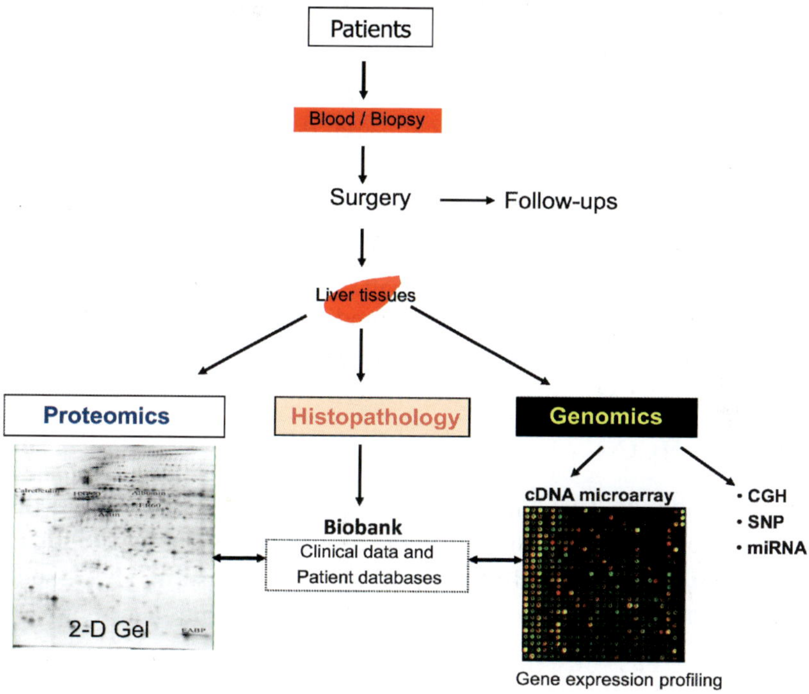

Figure 2. Biobank as the interface between tissue donors and research scientists. Blood and liver tissue samples are collected from patients. Clinical data such as demographic information (e.g., gender, age, race), clinico-pathological information (e.g., HBV or HCV infection, serum AFP level, tumor stage), and clinical outcomes (e.g., survival times) are collected from patients as well. Various technologies such as comparative genomic hybridization (CGH) array, single nucleotide polymorphism (SNP) array, miRNA microarray, cDNA microarray, and two-dimensional (2D) gel electrophoresis are used to reveal genetic or proteomic changes underlying HCC.

In addition to protein biomarkers research, extensive efforts have focused on identifying genetic biomarkers. In this chapter, we discuss gene and microRNA signatures that are diagnostic and prognostic for HCC. Years after the development of cDNA microarray technology, which can analyze the expressions of thousands of genes at a time, researchers have found gene signatures of HCCs and their associations with distinctive clinicopathological features. These findings suggested that the gene signatures could be used as molecular classifiers. During the past few years, the field of genetic biomarkers research has been enriched by the discovery of microRNAs. Owing to the escalating interest in microRNAs and cancer development, microRNA microarray and real-time quantitative PCR (qPCR) for microRNA profiling have been developed (Figure 3). Accumulating evidence has shown the aberrant expression of microRNAs in HCC, and demonstrated their roles in regulating cancer-related genes. As microRNAs are essential for transcriptional regulation, an integrated evaluation of mRNA and microRNA expression profiles may give more informative molecular signatures; these could be used to detect and classify liver cancer tumors and distinguish them from other entities, and to predict patients' survival as well as risk of metastasis and post-operative tumor recurrence.

Detection of HCC

Early detection of HCC allows prompt therapeutic interventions and should improve patients' survival.[12] In view of this, surveillance for HCC development is encouraged in populations at high risk of HCC, such as hepatitis B virus (HBV) carriers, and cirrhotic patients. Currently, most surveillance programs rely on the use of ultrasonography and serum α-fetoprotein (AFP) level measurement as the standard methodologies for detecting HCC.[13] However, growing numbers of studies suggest that both these techniques sometimes fail to identify early HCC tumors. Many early HCC cases are clinically asymptomatic and are negative for AFP, and many of the radiological findings cannot enable even experienced radiologists to discriminate early tumors from benign dysplastic nodules.[14]

To help physicians accurately detect early tumors, initial attempts have been made to identify specific gene signatures that discriminate

Table 1. Gene signatures for HCC early detection and classification.

	Study	Gene marker/signature	Potential application
Early detection	Nam *et al.* 2005	240-gene signature	Discriminate early HCC tumors from benign low- and high-grade nodules (HGDNs)
	Llovet *et al.* 2006	3-gene set (*GPC3*, *LYVE1*, and survivin)	Discriminate early HCC tumors from benign nodules
	Jia *et al.* 2007	5-gene set (*GPC3*, *PEG10*, *MDK*, *SERPINI1*, and *QPC*)	Detection of HCC in patients negative for APF
	Chen *et al.* 2008	Circulating hypermethylated *RASSF1A* sequence	HCC surveillance in HBV carriers
	Kaposi-Novak *et al.* 2009	35-Myc regulated gene set	Discriminate early HCC tumors from benign nodules
Classification	Boyault *et al.* 2007	Six HCC grouping signatures	Six HCC subgroups: G1: low HBV copy number G2: high HBV copy number and TP53 mutations G3: TP53 mutations G4: TCF1-mutated hepatocellular adenomas and carcinoma G5: β-catenin mutations and Wnt pathway activation G6: Wnt pathway activation and presence of satellite nodules
	Yamashita *et al.* 2008	Epithelial cell adhesion molecule (EpCAM)	Two HCC subgroups: EpCAM-positive: hepatic progenitor cell features EpCAM-negative: mature hepatocyte features
	Hoshida *et al.* 2009	Three HCC grouping signatures	Three HCC subgroups: S1: Aberrant Wnt pathway activation S2: Myc and Akt activation S3: hepatocyte differentiation

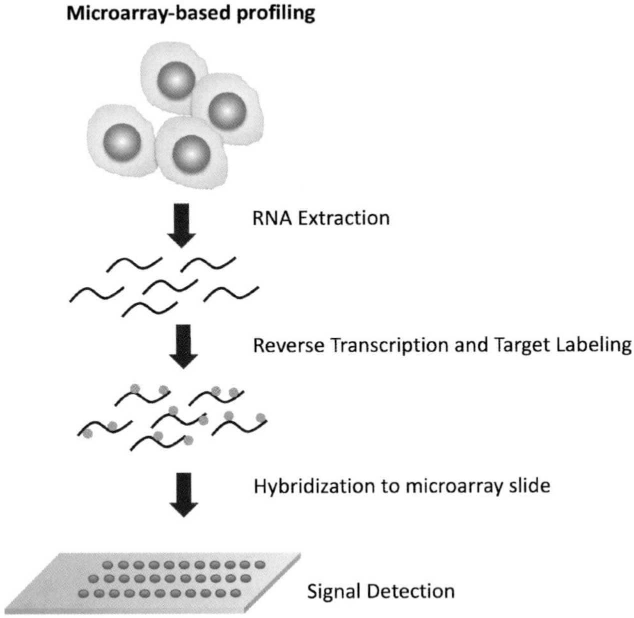

Figure 3. Principles of microarray technology used for profiling studies. Profiling of mRNAs or microRNAs using microarray-based technology involves four main steps: (1) RNA extraction, (2) RNA labeling, (3) hybridization, and (4) signal detection. During the RNA extraction of RNA from tissues, particular care must be taken with miRNAs because of their small size (mature microRNAs are 19–22 nucleotides long). The RNAs are then reverse transcribed into cDNAs, which are subsequently labeled with a reporter molecule, which in turn generates the signal for the later cDNA quantitation. The cDNA probes are quantified by hybridizing them to an array that contains hundreds of spots, and each of which contains a specific DNA oligonucleotide. After hybridization, the array is scanned using a laser scanner to measure signal intensity.

early HCC tumors from other entities. First, a Korean group reported a 240-gene signature that could discriminate early HCC tumors from benign low- and high-grade nodules.[15] About a year later, Llovet *et al.* reported another encouraging study on HCC patients positive for hepatitis C virus (HCV). In their study, expression patterns of 55 hepatocarcinogenesis-related genes were profiled in 37 patients, and the group whittled down the genes to three — *GPC3*, *LYVE1*, and *survivin* — which could discriminate early HCC from nodules with an accuracy rate of 94%.[16]

Table 2. microRNAs that have potential use in clinical settings.

Potential uses	microRNA Biomarkers	Remarks	References
Subtype Classification	miR-96, miR-126, miR-107, miR-375	* microRNAs were associated with genetic or clinical characteristics, such as HNF1-α mutations, β-catenin mutations, HBV-associated HCC, and alcohol-related HCC	30
	miR-190, miR-134, miR-151, miR-193, miR-133b, miR-324–5p, miR-182*, miR-105, miR-211, miR-20, miR-191, miR-340, miR-194, miR-23a, miR-142–5p, miR-34c, miR-124b, let-7b, miR-27a	* microRNAs were differentially expressed between HBV and HCV associated HCC	31
	miR-204, miR-34a, miR-148a, miR-122, miR-148b	* microRNAs that were involved in β-catenin mutation	33
Screening	miR-500	* An oncofetal microRNA in liver cancer * Detected in the sera of HCC patients (3 out of 10) * The miR-500 levels returned to normal after the surgical treatment	23
Monitoring for recurrence/ metastasis	miR-338, miR-219–1, miR-207, miR-185, miR-30c-1, miR-1–2, miR-34a, miR-19a, miR-148a, miR-124a-2, miR-9–2, miR-148b, miR-122a, miR-125b-2, miR-194, miR-30a, miR-126, let-7g, miR-15a, miR-30e	* This set of microRNAs helped to predict patients who are likely to develop metastasis/recurrence.	38
Estimation of prognosis	miR-125b	* High expression of hsa-miR-125b was correlated with longer survival of HCC patients	45
	miR-99b, miR-200c, miR-221, miR-31, miR-150, miR-220, miR-26b, miR-345, miR-29c, miR-372, let-7g, miR-30e-3p, miR-148a, miR-377, let-7c, miR-100, miR-99a, miR-125b, miR-139	* A set of 19 microRNAs was associated with patient survival	46
	miR-26	* Low expression of miR-26 is associated with shorter survival, but better response to interferon alfa therapy	47

Subsequently, a research group led by Snorri S. Thorgeirsson from the National Institution of Health, USA, reported for the first time that the Myc oncogene was one of the driver genes for the malignant conversion of dysplastic nodule into tumor, and a set of 35 Myc-regulated genes could be used to detect early HCC.[17]

HCC tumors with normal or low serum AFP levels have also drawn much attention. A Shanghai-based research group has studied mRNA expressions of 218 HCC specimens from patients with either high or low serum AFP,[18] and found that a combined score of five genes, namely *GPC3*, *PEG10*, *MDK*, *SERPINI1*, and *QPC*, could be used to classify cancerous tissues from patients negative for AFP. More interestingly, among the five candidate genes, *GPC3*, *MDK*, and *SERPINI1* encode extracellular proteins. Serum levels of these proteins may be easily measured using simple, clinically accepted methods like enzyme-linked immunosorbent assay.

Indeed, another research group from Hong Kong has demonstrated that a gene fragment that is freely circulating in the bloodstream could be used as a biomarker for HCC. By measuring the levels of hypermethylated *RASSF1A* sequences in blood from HBV carriers, researchers showed that the serum content of such sequences increased from the time of study recruitment to the time of HCC development in a cohort of HBV carriers who subsequently developed HCC.[19] Importantly, the hypermethylated *RASSF1A* sequence was detected in HCC patients negative for AFP.

Among blood-based biomarkers, microRNAs have been suggested as a superior type of circulating biomarker for cancer diagnosis. MicroRNAs are very stable in blood serum and plasma, and their quantities in serum are affected by the cancer status, although it remains largely unknown how microRNAs are released into the bloodstream from the cancer.[20,21] The first blood-based microRNA biomarker was miR-21. Lawrie *et al.* determined that the serum level of miR-21 was elevated in patients with diffuse large B cell lymphoma, and was associated with relapse-free survival of patients.[22] Around the same time, Mitchell *et al.* used a mouse xenograft model, into which a human prostate cancer cell line was inoculated, to show that circulating microRNA could be released from the tumor.[21] In HCC, identification of circulating microRNA as a biomarker has only just begun. To date, only miR-500 has been identified as a potential circulating biomarker for HCC.[23] The study found that miR-500 was expressed in several human liver cancer cell lines and up-regulated in 45% of HCC tissues. The serum levels of miR-500 were elevated in 3 out of 10 HCC patients, and returned to normal after surgical treatment. The data were encouraging, but a larger patient cohort is required to prove that miR-500 is a reliable biomarker.

HCC subtype classification

Genetic signatures that are distinctive of tumor behaviors such as drugs responses and oncogenic pathway activation are under intense investigation. This kind of genomic-based classification is clinically useful because it helps physicians to determine which therapeutic drugs or interventions would benefit patients most. Indeed, gene signatures have been developed for monitoring drug response among patients with breast[24] and lung[25,26] cancers. For HCC, development of such a molecular taxonomy system remains in its infancy. Nevertheless, there are examples showing how HCCs can be classified into distinct subgroups by gene or microRNA signatures.

A pioneering study of how mRNA expressions are linked to tumor phenotypes was reported by Chen *et al.*[27] In this study, mRNA expressions of HCCs were categorized into six major clusters: proliferation cluster, liver-specific cluster, T-lymphocyte cluster, B-lymphocyte cluster, stromal cell cluster, and endothelial cell cluster. Furthermore, by comparing the mRNA expressions of tumors sharing the same clinicopathological features, researchers identified two signatures that were associated with venous invasion and with nuclear p53 accumulation in cancerous tumor. A few years later, a French research group classified HCC into six groups using a combined score of mRNA expression, genetic alternations (e.g. loss of heterozygosity), and tumor phenotypes.[28] HCCs belonging to the six different groups displayed distinct clinical features, genetic abnormalities, and oncogenic pathway activations. Surprisingly, despite these differences, half of the HCC tumors were shown to have activated Wnt and Akt signaling pathways. In fact, Wnt and Akt pathways play key roles at various stages of hepatocarcinogenesis, and are now being targeted for the treatment of HCC[2].

Table 3. Prognostic gene signatures for hepatocellular carcinoma.

Clinical parameter	Study	No. of patients		Ethnic group	Array platform	No. of genes		Validation methods
		Training	Validation			Array	Signature	
Recurrence	Wang *et al.* 2009	23	25	Asian	Affymetrix Human HG-U133A	44760	57	qPCR
Metastasis	Ye *et al.* 2003	40	30*	Asian (Chinese)	In-house custom-made	9180	157	Statistic methods
	Budhu *et al.* 2006	20	95	Asian	In-house custom-made	9180	17	qPCR, IHC, ELISA
Survival	Lee *et al.* 2004	45	44	Asian & Caucasian	The Human Array-Ready Oligo Set	21329	406	qPCR, IHC
	Hoshida *et al.* 2008	106	234	Asian & Caucasian	DASL Assay	6000	186	DASL Assay

* Validation was done on patients of the training group.

Abbreviations: DASL assay, cDNA-mediated annealing, selection, extension, and ligation assay; ELISA, enzyme-linked immunosorbent assay; IHC, immunohistochemistry; qPCR, quantitative polymerase chain reaction.

Classification of HCC into subtypes can also be achieved using a single gene classifier such as epithelial cell adhesion molecule (EpCAM).[29] HCC tumors positive for EpCAM mRNA (tumor/non-tumor ratio ≥2) displayed features of hepatic progenitor cells (e.g. stem cell marker staining, Wnt-β-catenin signaling activation), whereas those negative for EpCAM mRNA (tumor/non-tumor ratio <2) presented features of mature hepatocytes. More strikingly, further stratification of the $EpCAM^+$ and $EpCAM^-$ groups by AFP status (cut-off value, 300 ng/mL) was prognostic for patient survival; patients in the $EpCAM^-$ AFP^+ subgroup had a shorter survival time.

MicroRNA profiling is another technique that has been used for HCC subtype classification. Ladeiro *et al.* reported that distinctive microRNA signatures are associated with clinical features, such as alcohol consumption, and HBV or HCV infection.[30] Around the same time, another group also reported a distinctive microRNA signature for HBV- or HCV-infected patients with HCC,[31] indicating a role for microRNA in regulating viral replication. In fact, miR-122, a liver-specific microRNA, has been shown to regulate HCV replication.[32] Ladeiro *et al.* also identified specific microRNAs that are associated with oncogene or tumor suppressor mutations. For example, low expression levels of miR-375 and miR-107 were associated with β-catenin and hepatocyte nuclear factor 1α mutations, respectively. Two years later, other microRNAs that are associated with β-catenin mutation were reported; these included miR-204, miR-34a, miR-148a, miR-122, and miR-148b.[33]

Despite these interesting findings, genetic classifiers are not yet being used in clinics to categorize HCC, partly because there is no consensus classification framework for HCC. However, progress has been made by Hoshida *et al.* who uncovered common molecular subclasses that were applicable to eight independent HCC cohorts from different studies.[34] Regardless of the microarray platforms used, each HCC cohorts could be robustly classified into one of the three subclasses: S1, aberrant activation of the Wnt signaling pathway; S2, Myc and Akt activation; and S3, hepatocyte differentiation. There is hope, therefore, that genetic classifiers for HCC will be available to physicians in the near future.

Signatures for predicting patients' prognosis

Perhaps the most extensively studied HCC signatures are those aimed at predicting patients' prognosis (e.g. survival time and risk of metastasis and recurrence). The first systemic study dates back to 2003, when Ye *et al.* reported a prediction of intra-hepatic metastasis by a 157-gene signature.[35] A better-defined metastasis-associated signature was subsequently reported.[36] In this study, a 17-gene predictor consisting mainly of the Th2 cytokine genes (e.g. tumor necrosis factor, colony-stimulating factor, interferon-γ, and interleukin-4, -5, and -10) identified the presence of venous metastasis in 87 of the 95 HCC samples in the validation set. For the prediction of recurrence after primary treatment of HCC, a Singaporean group described a 57-gene signature that was derived from a training set of 23 HCC patients with either vascular invasion or cirrhosis. This signature identified recurrence in 21 of 25 HCC patients in an independent test set.[37]

MicroRNAs may also be powerful tools for predicting HCC metastasis and recurrence. In 2008, Budhu *et al.* identified 20 metastasis-related microRNAs in HCC.[38] They tested a cohort of 131 cases, and used 110 additional cases for validation. The authors demonstrated that metastatic HCC tumors have a different microRNA expression signature compared with non-metastatic HCC tumors. The 20 metastasis-related microRNAs described in this study may help to identify patients with HCC who are likely to develop metastasis or recurrence.

Gene signatures that predict patients' survival time are under investigation as well. By profiling the mRNA expressions of 45 pairs of HCC tumors and matched nontumoral tissues, Lee *et al.* uncovered 406 unique genes whose expressions were predictive of patients' survival time.[39] Interestingly, the signature associated with poor patient survival was enriched for genes involving cell proliferation, anti-apoptosis, ubiquitination, and histone modifications. These biological processes could be the targets for new drugs that aim to lengthen patients' survival. Later, Hoshida *et al.* reported a 186-gene signature, which was derived from profiling data of formalin-fixed, paraffin-embedded adjacent nontumoral liver tissues; this signature accurately stratified 225 patients in the test data set into two groups of good and poor survival times.[40] The significance of this work was twofold. The data suggest for the first time that the prognoses of patients with small HCCs are determined largely by the gene expressions of nontumoral tissues but not by those of tumors. Furthermore, this study illustrated that mRNA expressions could be profiled in formalin-fixed, paraffin-embedded tissues, even those that have been archived for a period of 24 years. From a technical point of view, this finding is important because in most clinical scenarios the vast majority of tissues are collected as formalin-fixed specimens.

Instead of a gene signature, our group has developed a single gene marker for HCC, called liver-intestine cadherin or cadherin-17 (CDH17). In our early study, over-expression of CDH17 mRNA was restricted to HCC tissues, and was present in neither adjacent nontumoral tissues nor normal liver specimens.[41] Later, our CDH17 genotyping revealed that patients who inherited a particular haplotype of CDH17 (651 C > T and IVS6 + 35A > G) were at an increased risk for HCC.[42] CDH17 is believed to be a promising therapeutic target. By silencing CDH17 in an HCC xenograft using RNA interference, we could inactivate Wnt signaling and inhibit tumor growth.[43]

In addition to CDH17, our group has also discovered eukaryotic translation elongation factor 5A (eIF5A) as a prognostic factor for HCC patients.[44] There are two isoforms of eIF5A: eIF5A1 and eIF5A2. By determining their expression levels in a cohort of 258 HCC tissues using a microarray, our group has found that high expression levels of eIF5A1 in tumors was correlated with a large number of tumor nodules, whereas a high expression level of eIF5A2 was associated with the presence of venous infiltration in HCC patients. Given that both these associated clinicopathological features substantially affect the degree of HCC disease severity, eIF5A appears to be a promising tool for predicting patients' prognosis.

Researchers have also attempted to identify microRNAs that are predictive of patients' survival times. Li *et al.* showed that a high expression of hsa-miR-125b was correlated with longer survival of HCC patients,[45] and further investigation showed that this microRNA is involved in the suppression of cell growth and phosphorylation of Akt. In a separate study, a set of 19 microRNAs, including miR-125b, were found to correlate significantly with patients' survival time.[46] Subsequently, miR-26 was reported to be associated with disease outcome. This study included 214 patients and demonstrated that patients whose tumors had a low miR-26 expression level had a shorter overall survival.[47] An important finding of the study was that it also demonstrated the association of microRNAs with response to therapy with interferon alfa. Although patients with a low miR-26 expression level had a shorter survival, they had a better response to interferon therapy.

Conclusion

Recent advances in genetic biomarkers for HCC will potentially revolutionize the early detection and classification of HCC in clinics, and will enable prompt identification of patients at high risk of metastasis, recurrence, and with poor survival outcome. This will allow intensive follow-up and targeted interventions in such groups of patients. Nevertheless, before genetic biomarkers can be practically used in clinics, efficacy studies must be conducted across heterogeneous groups of HCC patients. With advances in technology, mRNA and microRNA profiling is becoming more cost-effective and easier, and the future looks promising for the use of genetic biomarkers in HCC.

References

1. El-Serag HB, Marrero JA, Rudolph L *et al.* (2008) Diagnosis and treatment of hepatocellular carcinoma. *Gastroenterology* **134**:1752–63.
2. Spangenberg HC, Thimme RBlum HE. (2009) Targeted therapy for hepatocellular carcinoma. *Nat Rev Gastroenterol Hepatol* **6**:423–32.
3. Laurent-Puig PZucman-Rossi J. (2006) Genetics of hepatocellular tumors. *Oncogene* **25**:3778–86.
4. Aravalli RN, Steer CJ, Cressman ENK. (2008) Molecular mechanisms of hepatocellular carcinoma. *Hepatology* **48**:2047–63.
5. Sun S, Lee NP, Poon RT *et al.* (2007) Oncoproteomics of hepatocellular carcinoma: From cancer markers' discovery to functional pathways. *Liver Int* **27**:1021–38.
6. Sun S, Poon RT, Lee NP *et al.* (2010) Proteomics of hepatocellular carcinoma: Serum vimentin as a surrogate marker for small tumors (< or = 2 cm). *J Proteome Res* **9**:1923–30.

7. Xu MZ, Yao TJ, Lee NP *et al.* (2009) Yes-associated protein is an independent prognostic marker in hepatocellular carcinoma. *Cancer* **115**:4576–85.
8. Yi X, Luk JM, Lee NP *et al.* (2008) Association of mortalin (HSPA9) with liver cancer metastasis and prediction for early tumor recurrence. *Mol Cell Proteomics* **7**:315–25.
9. Luk JM and Wong KF. (2006) Monoclonal antibodies as targeting and therapeutic agents: Prospects for liver transplantation, hepatitis and hepatocellular carcinoma. *Clin Exp Pharmacol Physiol* **33**:482–8.
10. Hu MY, Lam CT, Liu KD *et al.* (2009) Proteomic identification of a monoclonal antibody recognizing caveolin-1 in hepatocellular carcinoma with metastatic potential. *Protein Pept Lett* **16**:479–85.
11. Tsang FH, Lee NP, Luk JM. (2009) The use of small peptides in the diagnosis and treatment of hepatocellular carcinoma. *Protein Pept Lett* **16**:530–8.
12. Poon RT-P, Fan ST, Lo CM *et al.* (2002) Long-term survival and pattern of recurrence after resection of small hepatocellular carcinoma in patients with preserved liver function: Implications for a strategy of salvage transplantation. *Ann Surg* **235**:373–82.
13. Sun S, Day PJR, Lee NP *et al.* (2009) Biomarkers for early detection of liver cancer: Focus on clinical evaluation. *Protein Pept Lett* **16**:473–8.
14. Sakamoto M. (2009) Early HCC: Diagnosis and molecular markers. *J Gastroenterol* **44**(Suppl 19):108–11.
15. Nam SW, Park JY, Ramasamy A *et al.* (2005) Molecular changes from dysplastic nodule to hepatocellular carcinoma through gene expression profiling. *Hepatology* **42**:809–18.
16. Llovet JM, Chen Y, Wurmbach E *et al.* (2006) A molecular signature to discriminate dysplastic nodules from early hepatocellular carcinoma in HCV cirrhosis. *Gastroenterology* **131**:1758–67.
17. Kaposi-Novak P, Libbrecht L, Woo HG *et al.* (2009) Central role of c-Myc during malignant conversion in human hepatocarcinogenesis. *Cancer Res* **69**:2775–82.
18. Jia H-L, Ye Q-H, Qin L-X *et al.* (2007) Gene expression profiling reveals potential biomarkers of human hepatocellular carcinoma. *Clin Cancer Res* **13**:1133–9.
19. Chan KCA, Lai PBS, Mok TSK *et al.* (2008) Quantitative analysis of circulating methylated DNA as a biomarker for hepatocellular carcinoma. *Clin Chem* **54**:1528–36.

20. Chen X, Ba Y, Ma L *et al.* (2008) Characterization of microRNAs in serum: A novel class of biomarkers for diagnosis of cancer and other diseases. *Cell Res* **18**:997–1006.
21. Mitchell PS, Parkin RK, Kroh EM *et al.* (2008) Circulating microRNAs as stable blood-based markers for cancer detection. *Proc Natl Acad Sci USA* **105**:10513–8.
22. Lawrie CH, Gal S, Dunlop HM *et al.* (2008) Detection of elevated levels of tumour-associated microRNAs in serum of patients with diffuse large B-cell lymphoma. *Br J Haematol* **141**:672–5.
23. Yamamoto Y, Kosaka N, Tanaka M *et al.* (2009) MicroRNA-500 as a potential diagnostic marker for hepatocellular carcinoma. *Biomarkers* **14**:529–38.
24. Slamon DJ, Leyland-Jones B, Shak S *et al.* (2001) Use of chemotherapy plus a monoclonal antibody against HER2 for metastatic breast cancer that overexpresses HER2. *N Engl J Med* **344**:783–92.
25. Paez JG, Janne PA, Lee JC *et al.* (2004) EGFR mutations in lung cancer: Correlation with clinical response to gefitinib therapy. *Science* **304**:1497–500.
26. Lynch TJ, Bell DW, Sordella R *et al.* (2004) Activating mutations in the epidermal growth factor receptor underlying responsiveness of non-small-cell lung cancer to gefitinib. *N Engl J Med* **350**:2129–39.
27. Chen X, Cheung ST, So S *et al.* (2002) Gene expression patterns in human liver cancers. *Mol Biol Cell* **13**:1929–39.
28. Boyault S, Rickman DS, de Reynis Al *et al.* (2007) Transcriptome classification of HCC is related to gene alterations and to new therapeutic targets. *Hepatology* **45**:42–52.
29. Yamashita T, Forgues M, Wang W *et al.* (2008) EpCAM and alpha-fetoprotein expression defines novel prognostic subtypes of hepatocellular carcinoma. *Cancer Res* **68**:1451–61.
30. Ladeiro Y, Couchy G, Balabaud C *et al.* (2008) MicroRNA profiling in hepatocellular tumors is associated with clinical features and oncogene/tumor suppressor gene mutations. *Hepatology* **47**:1955–63.
31. Ura S, Honda M, Yamashita T *et al.* (2008) Differential microRNA expression between hepatitis B and hepatitis C leading disease progression to hepatocellular carcinoma. *Hepatology*.
32. Jopling CL, Yi M, Lancaster AM *et al.* (2005) Modulation of hepatitis C virus RNA abundance by a liver-specific MicroRNA. *Science* **309**:1577–81.

33. Pineau P, Volinia S, McJunkin K *et al.* (2010) miR-221 overexpression contributes to liver tumorigenesis. *Proc Natl Acad Sci USA* **107**:264–9.
34. Hoshida Y, Nijman SMB, Kobayashi M *et al.* (2009) Integrative transcriptome analysis reveals common molecular subclasses of human hepatocellular carcinoma. *Cancer Res* **69**:7385–92.
35. Ye Q-H, Qin L-X, Forgues M *et al.* (2003) Predicting hepatitis B virus-positive metastatic hepatocellular carcinomas using gene expression profiling and supervised machine learning. *Nat Med* **9**:416–23.
36. Budhu A, Forgues M, Ye Q-H *et al.* (2006) Prediction of venous metastases, recurrence, and prognosis in hepatocellular carcinoma based on a unique immune response signature of the liver microenvironment. *Cancer Cell* **10**:99–111.
37. Wang SM, Ooi LLPJ, Hui KM. (2007) Identification and validation of a novel gene signature associated with the recurrence of human hepatocellular carcinoma. *Clin Cancer Res* **13**:6275–83.
38. Budhu A, Jia H-L, Forgues M *et al.* (2008) Identification of metastasis-related microRNAs in hepatocellular carcinoma. *Hepatology* **47**:897–907.
39. Lee J-S, Chu I-S, Heo J *et al.* (2004) Classification and prediction of survival in hepatocellular carcinoma by gene expression profiling. *Hepatology* **40**:667–76.
40. Hoshida Y, Villanueva A, Kobayashi M *et al.* (2008) Gene expression in fixed tissues and outcome in hepatocellular carcinoma. *N Engl J Med* **359**:1995–2004.
41. Wong BW, Luk JM, Ng IO *et al.* (2003) Identification of liver-intestine cadherin in hepatocellular carcinoma — a potential disease marker. *Biochem Biophys Res Commun* **311**:618–24.
42. Wang XQ, Luk JM, Garcia-Barcelo M *et al.* (2006) Liver intestine-cadherin (CDH17) haplotype is associated with increased risk of hepatocellular carcinoma. *Clin Cancer Res* **12**:5248–52.
43. Liu LX, Lee NP, Chan VW *et al.* (2009) Targeting cadherin-17 inactivates Wnt signaling and inhibits tumor growth in liver carcinoma. *Hepatology* **50**:1453–63.
44. Lee NP, Tsang FH, Shek FH *et al.* (2009) Prognostic significance and therapeutic potential of eukaryotic translation initiation factor 5A (eIF5A) in hepatocellular carcinoma. *Int J Cancer* **127**:968–76.
45. Li W, Xie L, He X *et al.* (2008) Diagnostic and prognostic implications of microRNAs in human hepatocellular carcinoma. *Int J Cancer* **123**:1616–22.

46. Jiang J, Gusev Y, Aderca I *et al.* (2008) Association of MicroRNA expression in hepatocellular carcinomas with hepatitis infection, cirrhosis, and patient survival. *Clin Cancer Res* **14**:419–27.
47. Ji J, Shi J, Budhu A *et al.* (2009) MicroRNA expression, survival, and response to interferon in liver cancer. *N Engl J Med* **361**:1437–47.

Section V

Summary

Chapter 17

Current Therapy and Future Perspectives for Inflammation-Associated Cancer

L. Zhang and C. H. Cho*

School of Biomedical Sciences, Faculty of Medicine, The Chinese University of Hong Kong, Hong Kong, China

Inflammation is a self-defense biological process against various challenges, such as biological invasion, chemical and physical injuries. However when it becomes unsolved it could progress to chronic inflammation and further develop into cancer. Indeed, the relationship between inflammation and cancer has been well established. It involves different inflammatory cells including macrophage recruitment and neutrophil infiltration at injurious sites. All these could reciprocally stimulate various cytokines and chemokines secretion and also expression of some important transcriptional factors, namely NF-κB, STAT3 and HIF1γ into the microenvironment of tumors. These would activate different oncogenic processes including increase in proliferation and survival of cancer cells, promotion of angiogenesis at cancer sites, and enhancement of metastasis and invasion of cancer cells in distant organs. It is envisaged that concurrent inhibition of these pathological pathways or blocking several inflammatory mediators in the whole inflammatory cascade represents the current therapy and future targets for inflammation-associated cancerous diseases.

Introduction

Inflammation to start with is a host defense mechanism against invading pathogens, damaged tissues and cellular irritants. Both macrophages and

* Corresponding author. E-mail: chcho@cuhk.edu.hk

neutrophils are activated and represent the most important innate immune system that constitutes a first line of host defense against cancer cells. The outcomes of acute inflammation are either resolved or progressed to chronic inflammation, which leads to T cells activation, cytokine and chemokine secretion, and accumulation of macrophages at the sites of infection or injury. It is evidenced that inflammation and cancer are concurrently regulated. In some types of cancer, inflammatory conditions are present before a malignant change occurs. Conversely, in other types of cancers, an oncogenic change induces an inflammatory microenvironment that promotes development of tumors. Indeed there are evidences that inflammatory diseases increase the risk of many types of cancers, including bladder, cervical, gastrointestinal, ovarian, prostate, and thyroid cancers.[1] However, chronic inflammatory diseases, such as psoriasis and rheumatoid arthritis, do not increase cancer risk. Therefore, exposure to dietary and environmental carcinogens may be responsible for these differences.[2] It is envisaged that decreased exposure to these environmental stimuli and approaches to reduce inflammatory reactions would be crucial in the prevention and treatment of cancers. This chapter describes the causal relationship between inflammation and cancers and provides perspectives on how they could be treated.

Inflammation and cancer

Dr Virchow in 1863 first described the presence of infiltrating leukocytes in tumor tissues and suggested a relationship between chronic inflammation and carcinogenesis. In this respect, transcription factors such as NF-$\kappa\beta$, STAT3, and HIF1γ and their gene products such as pro-inflammatory cytokines TNF-α, IL-1, IL-6 and chemokines, COX-2, 5-LOX, MMP, VEGF, adhesive molecules, and others have provided the molecular basis for the role of inflammation in cancer.[3]

There are two pathways that connect inflammation and cancer, namely the extrinsic pathway, driven by inflammatory conditions, and the intrinsic pathway, driven by genetic alternations that cause inflammation and neoplasia. The two pathways usually converge, resulting in the activation of transcriptional factors (NF-$\kappa\beta$, STAT3, and HIF1γ). These factors will be described in the later part of this chapter. In this regard, drugs are developed to target cancer-related inflammation, for example, chemokine- and cytokine-receptor antagonists and COX inhibitors,[1] because these pathways have been implicated in angiogenesis, transformation of normal cells to cancer cells, survival and proliferation, invasion and metastasis of cancer cells. Also, it has been shown that these inflammatory pathways are activated by environmental stimuli such as tobacco, stress, dietary agents, obesity, alcohol, infections, and irradiation. All these account for as much as 95% of all cancers.[3] These findings indicate that inflammation-associated cancer is one of the most preventable diseases in humans.

The following is the plausible pathogenic mechanisms of how inflammatory microenvironment can do in cancer:

1. It can increase mutation rates and proliferation of mutated cells, and
2. It activates inflammatory cells which serve as sources of reactive oxygen species (ROS) and reactive nitrogen intermediates (RNI). This causes DNA damage and genomic instability and thereby promotes tumorigenesis.

Vice versa what tumor microenvironment can do in inflammation:

1. It shapes the differentiation and functional orientation of tumor-associated macrophages (TAM), and
2. It increases protumoral functions, such as promotion of growth factor and protease expression, increases of angiogenesis but decrease in adaptive immunity.

Adaptive immune system and tumor development

It is known that adaptive immune system carries out surveillance and can eliminate nascent tumors. In overt neoplasia, effective immune responses are suppressed through inhibition of dendritic cells (DC), the key initiator of adaptive immune responses. There are various cytokines (M-CSF, TGF-β, IL-6 and IL-10) present in the tumor microenvironment that contribute to blocking DC maturation in tumors.[4] They also have the potential to promote the differentiation and polarization of recruited monocytes into M2 macrophages.[5] TAMs as M2-polarized macrophages are also a potent suppressor of anti-tumor immunity.[1] It is the most frequently found immune cells within the tumor microenvironment. They promote tumor growth and may be obligatory for angiogenesis, invasion, and metastasis through the induction of different growth factors (EGF, TGF-β, VEGF, MMPs). To this end, TAMs are the most important players in inflammation and cancer arena and an important source of cytokines and also the hallmarks of inflammation-associated cancer.[4,6,7] Modifications of these inflammatory cells would be one of the therapeutic targets for cancer treatment.

The following are the three important transcriptional factors that play a pivotal role in the tumorigenesis of different solid tumors. They could be the major targets for future cancer therapy.

Hypoxia-inducible factor-1 (HIF-1) and tumor growth

Hypoxia is a common feature of solid tumors associated with decreased therapeutic response, malignant progression, local invasion, and distant metastasis. HIF-1 is a major regulator of cell adaptation to hypoxic stress and therefore a potential target for anticancer therapies. HIF-1 also mediates switch from aerobic to anaerobic metabolism to ensure their energy requirements, therefore facilitating survival in a hostile environment. It also plays a role in the recruitment in activation of TAM into solid tumors and may be instrumental to TAM-mediated angiogenesis and tumor metastasis.[4] Activation of HIF-1α-dependent genes has been associated with increased patient mortality. In pre-clinical studies, inhibition of HIF-1 activity has marked effects on tumor growth.[7]

Nuclear factor-κβ (NF-κB) and signal transducer and activator of transcription 3 (STAT3) in oncogenesis

NF-κB and STAT3 are activated in the majority of cancers and act as non-classical oncogenes. They may be promoted by either microenvironmental signals, including cytokines, hypoxia, and reactive oxygen reactive intermediates, or by genetic alternations.[7] They activate genes that control cell survival, proliferation and growth as well as angiogenesis and invasiveness. They are critical for both inflammation and tumor growth. The expression of antiapoptotic proteins Bcl2 and Bcl-XL is promoted by both

NF-κB and STAT3. NF-κB stimulates angiogenesis along with VEGF and IL-8 in tumor spread.[4] STAT3 also controls expression of cyclins D1 and D2 as well as proto-oncogene c-Myc in cancer cell proliferation.[6] Inhibition of these transcriptional factors represents novel therapeutic targets for inflammation-associated cancer.

Conclusions

Table 1 summarizes the causal relationship between inflammation and cancer. Agents that suppress all the inflammatory mediators or the pathways activated by them have a potential for the prevention and treatment of cancers. In this respect, inflammation-promoting tumorigenesis can be targeted in different ways: (a) inhibition of inflammatory signal transducers and transcriptional factors that mediate survival and growth of malignant cells, (b) blocking the action of chemokines and cytokines would decrease the recruitment of inflammatory cells, in particular TAM into the tumor microenvironment, and (c) depletion of immune and inflammatory cells that promote tumor development and progression.

Although a single anti-inflammatory agent may be effective in certain tumors, e.g. lymphoid tumors, it would be more effective if combined with more conventional anti-cancer drugs. It is because anti-inflammatory therapy is not cytotoxic on its own and needs to be combined with conventional therapies that kill cancer cells. Furthermore, cytotoxic therapies often lead to NF-κB activation in the remaining malignant cells to cause drug resistance. Therefore it makes sense to combine genotoxic drugs with NF-κB inhibitors as a way to overcome drug resistance and enhance anti-cancer efficacy.[6]

Table 1. Summary of inflammation and cancer

- Inflammation-associated cancer is the result of genomic instability and environmental insults
- ROS and RNI derived either from immune cells and external stimuli further increase DNA damage in cells
- Immune responses including cytokines and chemokines secreted from TAM and T cells further promote cancer cell proliferation, angiogenesis, invasion and metastasis

In conclusion, anti-inflammatory drugs can be used to reduce tumor incidence when used as prophylactics as well as to slow down progression and reduce mortality when used as therapeutics. It is also true that complete inhibition of a single biomarker is more likely to be toxic and unlikely to effectively cure diseases. Thus, it is plausible that concurrent downregulation of several biomarkers is more efficient to inhibit the dysregulated inflammation and produce less multi-drug resistance and systemic side effects in the treatment of inflammation-associated cancer.[3]

References

1. Mantovani A, Allvena P, Sica A *et al.* (2008). Cancer-related inflammation. *Nature* **454**:436–443.
2. Maletzki C, Emmrich J (2010). Inflammation and immunity in the tumor environment. *Dig. Dis* **28**:574–578.
3. Greer JB, Whitcomb DC (2009). Inflammation and pancreatic cancer: An evidence-based review. *Curr Opinion Pharmacol* **9**:411–418.
4. Mantovani A, Schioppa T, Porta C *et al.* (2006). Role of tumor-associated macrophages in tumor progression and invasion. *Cancer Meta Rev* **25**:315–322.
5. Allavena P, Sica A, Solinas G *et al.* (2008). The inflammation micro-environment in tumor progression: The role of tumor-associated macrophages. *Crit Rev Oncology Hematology*. **66**:1–9.
6. Grivennikov SI, Greten FR, Karin M (2010). Immunity, inflammation, and cancer. *Cell* **140**:883–899.
7. Sica A, Allavena P, Mantovani A (2008). Cancer related inflammation: The macrophage connection. *Cancer Lett* **264**:204–215.

Index